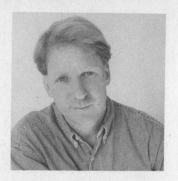

MICHAEL WINERIP

9 HIGHLAND ROAD

Michael Winerip was born in Quincy, Massachu-
setts, attended the public schools there, and graduated
from Harvard College in 1974. He has worked as a reporter for several newspapers, covering Appalachia for
the *Louisville Courier-Journal*, then moving to the
Miami Herald. For the last ten years he has been a
columnist and national correspondent for *The New
York Times*. He lives in Lido Beach, New York, with
his wife, three sons, and a daughter. This is his first
book.

9 HIGHLAND ROAD

9 HIGHLAND ROAD

MICHAEL WINERIP

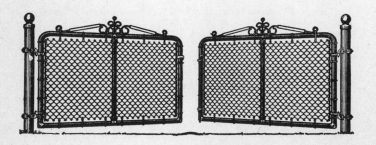

VINTAGE   BOOKS

A DIVISION OF RANDOM HOUSE, INC.   NEW YORK

FIRST VINTAGE BOOKS EDITION, JUNE 1995

The Library of Congress has cataloged the Pantheon edition as follows:
Winerip, Michael.
9 Highland Road/Michael Winerip.
p. cm.
ISBN 0-679-40724-3
1. Group homes for the mentally ill—New York (State)—Case
studies. I. Title. II. Title: Nine Highland Road.
RC439.55.W56 1994
362.3'23—dc20
93-38464 CIP
Vintage ISBN: 0-679-76160-8

Book design by Cheryl L. Cipriani
Author photograph © Jerry Bauer

Manufactured in the United States of America
10 9 8 7 6 5 4 3 2 1

To Sandy, who gave up London for this

A NOTE ON THE REPORTING OF THIS BOOK

IN *9 HIGHLAND ROAD*, I've employed the same journalism standards that I relied on as a reporter at *The New York Times* these last ten years. Whenever possible I have used an individual's real name. There are 150 people mentioned in this work of nonfiction; 124 are identified by their proper names; the 26 other names have been changed. Most individuals whose names I've changed are either the mentally ill or their immediate family members. Several group home residents are now back in the community and don't want employers or neighbors to know their pasts. In four cases I've changed the names of mental health professionals closely associated with group home residents, again to protect the privacy of those residents.

There are no facts altered in *9 Highland Road*. Occasionally, for privacy reasons, I have omitted the name of a hospital or town. But I have not changed these names. Any hospital, school, rehabilitation program, or municipality specified is the actual locale.

As a writer I've always relied extensively on quotes to tell a story. I began reporting this book in 1987, spent two years at the group home on a daily basis from 1990 to 1992, and was permitted access to all staff meetings. In the vast majority of cases, I've been present for comments appearing in direct quotations in this work.

The reader will notice in some scenes there is only one character in a room, yet there are quotes. Usually I am there too, although I do not say so explicitly in the text. In a few cases—for example, when Anthony and his father Dom are talking on one of their outings—people's comments are directed to me. That should be clear from context as well.

There are occasional scenes described here in which quotes are used though I was not present. In some instances—like Heather Martino's commitment hearing—I've relied on a court transcript and interviews with key participants. For other scenes I've culled comments from thousands of pages of group home and hospital records. A few times I have relied on reconstructions after verifying the exchanges with those present.

Michael Winerip
January 1994

CONTENTS

9 HIGHLAND ROAD

BY DECEMBER of 1990, the ordinary-looking colonial at 9 Highland Road had been forgotten by the people of Glen Cove, New York. In the two years since it had opened as a group home for a dozen adults with serious mental illnesses—schizophrenia, manic depression, major depression, borderline personality disorder—neighbors on the quiet suburban street had no cause to call the police. The dentist living across the way at 11 Highland, Dr. Edward Woodman, told his patients, "The group home's a great neighbor. They don't bother anybody. They do their thing, I do mine." The home had been so unobtrusive, some neighbors didn't realize it was still there. No sign stood out front, not even a little placard on the door identifying it as a group home. Just the normal three-inch-high number to the right of the front door: 9 Highland. New residents often got lost looking for the place. Long after it opened, Dr. John Imhof, a therapist making his first visit, knocked next door at 7 Highland and was told by the woman answering that she was sorry, but she didn't know anything about a group home on Highland Road.

In 1975 there were just 209 group homes for the mentally ill in the entire country. By the late 1980s there were 700 in New York State alone, thousands in America. And by 1994 more New Yorkers were living in state-funded group homes and apartment programs (12,536) than in state mental hospitals (9,726). For the first time since state lunatic asylums were opened in the early 1800s, government had radically changed the way it cared for the chronic mentally ill. The group home had replaced the state hospital as the backbone of the nation's mental health system.

In an era of tight budgets and high taxes, government had a strong financial motive: the State of New York spends $120,000 a year to care for a patient in a mental hospital; $35,000 in a group home.

A GROUP HOME is basically a good-sized house that is supervised by counselors twenty-four hours a day. The idea is not new. In the thirteenth century, residents of Gheel, Belgium, opened their homes to the tormented souls who made pilgrimages to the local waters to be healed. State mental hospitals in this country started boarding out their healthiest patients at the turn of the century, and with the introduction of antipsychotic medications in the 1950s, professionally supervised group homes made their first appearance.

The Glen Cove house has two single bedrooms, five doubles, four bathrooms, a living room, TV room, dining room, and kitchen. The only room that makes it different from other houses on the block is a small office on the first floor at the end of the entry hallway. There the residents' medications are kept locked up, along with their psychiatric records and the daily log sheets reporting any noteworthy incidents. The office has two desks and a bed where the counselor working overnight sleeps. This staff room is the size of a walk-in closet.

No one wears a uniform or walks around with keys on his belt. Staff and residents dress informally, in street clothes. If a stranger were suddenly dropped in the middle of the house, it's unlikely he'd figure out where he was. This did happen, to a fellow dating Julie Callahan, one of the original residents of 9 Highland. Julie was late returning from the beach one summer afternoon and was just stepping out of the shower when the young man, a medical student, rang the front door-bell. She'd been out with him only a few times and had never quite explained about 9 Highland. Julie grabbed a girlfriend at the house, directed her to let the guy in—but hold him at the door—then raced to her bedroom and threw on some clothes. Her hair was soaking wet. Still dripping, she ran down the stairs and led him into the living room. "Take a seat," she said, "I'll be right back. I have to do something with my hair." He waited on the couch by the TV and from the back-and-forth movement of his head it was soon plain that he was having trouble figuring out why there were so many people walking around in Julie's house. Finally his curiosity got the best of him and he asked Paula Marsters if she'd been at the beach with Julie, too.

"No, I work here," said Paula.

"Work here?" he said. "Oh, really."

As Julie led him out the front door and down the driveway to his car, she said, "So I guess you're wondering what that was."

IF, AFTER TWO YEARS, the group home appeared quiet and ordinarily suburban from the outside, on the inside there was turmoil daily.

As the state bureaucrats wrote in their memorandums, residents of 9 Highland were SPMIs, "seriously and persistently mentally ill." Their illnesses covered the spectrum from neurological in origin to man-made. Some of these men and women came from impressive, robust nuclear families with no other sick members. Others, the women in particular, had mental health problems that stemmed from being brutalized as children.

At public meetings, neighbors spoke of the home's residents as if they were aliens from another planet. Suburban Long Island leaders fought efforts to house the mentally ill in the community more fiercely than in any other part of the state. During the 1980s and early 1990s, six group homes on Long Island were firebombed.

The truth was, house residents were products of these very same suburban neighborhoods. Nassau County is a primarily white, middle-to-upper-middle-class suburb of 1.3 million with a few pockets of poverty, bordering the Queens section of New York City. When 9 Highland was being proposed, Glen Cove civic leaders warned that there were no laws preventing it from being filled with City people. (At suburban public meetings this is usually a euphemism for homeless blacks.) In fact, of the twelve living at 9 Highland as the group home entered its third year, one was black (she'd studied at Howard University and had lived in Great Neck, Long Island), and one was Latino, a Puerto Rican man from Glen Cove. Most were mainstream Nassau County, either Jewish or Italian American. Eleven of the twelve grew up in the county. Economically they ranged from a homeless runaway to a man whose parents lived in a million-dollar house that had polished oak floors, throw rugs, and antique furniture too valuable to sit on. Another came from a family that owned one of the largest businesses in Glen Cove.

All twelve at 9 Highland, from poorest to richest, lived off Social Security disability checks and Medicaid, the government's basic welfare programs for the mentally ill. Given the cost of a long-term psychiatric hospitalization, only an extraordinarily wealthy family could afford to keep a seriously ill adult child off the public dole. There was a good aspect to this forced egalitarianism. The middle- and upper-middle-class residents and their families tended to be more demanding of public community mental-health programs. They lived in suburbs where the public services—the schools, the parks, the beaches, the trash pickup—were first-rate. If they were being forced to rely on public care, they were going to do what they could to make sure it wasn't second-class.

THE RESIDENTS' problems didn't spill into the streets of Glen Cove in part because there was staff around twenty-four hours a day. Counselors at 9 Highland were well aware of each resident's trouble signs. It wasn't that these counselors were great psychiatric scholars. Some hadn't finished their bachelor's degrees and had never taken a course in the field. But staff and residents ate, watched TV, played cards, listened to music together, shared the same newspaper, slept under the same roof. They understood each other.

Supervision was more formal than it appeared at first glance. Every Tuesday evening the house manager met with the staff for two hours and reviewed each resident's condition. Any incident during the week was chronicled in a book of progress notes kept in the group home office. At the start of a shift, staff reviewed these notes. Most residents were on medication—antipsychotics, antidepressants, tranquilizers— prescribed by their psychiatrists. Until they earned the right to take meds on their own, they had to do it in the office, in front of a counselor, and it was recorded in the medication book.

A group home wasn't magic. It might reduce the number of hospital stays, but could not prevent them altogether. Some illnesses were just too severe. Even so, group home residents rarely had to be committed involuntarily. They usually talked it over with a counselor, packed a suitcase, then went in quietly. Civil liberties was not an issue.

AMERICA'S MENTAL HEALTH system is renowned for losing people through the cracks. The evidence is strewn through the streets. Between a quarter and a third of the homeless in cities are mentally ill. Twice as many mentally ill live on our sidewalks as in our state hospitals.

The group home was designed to give these people a middle ground between the hospital and street. Its tack was neither lenient nor authoritarian. Residents could come and go as they pleased without signing in or out. The front door was locked only late at night. They went off on overnights and vacations, could keep a car at the house if they had one. They were there voluntarily—they were not confined, remanded, incarcerated, or committed—and could move out at any time. On the other hand, there were curfews. Drinking and drugs were prohibited. People couldn't just hang around on weekdays; they had to go to a treatment or training program, school, or volunteer work, hold a job, or be looking for one. Everyone had to do house chores and took turns cooking meals.

Residents regularly complained there were too many rules.

Counselors complained there were no consequences when residents broke the rules. The rank-and-file staff griped that the house supervisors let residents get away with murder, that they were too quick to dismiss an outburst as a product of illness.

The supervisors knew that it would have been clearer and simpler to have specific punishments for each broken rule. Some group homes are run this way. But a strict system of punishments had to end with expulsion from the house. This the supervisors at 9 Highland wanted to avoid if at all possible. Most residents voluntarily took powerful psychiatric medications that helped with their illnesses but had humiliating side effects: drowsiness, weight gain, impotency, the shakes. Admitting they needed the group home was hard enough.

The biggest incentive to abide by the rules was the alternatives out there. The newspapers the residents read, the TV news they watched were constantly doing stories on the horrors of New York City's huge homeless shelters: the drugs, the violence, the disease. Those places were a forty-five-minute ride away.

For many this was a place of last resort and they weren't exactly ecstatic about it. As a resident said one not-so-great day when a counselor inquired about his health, "How'm I feeling? How do you think I'm feeling? I live in a group home."

ON A COLD, starry December night in 1987, I walked up the hill from Glen Cove's main street to take a look at the vacant house on the corner of Highland Road and Douglas Drive. I was on assignment for *The New York Times*, in town to cover a public meeting on a proposed group home, and wanted a peek at what I was writing about. Standing in the dark, staring at that empty house, I couldn't find anything to put in my notebook. What struck me most about the house was that nothing struck me about the house.

The public meeting later that night at town hall was a different matter. I knew people weren't going to welcome a group home to their town, but I hadn't anticipated so much anger, prejudice, and misinformation from such a well-educated, upper-middle-class audience. Speaker after speaker made it sound like a home for the mentally ill would turn life on Highland Road into one big, long shower scene from the movie *Psycho*. By 11 P.M., when the last vestiges of decorum had degenerated into shouting and threats, I'd filled every page of my notebook on both sides.

Over the next year, I covered the battle to open 9 Highland, doing a final story when the first residents arrived in December 1988.

Then I moved on to other things, though I continued to write about group homes and their battles. You didn't have to be a genius to detect a pattern. No matter what city, burg, or state I was reporting from, the neighbors at these public meetings—rich, poor, black, white—all sounded the same. Group homes were spreading across the nation, but because the houses were scattered and small, the general public did not have an inkling of what they were. Most psychiatrists and psychologists I meet have never stepped inside one.

In early 1991, I took a leave from the *Times* and for the next two years camped out at 9 Highland, to learn.

This book opens in the late 1980s with the battle to establish 9 Highland. But the heart of my story is the day-to-day life of the home in 1991 and 1992, the third and fourth years of its operation, when the public had forgotten it and I came to know the residents so very well.

chapter 1

JULIE CALLAHAN, FALL 1988

TUESDAY, SEPTEMBER 20, 1988, Julie Callahan made the long trip by train from the mental hospital where she'd been living the last sixteen months to Glen Cove, Long Island. She was in a sweet frame of mind. It was great just being off the psych ward. Julie rarely requested a pass to leave the mental hospital, didn't have the money to go anywhere—or anyone to visit, for that matter. She wouldn't have been able to go for this interview at the group home if the hospital social worker hadn't taken pity on her and dug up the thirty-dollar carfare from a special charity case fund.

The midmorning off-peak train was empty. The suburban business-men and lawyers who'd filled the seats a few hours before reading *The Wall Street Journal* and *The New York Times* were in their Manhattan high-rise offices now. The conductor, an older man, moved leisurely through the car and as he punched her ticket, he teased her about what sort of adventure she was heading off to. Strange men were always talking to her. She was twenty and very pretty and usually alone. Julie told him she had the day off from college and was traveling home to visit her family on Long Island. She liked it that he actually believed her. A good sign. She needed to be able to dish it today.

Most of the trip she stared out the window at the rain. The leaves were beginning to change, though it felt like summer still, eighty degrees and muggy. She wanted this group home in Glen Cove. She'd looked it up on the map and it was the perfect location. This was her plan: Get into the Glen Cove house; enroll nearby at North Shore Hospital's outpatient day-treatment program, which was "quote-unquote the best on Long Island"; and get back her old psychiatrist so she didn't have to start over with some new idiot.

She was excited about the prospect of moving back to suburban Long Island. Except for this hospitalization, she'd been off the Island only once, for a school field trip to the United Nations. Until she was sixteen, the farthest she'd been from home by herself was her high school.

Julie had studied the train schedules endlessly, allowing extra time in case she missed her connections. At a young age she'd been forced to fend for herself and learned not to leave anything to chance. She had set off five hours early, taking the commuter train into New York City, two subways across Manhattan (her first subway rides), and then the Long Island Rail Road eastbound from Pennsylvania Station to Glen Cove. The trip lasted three hours. She had so much time before the appointment, she stopped for a hamburger at the Mykonos diner, then rode a taxi to the Angelo J. Melillo Center, a mental health clinic in Glen Cove, where she asked for somebody named Linda Slezak.

There was another young woman ahead of her. Julie thought of this screening as a college interview for mentally ill achievers. They'd want her to perform, give them something so they could fill their little notebooks. These social workers always acted very concerned if you didn't supply a few new juicy details. They'd have a stack of her hospital records that reached the ceiling, but they'd want to hear it all over again, in her own words, the Julie Callahan story. She hoped she'd be able to talk. Sometimes she tried but nothing came out.

The waiting lists were long for these homes. At the hospital they told her to apply for every one on Long Island, and maybe she'd get lucky. She had already interviewed at one other, and when it was over asked how long before she'd get in. A year, they said, maybe two.

Everything she'd taken on in her young life, she'd excelled at. She was the star of her Future Business Leaders of America club in high school, typed eighty words a minute, and was selected to compete in the New York State scholastic championships for business students.

She'd been picked for the all-county orchestra and was a fine athlete.

Now she needed to be a star mental patient.

JULIE WAS ONE of forty applicants for the twelve-bed house scheduled to open soon in Glen Cove. All that fall, while the vacant colonial at 9 Highland was being remodeled, Linda Slezak, the director of the mental health clinic's new group-home program, interviewed prospective residents. Linda was being very careful. The Glen Cove house would be only the sixth group home for the mentally ill in a county of 1.3 million people. The first had opened in 1983, five years before. So far, there had been no public slipups at the other homes, but opposition to them had been loud and vicious and Linda Slezak knew it would take only one sensational incident—one violent front-page story (GROUP HOME INMATE GOES BERSERK!)—to destroy the group home movement on Long Island. In her twelve years as a social worker Linda had labored at several rungs of the mental health system, and she knew all the failures. She'd worked at Creedmoor state psychiatric hospital in nearby Queens in the late 1970s. As homelessness worsened and the public began complaining about too many crazy people in the streets, social workers like Linda Slezak were hired by the state to do discharge planning. But where was Linda supposed to send the released mental patients? To the big, for-profit adult homes and run-down hotels in Long Beach or Far Rockaway, where they did nothing all day, stopped taking their medication, and soon suffered relapses? How could you do discharge planning when there was no destination to plan for? This was why Linda had jumped at this new job developing group homes. She saw them as the future.

Julie Callahan's file worried her. The private psychiatric hospital where Julie currently was being treated had sent a referral packet of evaluations that was so thick, its heft alone was cause for concern. At twenty, Julie already had a history in the mental health system. She'd spent the previous twenty-two months in two different mental hospitals, had her first hospitalization at seventeen. On page 3 of the referral form, a hospital social worker had crossed out "emergency family contacts" for Julie and written "estranged from family; ward of the state."

The personal and family history sections described a brutal, chaotic life. Julie grew up in a poor, working-class family. Her father was a laborer, her mother a homemaker. The Callahans had no car, which, the report noted, is highly unusual for suburban Long Island, where almost everyone drives. The family was described as abnormally insular. The report said the mother left the house only a few times a year. Growing up, the children were not allowed to go to friends' houses, visit malls or pizza shops, or date. They were under strict orders to come right home after school, and if they didn't their mother became enraged. No one slept alone. They paired up, sleeping two brothers and two sisters to a bed. Falling asleep in the parental bed was encouraged, a psychologist had noted in the file.

Starting as a young teenager, Julie was physically and sexually abused regularly by her father, the reports said. While still in high school, she was removed from the home by the county and placed in foster care. She had always been an honor roll student and continued to do well in school despite her trouble.

The psychological reports mentioned "episodes of sexual promiscuity shortly after leaving her home." Linda Slezak looked for more detail, but there was nothing else.

When county Child Protective Services began investigating her natural parents, the caseworkers were skeptical of the incest at first. One hospital report noted, "The family has unanimously bonded in their denial of the patient's story." However, after an investigation and hearing, a family court judge sided with Julie and ordered that she be permanently removed from her home, warning her father that any further complaints would result in criminal prosecution. An investigator testified, "There's nothing I've seen that wouldn't back Julie's assessment 100 percent." Child Protective Service workers continued to visit the Callahan house after Julie was removed, to check on the other children.

While living at the foster home, as a high school senior, Julie started seeing a therapist for the first time. Eventually she told the therapist that she was having sexual relations with her new foster father. Julie's account of the sexual activity made her sound quite passive. "He just told me what to do and I did it." The therapist acted quickly to get Julie removed from the foster home. Abuse charges were brought against the foster father.

Evaluations noted that though Julie had never been a behavior problem in school, had not done anything criminal or violent, was not a drug or alcohol user—in short, she was no delinquent—she was next placed in a school for delinquent girls. There, for the first time, she began making suicidal gestures, swallowing Ajax and putting plastic bags over her head. She was removed and placed in a second foster-care home, run by a woman. There she was fine for a time, but then lapsed into depression. As awful as her childhood had been, she missed her family. Julie was particularly close to a younger brother and sister, and the reports noted that she was devastated when her parents wouldn't let her visit them anymore. She grew intensely suicidal, the report said, turning up at her therapist's office to say good-bye.

In the spring of 1986 she was admitted to the psychiatric wing of a local private hospital and spent a month there. Doctors discussed a long-term hospitalization, but Julie insisted on being discharged to her foster mother's home. That fall she enrolled in college, but was soon institutionalized again. Her parents had been phoning Julie at the foster home, threatening her, accusing her of making up the sexual abuse stories to destroy them. Julie was suicidal, panicky, depressed, the reports noted. When she did sleep, she had a recurring nightmare that her father was raping her.

She spent the next seven months at the Long Island hospital, where she was diagnosed with depression and a borderline personality disorder. In May 1987 she was transferred to another private hospital in the New York area, which had a program specializing in borderline personality disorder. Linda Slezak knew its reputation well. By the time the referral packet arrived on Linda's desk, Julie had been hospitalized on that borderline unit fifteen months. Linda Slezak saw patterns in the hospitals' behavioral and testing reports that made her uneasy about Julie Callahan as a group home resident, and other things that were just plain puzzling.

Julie appeared to do miserably adjusting to new places. In her first three months at the Long Island hospital, she'd been suicidal and at one point escaped from the locked ward. During her first six months on the borderline unit, the psychiatrist was so concerned about Julie's resistance to therapy that a special evaluation was ordered to determine if Julie's "isolative, uncooperative, oppositional behavior" might be a defense against "a psychotic core." Borderline personality disorder is a broad term that describes a person sicker than a neurotic, but not ill enough to be classified psychotic. The psychiatrist was concerned that maybe Julie was sicker than they thought—psychotic, and perhaps even schizophrenic.

Did a new group home want someone who might not be stabilized yet?

Her IQ test scores intrigued Linda Slezak. Julie had taken the test three times in a year and a half, with a variety of results. Her performance IQ had been as low as 102 and as high as 126; her verbal IQ had ranged from 99 to 111. Her range of scores on various sections of the test was huge; in the picture completion section she'd scored near genius; in vocabulary, not much above retarded. Assuming the test was reliable, something substantial was interfering with Julie's thinking at times.

There was another oddity. "Julie possesses a very confused sense of self," one psychologist had written. She has "a poor sense of her body, mixed with anxiety and confusion as to which parts are where and what is visible and what is hidden." Here was a person of superior intelligence, an honor roll student who was sexually active, and at the same time she didn't know where her body parts were?

The report also mentioned a post-traumatic stress disorder, but did not elaborate on whether this involved flashbacks, or what form it took.

Linda Slezak was struck too, by Julie's reactions to the Rorschach inkblots and the Thematic Apperception Test (TAT). For the TAT, a person is shown a series of evocative black-and-white illustrations and told to interpret what's going on in them. Try as she might to hold it in, young Julie's life came leaking out in her reactions to those blots and still-lifes. To a TAT card of a girl standing beside a door, weeping, Julie responded: "She's crying, but that doesn't matter because she did what she did." (The tester wrote: "absence of responsive caretakers in her harsh world.") To a card of a boy gazing downward at a violin on a table in front of him: "This kid was probably playing the violin and someone told him to stop playing probably because he wasn't playing that well." (The tester wrote: "criticism abounds in her life.") To one of the colored Rorschach cards, she answered: "I see a woman and her face is kind of being squashed by this green stuff and her face is dripping like bleeding . . . and it looks like they both have one leg chopped off, someone cut it off or something." (The tester wrote: "The patient experiences herself as a passive recipient of horrors too terrible for her to describe in other than a bland monotone . . . telling story after story where victims suffer beatings, murders and lascivious seductions.") She threw one card back, telling the tester, "I'm having this unnatural response to this picture that I can't deal with . . . I don't really feel like going on with this." (The tester wrote that there was evidence of "transient psychotic state at these moments marked by an inability to accurately perceive reality.")

The two most recent assessment reports that Linda Slezak had from the borderline hospital unit only added to the confusion. The July report was prepared for internal hospital use and was quite pessimistic.

The August referral was upbeat, written to encourage a group home to take Julie. The July report described Julie's prognosis as "guarded"; the August referral to group home agencies described her prognosis as "good." Her therapy still varied "between fluency [and] prolonged periods of silence when she is unwilling to divulge information."

The July report said she had a tendency to be defiant in subtle ways that caused confrontations with the hospital staff. She'd wear her housecoat and slippers beyond the time when she should've been dressed, miss appointments for her focus group, and act "dizzy and irresponsible when, in fact, she is quite competent."

On the other hand, Julie had recently been elected president of the hospital's patient council, serving "responsibly." In July she'd done well at a day camp volunteer job. Her thinking was described "as clear, well organized and quite articulate" with "no evidence of thought disorders at this time." She had never acted out suicidally on the borderline unit, despite ongoing "waves of passive suicide ideation." And there had been progress in psychotherapy. She'd opened up enough to talk some about the incest, the shame, the disgust she had for herself, and how dirty she felt. "Later in the treatment healthier elements such as anger began to emerge," a therapist wrote. Julie was beginning to understand where to place the blame.

After a first reading of the file, Linda Slezak phoned the social worker at the hospital borderline unit. Was this young woman really ready to live outside? What about the promiscuity? The borderline program was an all-female unit. Now she was being considered for a home where half the residents would be men. The reports all described her as "attractive and stylish." Would Julie forever be getting entangled with men in the house and away from it, and if so, how would that affect group home life? And what about Julie's family? Some of her worst problems came after contact with them. The borderline unit was a long way from her Long Island hometown, and she had not seen the family during her stay there. If she moved to Glen Cove, she'd be a short drive away. A group home couldn't control and monitor these visits the way a hospital could.

The social worker on the borderline unit didn't try to snow Linda

Slezak. Julie was a tough case, she acknowledged. But there'd been real progress, and after twenty-two months, Julie Callahan wasn't likely to benefit from more hospitalization. The bottom line: Julie had a chance of making it on the outside. Linda Slezak listened. She respected this hospital. Julie had been lucky that a private institution of this caliber had been willing to take her, considering her only insurance was Medicaid. The hospital knew its people. Patients attended group therapy daily and saw their therapist privately at least three times a week. This wasn't a state institution. Linda Slezak knew patients who'd gone for months at Pilgrim State Psychiatric Hospital, the biggest public institution on the Island, without seeing a therapist. Pilgrim State sent Linda patients to be interviewed for the group home who had psychotic episodes in the midst of their screenings.

Linda decided to ask Julie in for an interview.

She always reread a candidate's packet the day of the screening. At the top of the very first page of the hospital's referral there was a place for a patient to voice a "chief complaint." It was a perfect opportunity to show off, say something like "Hospital life is too constricting, I yearn for independence."

Julie had commented: "They admitted me to the first hospital because I was suicidal. I am not suicidal anymore but I think they sent me to the borderline unit because I don't have anywhere else to go."

SITTING IN THE small waiting room, Julie worried about how much she should tell. For all the therapists and social workers she'd met during her three years inside the system, she still found it hard. There were times she'd go through an hourlong therapy session at the hospital without saying a word. They thought she was obstinate. She just couldn't get anything out. She'd think what to say but it was as if her voice was frozen. She didn't even remember some of the sessions; they were a blank. Always they picked at her worst problems: the incest, running away, her supposed sexual promiscuity, her crazy family. There were pieces of her past she couldn't recall herself, and that was embarrassing and frightening and nothing to admit to strangers. She didn't remember something as major as running away from her parents' home. It made it harder to explain why she'd done it.

Yet if she didn't tell these group home people some of her problems, she might blow everything. She could envision it: "Tell us, Miss Callahan, do you perceive yourself having problems in the group home? No problems? Ah, yes, very good," and then they'd scribble, "In denial! Out of touch with reality!"

And if you say problems, maybe you have too many problems.

She knew she couldn't be totally truthful. You never could. She felt the therapeutic program on the hotshot borderline unit had been useless for her. She did not believe she had a borderline disorder. Living with borderline women for all those months, she knew the type inside and out—the rapid emotional swings from euphoric to suicidal. One minute they'd be talking about how much they hated someone, then it was how much they needed them. They felt they were the greatest, then suddenly they felt worthless. They'd brag about being on the most elite unit at the hospital. Then they'd try to outdo each other for who was sickest, cutting their arms up with razor blades and running to the counselors to show them. They were anorexic and bulimic, drug and alcohol users, and she wasn't any of those things. But she knew she couldn't say this. The one person who wasn't borderline on the esteemed borderline unit. Right.

SHE WAS interviewed by Linda Slezak and two other people in a windowless conference room with beige walls. Everyone sat in cloth swivel chairs around a coffee table. One of them had a yellow legal pad and made notes whenever Julie said something. She could tell they were trying to be nice. She felt like she was on trial. She did not look at them and would not have been able to describe them afterward.

Most of what she told them was predictable: that she needed help living on the outside, that she hoped to learn these skills from the group home. "I'm really scared. I have a problem with dependency. I need something in between the hospital and living on my own before

I'm self-sufficient." She was looking to work on her two emotional goals, she said, depression and loneliness. She wanted a place where she'd feel safe.

Oh yes, she answered, she'd made excellent progress on the borderline unit.

They explained about everyone having assigned daily chores and asked if she'd be overwhelmed or feel too confined living in a house with eleven other people. Julie told them it wouldn't be a problem, that she'd grown up in a small house and came from a family where the kids shared the housework.

Did she plan to be in contact with her family?

She was silent for a long while. "I haven't seen my family in two years," she answered carefully. ". . . And don't expect to . . ." It was true. She hadn't the faintest idea how to get from the group home to her parents' house. She did not know how to drive, wasn't familiar with Long Island's parkways or expressways, became sick every time she was in a car. And the public transportation system on the Island was so bad, she grew nervous just thinking about how many buses it might take. The only group home on Long Island she hadn't applied to was the one nearest her parents' home. That was what she should have said, but all she could get out was, "I've had a lot of family problems . . . I don't feel comfortable talking about it." She stopped and waited. They let it go.

She needed to tell them one more thing, in case she was accepted. "I have flashbacks at night in the hospital. During these episodes I feel people may harm me." She said it would be best if the staff at the group home left her alone when this happened, didn't speak to her or touch her, let her withdraw and isolate. Several hours later she'd be able to talk. These episodes passed, she said, and they were only at night.

The interview took a half hour. At the end they thanked her for coming and said she'd be hearing soon. She walked out feeling like a real incompetent. It had been a long time since she'd done so poorly on an interview. Was she regressing? She hadn't been able to look up, didn't know if there were five people in the room or twenty-five. On the train ride back she felt weak and very dizzy. God, this was the one she'd wanted. "It's pathetic," she said to a friend at the hospital. "I applied to a group home, not Harvard, and you wait for them to make a decision like your life depends on it."

LINDA SLEZAK and her two assistants discussed the screening immediately after the applicant left. No one spoke for a while. Then Ron Auslander caught Linda Slezak's eyes—they were moist—and said, "She brings out all your mother instincts."

"And your father instincts didn't come out?" Linda Slezak shot back.

Laurie Nardo was the third member of the screening committee. "I'm not a mother or father, but I feel it."

What struck them most wasn't anything Julie had said. It was how she sat hunched forward the whole time, head down, her hair in front of her face, like she was trying to make herself invisible. In Linda Slezak's years as a social worker, she found that after about twenty minutes she could get even the very fragile to look her in the eye and smile about one thing. Not Julie Callahan. The best Julie did was a few quick glances out from behind her hair. No one had to say it. Something awful had happened to Julie that "abused as a young teenager" didn't fully cover. The evaluations had said attractive and stylish, but Linda Slezak was struck by how small, young, and physically immature Julie appeared. Laurie Nardo had mistakenly written in her notes that the twenty-year-old Julie was eighteen.

All three had gone easy questioning her. Often when they had concerns about someone, they'd probe to see how the person responded to a little pressure. None of them wanted to probe Julie's sexual or family history. The evidence was plain to see.

The three agreed that Julie came across as rational, intelligent, with insight into her problem. There were applicants at these screenings who sounded like car salesmen in fifth gear. Another woman from the same borderline unit had let her narcissistic self shine at the screening: "Take me . . . You'll never regret it . . . I'm coming from this top hospital . . . I'll be a group home star . . . I'll make your group home great!" Julie was direct: "I have problems . . . I am frightened . . . I want this . . . I will try." She didn't seem a typical borderline personality at all. In fact, that day, all three social workers commented that they saw nothing in Julie reflecting borderline behavior. They assumed the stress of the interview masked it.

After fifteen minutes skirting around the edges they reached the heart of the matter: How could they not take her? On her notes beside "Recommendation:" Laurie Nardo wrote: "Accept. Patient has a history of severe trauma and is still extremely distrustful and tentative with others."

There was a final hurdle. Julie had to be approved by an administrative review committee of psychiatrists, psychologists, and social workers. Linda Slezak would be responsible for arguing Julie's case before this committee.

The administrative committee usually gave Linda Slezak's choices a rubber stamp. Not this time. People had misgivings. These mental health professionals did traditional clinical therapy. They were in favor of group homes, but not with the same fervor as Linda Slezak. They'd watched the Glen Cove community rise in opposition to the home, knew the hate that was out there and how the civic association leaders were waiting for 9 Highland to fail. Julie had never lived successfully on her own out in the community, they pointed out. She'd been involved sexually with her foster father, tried to poison herself at the school for delinquent girls. Would her sexual promiscuity attract attention in Glen Cove? Glen Cove was a small town, twenty-five thousand people. Would she become the loose number from the group home?

Then Mildred Brodsky, a social worker supervisor, said, "Linda, what will happen to her if we don't take her?"

"Right," said Linda Slezak. Mildred hadn't meant it as a question. They all knew. This young woman might be trapped in a hospital all her life if some group home didn't give her a shot. The fancy borderline unit had done what it could. They were finished with her. She was aging out of foster care. The next hospital would likely be Pilgrim State, where a Julie might be broken.

Linda Slezak's best assurance was: "We feel there's a realistic possibility we can manage her." The committee went along, recommending a few trial overnights for Julie just to make sure.

A week after the interview, Julie heard. She was happy—actually she even felt better than that. She told her friends on the unit, "It's hard for me to keep my ecstaticness down."

Linda Slezak didn't know exactly when 9 Highland would be opening. The opposition had already delayed it over a year, and challenges were continuing in court. As the months passed, several accepted for the house had dropped off the waiting list.

Julie waited. Where else would she go? All her bridges had been burned, and they'd been rotten anyway. A few more months in a mental hospital wasn't going to kill her. Besides, she was terrified of being homeless again.

TWO DAYS BEFORE Christmas of 1988, Julie was scheduled for a trial overnight at the house. She walked past it a couple of times before finding the place. Inside, people were humming around the Christmas tree. Everything was so new. She couldn't tell the staff from residents. Julie noticed the wall-to-wall carpeting. There was a fireplace. She hadn't been in a house with a fireplace before. She'd always wanted to toast marshmallows in a fireplace.

Everyone was smiling too much. It had the feel of the first day at a new school, when no one knows anyone but everyone will pretty soon, and so they're all on their best behavior not to make any memorable mistakes. Julie toured upstairs and down. She didn't go into the kitchen. She didn't know if residents were allowed in the kitchen. In the hospital the kitchen was off-limits. You couldn't just roam around the hospital poking your nose everywhere.

She met the staff and some of the others who'd be living there. To prospective residents like Don Berlin, the house was small. He'd sat in the cramped staff office on the first floor taking his meds and been struck by how you could see in a line straight across to the kitchen on the other side of the house. He wondered, when there were twelve of them, how they'd stop from bumping into each other. Where would he go for privacy? Don was used to privacy and a fireplace. He had grown up in Garden City, one of the wealthier Long Island suburbs. Julie had grown up in a filthy, lice-infested shoebox of a house. She'd only seen one other house from the inside that was as nice as this.

The bedrooms were homey. She'd hoped to get one of the comforters decorated with flowers, but hers was a plain maroon. At night, the room was dark and quiet; few cars traveled Highland Road at that hour. It was the most comfortable bed she'd ever slept in. Another first! Listen to me, Julie thought, I'm turning into an advertisement for the friggin' mental health system. Night was her biggest fear. She was scared she might have a flashback and ruin everything. Get kicked out before she moved in.

But no one commented the next morning. Apparently she hadn't done anything embarrassing. Certainly they would have said something if she had. She and two others, Don and Mary Beth O'Rourke, strolled around the downtown area. Julie loved how close it was, just an easy walk down the hill from the house. The three went to a diner named Henry's for lunch. Both Don and Mary Beth seemed gentle and soft-spoken. Julie didn't think either was likely to be a close friend—they seemed a little too straightforward for her—but she appreciated their pleasantness and thought they'd be easy to get along with. Don, a sweet, plump man with glasses and a precise, sincere way of speaking, looked like a librarian.

After lunch Don walked Julie to the Long Island Rail Road station, about ten minutes from the house, and waited with her for the train back to the hospital. It was a nice gesture, Julie felt. When it was time to say good-bye, Don leaned forward and suddenly gave her a huge, wet, passionate kiss on the lips. Julie froze. Before she had time to be upset, the train doors slid shut. What the hell was that? Julie wondered as the train pulled off. Why'd he do it? Had she done something to lead him on? Was she developing a pattern, like they said? Just what she needed, a promiscuity charge even before she'd moved in.

Her hospital pass was good until 5 P.M. She arrived back on the ward as night fell, Christmas Eve, her third straight Christmas at a mental hospital.

chapter 2

WE LOVE MENTALLY
ILL PEOPLE

LINDA SLEZAK'S search for a home had started in early 1987. That winter and spring she looked at fifty houses. After a while she'd seen so many they blurred in her mind. The state was vague about how much she could spend. Linda figured it would take between $300,000 and $400,000 for purchase and renovations. It sounded like a lot, but the real estate market was booming in New York's suburbs, prices were at record highs, and she needed six bedrooms, four bathrooms, and three thousand square feet to meet state standards. Plus, Glen Cove, New York, is an upper-middle-class community. There are poorer areas on the Island where she could have found a house for half that price, but the state's policy was to spread these houses around so there would be no group home ghettos.

A realtor showed her a house on Pearl Street with an unattached cottage that seemed a good bet. The price was in the ballpark. She called an appraiser, arranged for an architectural feasibility study, and brought her supervisor, Dr. Dan Vogrin, to see it. The house could be adapted to sleep twelve. For two months she dealt with an agent at Sound Real Estate, visiting the house several times. The agent seemed casual for someone who stood to make 7 percent of $350,000. The woman's answers were a little vague. She kept saying she *thought* the owner would be interested in selling. Then she stopped returning calls. Finally Linda got her on the phone to ask, "Is something wrong?"

"My boss won't let me sell to you," the agent said. Linda found a house, on LeMarcus, up the hill from the mental health clinic. The owners had a retarded daughter and were sympathetic. The house was nearly one hundred years old and would need major renovations, but it was large and had been a nursing home in an earlier time, so there was a precedent for a nontraditional residential use. State construction analysts inspected the home and approved. On June 10, Linda notified the city of her intent to open a group home there. The day before they were to go to contract, the lawyer for the owners called to cancel. Another buyer made a cash offer for the house, the lawyer said.

She made hundreds of calls. Always she'd explain up front that this was to be used as a group home for the mentally ill. Many people were quite honest. "Oh, no way. I'm moving out of town, but I still wouldn't do that to my neighbors." She never considered bringing a civil rights suit. Even if she won, it would take years, and the point was to open a group home fast, not make new law.

She and Dan Vogrin met with Glen Cove mayor Vincent Suozzi to let him know of their hunt for a house. Under state law they had no obligation to do so, but they wanted to be good neighbors and keep the mayor informed. Mayor Suozzi was sixty-one at the time and in his eleventh year as mayor. He was a pragmatic, old-fashioned Glen Cove pol, the son of immigrants who knew everyone in town by name and tended to think of politics in ethnic terms. The mayor acted friendly, but never was quite satisfied with Linda's site selections. He said he wouldn't recommend buying the house Linda had seen on Landing Road; that was a Polish neighborhood and the people would put up ferocious resistance. He also felt it was too close to a home for the retarded. At another point he advised against a house in Strathmore Glen, a modern section of single-family homes. He felt that heavily Jewish community would band together and resist.

Finally, in early summer, an agent from Gil Realty took Linda to see a colonial-style home being sold by a couple getting divorced. The divorce was so stormy, a receiver had been appointed by the courts to sell the house. The house *had* to be sold. Linda Slezak was delighted with what she saw. The location was perfect. From the house, it was an easy walk down the hill one block to Glen Cove's main shopping district. The principal bus depot in Glen Cove was just two-tenths of a mile away. The Long Island Rail Road train station was a ten-minute walk. Linda pulled out her tape measure and went from room to room. The house met state standards; they'd be able to sleep twelve. The price was reasonable, $320,000. It would have been nice if the backyard were bigger, but all in all Linda could not have been more pleased. It was located on a corner lot, abutting just two homes, which would minimize impact on the street. A ten-foot-high hedge surrounded much of the property, blocking out one of the neighboring homes completely.

When Linda notified Mayor Suozzi's office about 9 Highland, a City Hall aide asked if she could hold off until after the primary in September. The mayor had a tough reelection bid coming. He felt that no matter what position he took, he'd alienate people and lose votes. Linda was inclined to give him the benefit of the doubt on this. She realized group homes didn't bring out the best in local politicians, but he seemed to be a decent person and was fairly straightforward about what was on his mind. Like Linda, he was a Democrat in an overwhelmingly Republican county. She felt he was asking for a trade-off: Put this thing off until after the primary and you'll get help with the group home.

She was willing to go along with the aide's request, and conveyed this to her superiors. Though the group home was state funded, had to meet state specifications, and was open to anyone no matter how poor, it would be run by the Angelo Melillo mental health center, a private, nonprofit agency in Glen Cove. Linda had been hired by the Melillo clinic in January of 1987 to create a group home program for the agency. She answered to Dan Vogrin, a psychologist who was the clinic's executive director, and also to the Melillo Center's board of directors. For twenty-five years the clinic had operated quietly in Glen

Cove, providing individual and family therapy as well as alcohol treatment. In New York State, private nonprofit agencies like Melillo run about 90 percent of the group homes for the mentally ill.

During the 1970s, when the public mental hospitals were being emptied into the streets, the state had little interest in creating group homes. Small nonprofit agencies stitched grants together and opened homes to meet their local problems. By 1980, when the state finally acknowledged the need for large-scale community development, there were already about forty homes for the mentally ill being operated by nonprofits across New York. Having nonprofits do it took some of the political heat off the state. It wasn't the big, bad state marching into Glen Cove to open a house; it was their fellow Glen Cove residents, Linda Slezak and the Melillo board members. And the nonprofit agencies could run a group home for about 40 percent less than it would cost the state to do the job itself. A state-run home had to hire its workers from the state psychiatric hospital system and pay them a union wage; the nonprofit agencies were nonunion and paid less. Personnel costs for a twelve-bed state-run group home were about $240,000 a year, versus $130,000 a year for a nonprofit like Melillo.

At the July 21, 1987, meeting the Melillo board of directors voted to honor the request from the mayor's office and hold off on 9 Highland until after the September primary. The only person present who disagreed was Melillo's new attorney, Seth Stein. Stein devoted much of his law practice to getting group homes opened. He told board members that in his experience delaying never helped, that politicians would oppose these houses regardless of how many hoops the agency jumped through. He wanted to say more, but this was his first Melillo board meeting. It would have been impolite to be too forceful. He didn't tell them that a few years earlier he'd represented an agency opening a group home for the retarded in a wealthy section of Great Neck, Long Island. Trying to be good citizens, Seth and the director of *that* agency had gone to *that* mayor and confided that they planned to soon buy 312 Melbourne Road. Forewarned, these wealthy, enterprising Great Neck neighbors banded together, formed a corporation, and bought 312 Melbourne first, so it could not become a group home.

The state attorney general had to drag them through the courts to get the house back. The opening of *that* group home was delayed years.

Seth Stein knew that Melillo's board members didn't have the vaguest idea of what they were about to get themselves into. Gil McGill, a local attorney who was the new president of the board, had voted in favor of a group home without really knowing what one was. He had never visited one. These board members had joined an agency that was perceived in Glen Cove as a do-gooder organization, along the lines of the Red Cross or Boy Scouts. The Melillo Center shared a building with the Boys' Club. Who could be opposed to alcohol treatment and family counseling? Melillo board members were professionals, businesspeople, government workers, hospital officials, anthropology professors. Many were quite conservative. Both Gil McGill and Dan Vogrin were involved in Republican politics in the towns where they lived. These were the kind of people active in the library and volunteer ambulance squad. They weren't prepared to be despised.

MAYOR SUOZZI easily won the Democratic primary on September 15, and on the sixteenth, at a special 8 A.M. meeting, the Melillo board unanimously approved the purchase of 9 Highland Road. Though a notice had been sent to all members announcing that the group home would be the focus of the board meeting, only eight of twenty-five showed, just one above the number needed to conduct business. Also attending that meeting were Linda Slezak, Seth Stein, and Karen Mankin, a state official in charge of group home development. Mankin told the board that the state considered 9 Highland an ideal location and that if the Glen Cove agency didn't approve it, the state would find another nonprofit agency to run a group home there. Dan Vogrin explained that expanding into group homes was a way to help the clinic grow and said he hoped the agency would run several someday. The meeting was quite upbeat.

Within three weeks the agency had put down $16,000—5 percent —and signed a binder for 9 Highland. The closing was scheduled for mid-December. On October 6, Linda Slezak personally drove to city hall to deliver the official notice required by state law, announcing the intention to open a group home. The mayor wasn't in, so she left the papers for him. When he returned Mayor Suozzi threw a fit. Were they trying to turn the group home into a political football? He didn't want word leaking out about a group home on Highland before the November 3 election. He was damn well going to get them to withdraw this stupid notice. The mayor asked Dan Vogrin to city hall. He intended to tell off this Vogrin guy, good.

Suozzi is a big-bodied man, well over six feet tall, an imposing figure. He was livid, pacing his office, gesturing, talking rapidly. When he calmed down enough to sit, he wiggled his foot ferociously. "What are you, a bunch of jackasses?" Mayor Suozzi shouted at the Melillo director. "This is a catastrophe." Didn't they understand it would be used against him in the election? This man Vogrin had a doctorate— he needed to go back to school. "You're an intelligent person," said the mayor. "What are you putting this on my desk?" These people had to be stupid. "I have to think of myself, too," the mayor said. "Can't this wait two or three months?" Didn't Vogrin understand that the election was mean-spirited enough without a group home being tossed in? Mayor Suozzi was up against Republican city councilman Donald DeRiggi, and they hated each other. All he needed was DeRiggi labeling him a group home lover.

As a matter of law, Melillo did not have to wait; the agency could begin the notification process whenever it desired. But Dan Vogrin was not looking for a confrontation. A quiet, reserved, conservative man, Dan had no desire to make an enemy of the mayor. He didn't want to turn the group home into an issue during the election either, and offered to withdraw the notice until November.

When Linda Slezak heard, she kept silent, but was disappointed by her boss. First Mayor Suozzi wanted to wait for the primary; now the election; next they'd all be waiting for Suozzi's reelection. She was coming to see Seth Stein's point. There never was a good time to announce a group home.

At the October 21 Melillo board meeting, members discussed the group home again. One of the board's anthropology professors, Dr. Jean Wagner, asked what they would do if there was "vigorous protest" from the neighbors. Could they get out of the contract for the Highland site in that event? On November 3, Mayor Suozzi was defeated. On November 4, Linda Slezak sent the mayor formal notice of the plans for 9 Highland. Under state law, the clock was now running; the city had forty days to decide whether to support or oppose the home.

All was quiet for a week.

THE LAW governing group homes in New York state has been damned as discriminatory, because it singles out group homes for a special hearing procedure. The law requires agencies to give municipalities notice before opening a group home. Critics of the law say if the mentally ill or retarded want to buy a house in a residential area, it is no one's business, and they shouldn't have to notify the municipality of their intent.

On the other hand, the New York law restricts the legal grounds for opposing a group home, limiting local political interference. As a result, it is credited with spurring group home growth. Seth Stein has repeatedly used the law to open homes in the face of overwhelming local opposition. Passed in 1978, it is known as the Padavan law, named for its sponsor, state senator Frank Padavan of Queens. Even its name is testament to the law's confusing, tangled roots. Senator Padavan often battled group homes and advocates for the handicapped, yet the Padavan law has fostered group home development.

Until the mid-1970s, group homes were so rare, there was no talk of a law to regulate them. Large numbers of retarded and mentally ill continued to live in crowded, run-down state institutions, just as they had in this country since the opening of the state asylums in the early nineteenth century. But on January 6, 1972, Geraldo Rivera, then a young reporter for the local ABC television station, took a camera crew into Building 6 of Willowbrook state institution for the retarded on Staten Island, New York. He filmed a ward of sixty emaciated children, many naked, some in straitjackets, a place with shit smeared on the walls and a single attendant to keep order. The shocking footage was the impetus for a federal lawsuit that in 1975 produced a remarkable consent decree. New York governor Hugh Carey and the federal judge agreed they would not simply settle for making Willowbrook a better institution. Instead, the fifty-four hundred residents of Willowbrook were to be moved out. At the time, the state had about 150 group homes for the retarded *and* mentally ill. Suddenly, just to meet the needs for the retarded at Willowbrook, New York was under court order to add over 500 group homes.

This push into the communities was nationwide. Forty states eventually came under similar court orders involving retarded adults. For the first time in the history of this country, large numbers of handicapped adult Americans would be living out in the neighborhoods in publicly funded housing.

Over the next three years the battle to establish group homes turned vicious. To local leaders, supporting a group home was political suicide. A typical opposition tactic in those days was for a zoning board to rule that a group home was legally a boardinghouse—a place where several unrelated people lived—and boardinghouses were prohibited in residential zones. An even cruder zoning tactic was for a town to pass a law retroactively prohibiting group homes. Governor Hugh Carey's administration defended group homes in about two dozen of these cases from 1975 to 1978. Such local laws were blatantly unconstitutional, but by the time courts overturned them group home agencies had often lost the houses they had an option to buy. A bad local law could still be an effective delaying tactic to kill a group home. As a result, Governor Carey's liberal Democratic administration wanted to pass a law that would bring some order to the process and help open the group homes they had pledged in the Willowbrook consent decree.

Opponents of group homes had their own reasons for wanting a law. Their efforts to stop homes from 1975 to 1978 had met with mixed results. The 1970s was a decade when courts were generally responsive to social change and group home advocates had won their cases several times in state courts. A case of particular importance was a home for retarded children opened in Senator Frank Padavan's Queens district. The agency, Working Organization for Retarded Children, signed a contract in 1975 to buy a house and *then* informed the Queens community. When the leaders of the local civic association learned, they challenged the house in court as a violation of single-family zoning. They got their local politician—Senator Padavan—involved. Senator Padavan argued that the home had been sneaked in and the community should have received prior notice. The lawsuit put a real strain on the Queens group home agency. With pending litigation, the agency couldn't secure a mortgage from a bank to buy the home, so it was forced to pay cash. After the purchase, the house sat vacant two years while the case wound its way through the courts. Finally, in 1977, the group home prevailed. Senator Padavan was peeved. The conservative Republican senator from Queens wanted a law that would require communities to be given prior notice.

Paul Litwak, an attorney in Governor Carey's office of Mental Hygiene who actually wrote most of the bill, believes Senator Padavan may not have fully understood the implications. "We sure knew this bill would facilitate group homes," says Litwak. "We knew, but we were not about to be real public about the power of the bill and certainly we weren't going to share our perception of the bill with Senator Padavan." Senator Padavan, chairman of the mental hygiene committee in the Republican-controlled state senate at the time, says he understood full well; he was simply looking for a law that would balance community rights with the rights of the handicapped.

If Senator Padavan did indeed misread the power of the bill he was lending his name to, he was not alone. The press certainly didn't catch it. Passage of the Padavan law attracted little notice. Longtime advocates for group homes were confused about it, too. Murray Schneps, the attorney for the group home in the Working Organization for Retarded Children case in Queens, opposed the Padavan law in 1978. He felt it was anti–group home and he had no love for Senator Padavan. Few advocates did. But in time most of them developed a fondness for "his" law.

· · ·

THE PADAVAN LAW killed opponents' most important means of blocking the homes: their friendly local zoning boards. Its key provision was to bypass local boards and appoint a state hearing officer to decide if a group home should be approved. The law mandated that the home had to be treated like a single-family residence for zoning purposes, as long as it housed no more than fourteen people. This guaranteed an agency the legal right to place a group home in any residential neighborhood in New York State.

The law set strict timetables for administrative action, making it easier for an agency like Melillo to get a mortgage for a house. Once the agency informs the city of a planned group home, the city has forty days to approve or challenge the home. During this period the city can (and usually does) hold a public hearing. Assuming the home meets state construction and square-footage guidelines, local officials can oppose it on only two grounds: that their town is being oversaturated with group homes, or that there is a better alternate site in their town for the group home. If the city decides to oppose the group home, an administrative hearing is to be held within fifteen days. The hearing is conducted by an official from the state Office of Mental Health. Within thirty days, the decision whether to approve the group home is to be rendered by the commissioner of the Office of Mental Health. Generally this has been good news for group home advocates. Since the late 1970s it has been the state's policy to fund and open group homes, so the state commissioner is likely to be a receptive judge. If the commissioner rules in favor of the group home, local officials have thirty days to appeal to the state courts. Appeals skip the first tier of courts and go directly to the state's appellate division. This higher court is less likely to be swayed by the pressures of local politics. Indeed, the courts have been extremely supportive of group homes, interpreting the Padavan law as having a strong, pro–group home orientation.

The Padavan law was a classic example of protecting an unpopular minority to achieve a public policy goal. In the 1960s, civil rights for black Americans was imposed on southern states by federal law and federal courts. In the 1980s, under Ronald Reagan, the federal government quit advocating for the disadvantaged. Civil rights for mentally ill and retarded New Yorkers seeking a home on a quiet street in the 1980s was imposed on local towns by state law and state courts.

From the advocate's point of view the Padavan law had only one major drawback: the prior notice provision often subjected an agency like Melillo to months of relentless pounding by neighbors and local politicians.

ON NOVEMBER 13, 1987, Mayor Suozzi responded to Linda Slezak's letter, saying he opposed the group home at 9 Highland. The site was neither "suitable" or "practical," he wrote, "and it is not located in a functional community setting." He noted that Highland Road traffic was "very heavy" at present and would be much worse if a proposed hotel was built downtown. He suggested a more isolated site in a wooded area, away from most people, similar to the Red Spring Lane site in Glen Cove, where a group home for retarded adults had opened in 1980. He emphasized that Melillo should not seek such a site in Glen Cove, but instead go to another town, maybe Lattingtown or Locust Valley or some other part of Oyster Bay. He accused the mental health agency of "insensitivity" and wanted to know why state officials hadn't "interacted with local government officials before a decision is reached." He blasted the Padavan law as a "travesty of moral justice" and sent copies of his letter to all the local newspapers.

Linda Slezak felt like someone had dropped a group home on her head. She was particularly infuriated at Suozzi's lines about not interacting with local officials. She wanted to tell the newspapers what nonsense it was. She felt it was ridiculous to protect this politician. Cooperation had gained them nothing, and now the mayor was making them look bad publicly. But Dan Vogrin, her supervisor, said no; it was dangerous calling a politician a phony in print.

Mayor Suozzi didn't say it at a public meeting, but he saw the need for group homes and wasn't unsympathetic. He also felt that by reject-ing 9 Highland he was doing what any normal mayor would do. Even back in 1979, with the isolated Red Spring Lane site for the retarded—which he now acknowledged was excellent—he had suggested alter-nate sites. You oppose these just to placate the closest nearby neigh-bors, he said. He knew that even the people living two blocks away weren't really affected. As for 9 Highland, the address didn't really matter, it would have been the same for any site. He didn't feel any mayor could approve any specific group home site, especially in an area of any density. Though he was in his sixties and had just been voted out, who knew what his political future might be? You support a group home, he said privately, voters don't forget that kind of thing.

WITHIN A WEEK of Mayor Suozzi's letter, a Highland Road civic association was formed and on November 20 neighbors filled City Hall to discuss how to stop the proposed home. The opponents' meeting was the lead story in the weekly Glen Cove *Record-Pilot* Thanksgiving morning, 1987, with the entire account devoted to strat-egies for killing the home. The story featured a front-page picture of the president of the newly formed civic association, identified as Dr. Roy Speiser of Stuart Drive. No Melillo official was quoted.

With each week the *Record-Pilot* stories grew stronger. The head-line Thanksgiving morning referred to the "Home For Transitional Mental Patients." A few issues later, the front-page headline was call-ing 9 Highland the "Mental Group Home." The November 26 issue pointed out that fire escapes would be mandated and "will definitively change the residential character of the neighborhood." In fact, group homes in New York look like any other residential home and do not have fire escapes, which Dan Vogrin and Linda Slezak pointed out in the December 3 *Record-Pilot.* However the *Record-Pilot* was not about to trust the likes of Dan Vogrin or Linda Slezak, and in the same December 3 story gave opponents the final word on fire escapes. The newspaper quoted "some residents of the area" who "claimed that architects with whom the Melillo agency had been in contact, had said there would be fire escapes." (The agency couldn't win; when people finally accepted that there would be no fire escape, local resident Harold Seidman warned they were creating a firetrap.)

Linda Slezak was growing more frustrated by the day. She didn't expect the members of the Highland civic association to like the group home; she just wanted them to have the facts straight. On December 2, at about 3:30, her office phone rang and it was a man who identified himself as Jim Iversen. He explained that he lived in the area and was a member of the Highland civic association. He said he was a private investigator doing pro bono work for the association. He was trying to get information about the home. The Melillo Center's policy was to be responsive to all inquiries. The more Linda talked to James Iversen on the phone, the more she liked him. He wasn't asking about fire escapes or mental inmates. Here was a guy who seemed intelligent and fairly open-minded, and was quite amiable. Linda saw the conversation as an opportunity to explain why group homes were needed. In particular, Iversen seemed very curious about Linda's contacts with Mayor Suozzi, especially the mayor's opinions on earlier sites and his feelings about the Highland Road site. Linda didn't mind telling him. She wanted the neighbors to know that the agency had tried its best to be a good citizen by keeping Mayor Suozzi informed from the start. When they finished, Linda felt the talk with Iversen had been productive.

The same week she took a call from city councilman Donald De-Riggi, who had defeated Mayor Suozzi and would be taking over as mayor in January. He wanted to meet to discuss the home. Linda suggested inviting her supervisor too, but the mayor-elect preferred seeing Linda alone. She thought that odd, but figured that as incoming mayor maybe he preferred a low-key briefing. Everything in the paper was so slanted, she was pleased to have the chance to get her views across to him. He suggested lunch Friday at Old Gerlich's, a popular spot with Glen Cove political types.

When she arrived at the restaurant, she did not see Mayor-elect DeRiggi. A man asked if she was Linda Slezak. It was James Iversen, the pro bono private investigator. "The mayor didn't tell you I was invited, too?" Linda was irritated. She was expecting a one-on-one with the new mayor. Donald DeRiggi arrived soon after. The mayor-elect made a big deal out of finding the right table, and sitting in a special way. He sat Linda down in the middle seat with her back to the wall. DeRiggi was on her right, Iversen on her left. DeRiggi insisted only this seating arrangement would do. Linda noticed that he kept parading back and forth to the buffet table, as if trying to show off their meeting. The mayor-elect wasn't asking questions about how group homes worked. All he seemed to care about was her past meetings with Mayor Suozzi and Melillo's decision to delay the home until after the election. Each time he asked her a question about Mayor Suozzi, he'd tell Linda, "You'll have to speak up, I have this very bad cold. My ears are stuffed up. Speak up." Linda spoke up. She was practically shouting. He kept trying to pour her wine. She refused, but he persisted. Iversen seemed to squirm in his seat, as if he was embarrassed. Every time Linda tried to talk about the group home, Councilman DeRiggi changed the subject to Mayor Suozzi.

The meeting dragged on for an hour. It was pointless. Linda was anxious to get back to work. She was tired of talking so loud.

Afterward, Dan Vogrin asked how it went. "It wasn't what I expected," she said. "I have such a funny feeling about it. I can't put my finger on it."

That night at 2 A.M. she woke from a nightmare, her heart and head pounding. She'd dreamed she was in a house with a sliding back door. The door opened and a little animal dashed out of the forest through the door, and began biting Linda's leg. She couldn't shake the animal loose. It was a specific animal, but its name kept eluding her. She awakened still trying to identify the animal. The dream had left her with such a frightening feeling. She was sweating and crying. Then it dawned on her: it was a ferret. "Oh my God!" she said. He kept telling her to talk louder. He was taping the conversation. Iversen had been taping the conversation at lunch. It had to be: The private investigator. Sit this way. Speak up. They should have just said, "Talk into the microphone, you fool!"

Linda climbed out of bed, went into the bathroom, washed her face, and took some aspirin for the pounding in her head. She went back to bed, but couldn't sleep. She kept hoping her husband Jim would waken so she could tell him. What had she gotten herself into? Where was this going to stop? She lay in the dark, waiting for morning.

THE PUBLIC HEARING was 7:30, December 9, at city hall. Before the meeting Linda, Dan Vogrin, agency attorney Seth Stein, and Karen Mankin, from the state office of mental health, met for dinner. Stein cautioned them not to take the opponents' comments too seriously. It didn't matter, he kept repeating; the law was on their side. He told Linda the same when she called him with her suspicions of being secretly tape-recorded: it didn't matter. "They can say what they say," Seth told her, "you haven't done anything wrong. You have a good site, you'll win at the hearing stage." These disputes had to run their course, like a fever, he said. The anger had been festering in the neighborhood for weeks, so the public hearing would be bad, and things would continue bad for a while. They just had to hang on until the fever broke.

Stein didn't like these meetings, but he had been to enough of them not to take them personally. He never allowed himself to show the slightest loss of control. He had to be able to answer everything, even at the expense of appearing to be a smart-ass know-it-all. He'd seen the alternative: once they sense you're on the defensive, they press you like a dog. Seth did not mind confrontation, he thrived on it. He'd been a star high school debater and a language major at Columbia, studying Greek and Latin.

During dinner, Karen Mankin took the official state line, saying that these meetings were a good chance to educate the public. Seth did not believe it for a second. You can't educate people while they're pounding you on the head. He did not believe there was enough education in the world to get the people of Highland Road to voluntarily accept a home on their street for twelve mentally ill people.

The four were the first to arrive at city hall and took seats together in the front row.

· · ·

BY THE TIME the meeting began, over one hundred people had squeezed into the oak pews in the council chambers, with the overflow standing in the rear and around the sides. They were an impressive-looking group. Several, in business suits, had come to city hall directly from their jobs in New York City. The city council, including Mayor Suozzi, and Mayor-elect DeRiggi, sat up on the elevated podium at the front of the hall. Behind them were teal-colored banners proclaiming Glen Cove's two-hundredth anniversary.

Mayor Suozzi welcomed everyone. "I would ask only that we are courteous to each other," he began. "Let's have some respect." In particular, he said, "I do not want any catcalling!"

Dan Vogrin and Linda Slezak talked first, standing and speaking from their seats in the audience, describing the Melillo agency and the proposed group home—what it is, how it runs. Then Roy Speiser, head of the civic association, took over the meeting. Speiser, a chiropractor whose office is around a corner two blocks from the home, began by making it clear that anything said that evening should not be construed as being unsympathetic to the plight of the mentally ill. "The thing is we all are considerate of these people. Mentally ill people certainly deserve proper treatment. I don't think anybody I have spoken to in the community is in any way insensitive to the needs. We all agree that these patients do need proper care."

He had concerns, though. "Well, according to the people I spoke to, which we will have the testimony here tonight from a doctor of psychology . . . he says in his professional opinion that not only have those programs failed, but they failed to achieve the goals they're set up to achieve. They do not really help these patients; in fact they are doing more harm . . . They want to take these patients out of these terrible institutional settings and I am sympathetic, I think it is a terrible place and the state should have thought of this a long time ago and should have taken care of it, or maybe they should have upgraded facilities they had. Maybe they should have managed it better."

And what about the people who would be living in the group home?

"Potentially," said the chiropractor, "they could have been dangerous to themselves, they might have committed some dangerous activities. In some cases they have schizophrenia, psychosis, other possible psychiatric problems, and now they are put under control by chemical means, . . . given severe doses of medication to chemically control them . . . Now they are saying we are going to take these people out of the psychiatric facility and put them into a residential house right in your neighborhood. They're going to tell us these patients are OK, they can function in society, we want to integrate them back into society. Well according to one psychologist I have spoken to . . . they may never integrate into society, they may never be able to hold jobs. . . . Are these patients really going to get well in a group residence house?"

He pointed out that group home members were going to have to walk down the hill to town to catch the bus. "A steep hill, a dangerous hill and there is a lot of traffic. These patients will come out, they're on heavy medication, somewhat disoriented, probably out of touch with reality . . . and have to walk down the steep hill. In the wintertime it is icy." He wanted to know if it was really fair to do this to the mentally ill.

"Are we as a community going to be served? To me it doesn't smell right." He questioned whether they wanted this "experimental program" on their street. He felt the house was too small. "Do you know anyone that has twelve people in a residential house?" he asked. "Really what you are creating here is a barracks."

And what about the little children? There was a school bus stop two hundred feet from the house. "Little children have to stand and wait for their bus to come along. I have a son that is two and a half. I spoke to many of the mothers on the block . . . and I will tell you that the mothers that I spoke to would absolutely not allow their child to stand on that corner with this facility in front of it, not one of them. Would you trust your five-year-old child to stand there by himself when you have twelve psychiatric patients twenty or thirty feet away from them? Would you? I certainly wouldn't."

A block away from 9 Highland is Saint Paul's Episcopal Church. "Right across the street you have a day nursery school, Saint Paul's," the chiropractor continued. "My wife has spoken with some of the mothers who have their children there. They don't feel comfortable about it at all. They already had one incident where somebody wandered in the school. The public schools have extraordinary security, they have passwords, they have TV cameras, they don't allow people in because of all the incidents with children getting kidnapped or injured or hurt. Is it safe to have a collection of twelve people right there at a school bus stop and right across the street from a nursery school? . . . The point I'm trying to make is why are we graced with this or blessed with this selection when other areas need to be served?"

In concluding, the chiropractor reemphasized his compassion. His speech was met by loud applause.

An older woman, Paula Kabnick, began, "I'm Mrs. Kabnick and I live at 39 Highland. I've been a wife of a doctor for forty years." She wanted to talk about traffic. "If anybody ever came down Highland Road, normal people like me, we take our lives in our hands." She was particularly concerned about the new city parking garage, on the edge of downtown, a block from the house. "They come out from there and going left or going right, coming down the hill, going left, going right, you have congestion there . . . It has become Thirty-fourth Street and Fifth Avenue—Christmas! How can you put these poor people in a place like that? Are you going to . . . tie them down, hold their hands like you walk the poor children who walk across the street on School Street that have a problem? The light goes fast, they don't go fast. I mean they are afraid they will be run over. Adults are run over. I have had several close calls myself. How can you put poor people in a neighborhood like that?"

The difficulty of placing a group home anywhere became apparent with the next speaker, Dr. Rocco Cirigliano, a psychologist in private practice who lives in the neighborhood. Dr. Cirigliano worried not about too much traffic, but that the street was too quiet—there wasn't enough traffic, apparently—and the house should be put on a *busier* street. "If I were God and in charge of this situation, I probably would have handled it much differently," Dr. Cirigliano explained. "I would want some neighborhood where there would be anonymity. I would want them to go and come without being identified. I would want to have it definitely on a larger street, a street where there would be people in the neighborhood that would not have to crisscross in front of this facility every day."

They had come together to discuss mental health, but the civic association's psychologist believed a key mental-health issue was being overlooked. "Someone should be caring about the people in the community and their mental health," he said. "There has been a violation of the people on a mental health level and my feeling is that— could not something else have been done differently?"

As Dr. Cirigliano spoke, it was hard to get a clear picture of exactly where he wanted these people to live, although he plainly did not want them in a group home on Highland Road. "I do not feel that they should be given a normal community environment," he said. "My contention as a professional is that what these people need is an enriched community environment." Where then? It sounded like they would be far away, and yet close at the same time: "Some kind of cluster community . . . a facility where they can live the rest of their lives with a total support system for them, with health facilities they need, with the rehabilitation program they need." In case anyone felt this sounded like a state mental hospital, Dr. Cirigliano elaborated. "Not Pilgrim State," he said. "But a community on their own where they could receive what support systems they need and yet be relative to the community."

He concluded by saying, "We have a name for fourteen people living in a house that was built for four, with five to twelve or fourteen people visiting them. We call it a slum." The audience burst into applause.

Roy Speiser wanted to know what would happen at night, from 11 P.M. to 6 A.M., when there was just one counselor on duty. "What if one of those patients wakes up and decides to wander off? Anyone can go into a psychiatric episode, no alarms on the doors, they can walk right out the door . . . One person, possibly a high school graduate that is trained who may have worked in the Burger King, is competent to watch these twelve psychiatric patients?"

Linda Slezak answered that staff would be a mix of professionals and paraprofessionals, and all would be given special training in mental health care. "In terms of the staff member who will be sleeping at the residence, there is really almost no such thing as a person having a sudden episode," she said. "That is not our experience." That brought sarcastic comments from the audience. "A trained staff will see signs and symptoms," she continued, "will know the trouble is coming and will know how to take care of it." Again there were sarcastic comments: "You expect us to believe this?"

People began shouting out questions at her.

"What are they going to do to get fresh air? Are they going to walk the streets? Are they going to go to facilities? They have to breathe."

Linda said they would do pretty much the same thing people in the neighborhood do.

"I have a garden," a woman shouted.

"This house has a backyard," Linda responded.

"No they don't," said the voice.

"It is bigger than mine," said Linda.

"For these poor people," a voice from the audience continued, "they'll be breathing in gasoline and oil and not fresh air. I think you should find a facility where you will have enjoyable green grass and animals."

Several times when Linda tried to answer, she was drowned out by comments or boos from the audience.

"Please don't," Mayor Suozzi said. "Especially this time of year." He hated to see catcalling at Christmastime.

''I HAVE BEEN on that street for thirty-two years," began Marilyn Goodman, another neighbor. "It is one of the most beautiful streets in all of Glen Cove. We have great pride. I also have great compassion for the patients, but this is not the place. . . . New York has many halfway houses and at those very halfway houses people are not in shackles, they are not in chains and nothing is there to keep them in that house. They are free. Many of those free people who wandered away from the halfway house on Thorazine neglected their medicine and they are sleeping on the street. I want to be honest with you. I have two daughters that are psychologists and before I came down here . . . I asked for some input. Both of them grew up in Glen Cove, both of them went to schools in Glen Cove. Look at Highland Road. You know very well what kind of people you are talking about. We do not have chains, we do not have shackled patients. If they are schizophrenic, my rights are being absolutely denied when I do not know who these people are because of the privacy and privilege of communication of doctor-patient relationships. I have no idea who my next-door neighbor is going to be, but if the patient wanders away and sits on my neighbor's front step, who is going to come and get them? Because they do, they are disheveled and they have problems and it is true, we know it. We know it very well. If a patient neglects to return home, who is going to put him on medication, who is going to go after him? It happens all the time. It shouldn't happen in our neighborhood. We have a very old, wonderful street and I really want to preserve that character."

Many of the audience questions were handled by Melillo's attorney. As Seth Stein spoke, he gazed around the room, making eye contact. They asked if instead of one house of twelve, Melillo would consider three small houses of four. No. They asked if they found an alternate site that was as good, would Melillo take it. Seth said the law only required them to take an alternate site considered *superior*, not simply as good. This had been upheld by the appellate division, he said. They asked about the group home budget. He explained the mix of state and federal funding. Alan Parente, a former mayor of Glen Cove, asked wasn't it possible the state could stop funding group homes. Seth said it was. What then? said Parente. Seth told him it was as likely as the state's ending funding for nursing homes or Medicaid. "How likely is that?" Seth asked him, and Parente changed the subject.

"Can we know the names of the private banks providing the mortgage?" Parente asked.

"No," said Seth, "that's private."

"Can we get that under the Freedom of Information Act?" asked Parente.

"You can request that," said Seth.

"I suggest that the city counsel request that information because I would like to know which bank or if the banks are aware what the money they are going to be lending is going to be used for."

"The banks are fully aware," said Seth.

Former mayor Parente then launched into a lengthy speech on the victimization of Glen Cove. This is what he couldn't understand: "Why Glen Cove? This community probably has done more to meet the social needs of its residents than any other community around . . . If they went into Brookville or Lattingtown or Locust Valley, because of the wealth and affluence and powers of those people, they would have a very difficult time, so they chose Glen Cove, and I take it as a personal affront when these people stand up and have the gall to tell the people in this audience and myself that that house up there is not going to have an effect on the property value of the people who live there, that it's not going to have an effect on that downtown area. We know it will . . . It will, no matter what!" He suggested the city hire special counsel to oppose the home, and became the first to pledge a donation.

Only a couple of speakers from the audience spoke for the home, and none were from the neighborhood. Gil McGill, the local attorney who is Melillo board president, talked briefly. Behind the scenes he had been working for the home, but he had made a decision to say as little as possible publicly. He ran a one-man law office and was afraid being too openly supportive would hurt business. By the time he was done speaking, his tone was so conciliatory, a man from the audience shouted: "Are you saying at this time you are going to establish a moratorium?" Seth took over and said they would do what was required by law.

Howard Rothenberg, the social worker on the eighteen-bed psychiatric wing at Glen Cove Hospital, spoke of the need. There were only six group homes for the mentally ill in Nassau County, he pointed out; the state estimated about fifty were needed. In the last year, he said, forty patients from Glen Cove Hospital could have used a group home; only one got in. "From where I sit and from my job, that is a shame. It creates a problem for me as a discharge person. I am the one who tries to help these people plan . . . So far I have only been able to successfully place one person in a community residence." While waiting for a group home, this person was rehospitalized four times, "because he did not have an adequate place to live and he came to my hospital basically because it got cold in November." A group home, he said would serve the community well.

Serve the community? said Eric Pasmatera, a member of the audience. "Serving six or twelve people from the community, you are not serving the community. This," he said gesturing toward the nicely dressed men and women in the packed room, "is the community."

No elected official spoke in favor of the site. The closest to being supportive was Joe Cassin, a city councilman who's a professor at a local college. Of course, he was as "disappointed" as anyone in this particular site, he said. But he went on to say, "I don't know about anybody else in this room, but I have a nephew who is in one of these facilities in California . . . He cannot function alone. He was out in a Jeep, bounced his head, was unconscious for two and a half months and finally was pieced back together and was a burden to his family in such a way that nobody could function at home. What were they going to do, put him in a jail somewhere? The philosophy of these community homes is correct . . . What about my nephew? Should he be kept under lock and key? He can function to a point, he is learning."

A voice from the audience called out, "How big is the place where your nephew is?"

It was twelve people, like the proposed Highland Road home.

The leader of the civic association shot up his hand. "In respect to your nephew, Mr. Cassin. Your nephew has traumatic brain damage," said Speiser, the chiropractor. "I have treated patients with traumatic brain damage where their heads went into a windshield or they collided with a vehicle. I'm not diagnosing it, I'm not qualified; however we are talking about in this facility psychiatric patients who are diagnosed as psychotic or schizophrenic."

Councilman Cassin looked pained. "He is in the company of other people with other mental disabilities," he answered softly. "I was hoping you would take my statement as being a statement. I do not want to get into an argument."

The rest of the night—the last hour—belonged to the politicians. It was like watching the entire defensive unit of the Chicago Bears pile on an opposing quarterback who'd had both legs broken three plays earlier.

In a bold voice, councilman Louis Giansante said, "I just want to go on the record as being against it," and the audience applauded enthusiastically. He said he supported some alternate site that would be isolated and separated from neighbors by plenty of fences and bushes. That way, he explained, a real estate agent selling another house in the neighborhood would be able to say to prospective buyers, "You see the fence? You see the gardens? You see the bushes? You won't see the people. *Then* explain the people in the house."

"I'm against it," said councilman Charles Dobrescu. "We are against it. We will take all reasonable actions for the purpose of opposing the establishment of the facility at 9 Highland Road . . . There is another place to put them . . . We are not saying we are against what you are going to do. It is the old syndrome, but it is for somebody else's backyard. We are for schooling."

Mayor-elect DeRiggi took control. A former Nassau County assistant district attorney, he bore down on Linda Slezak the way any hard-driving prosecutor would in a criminal matter. He began asking her all the things they had talked about at lunch at Old Gerlich's. Linda knew just where he was heading, and was miserable. He was going to try to get her to talk about Mayor Suozzi's involvement. When she couldn't remember a minor detail, a voice from the audience taunted her, "We don't like to remember." DeRiggi asked her about Landing Road, the Polish section that Mayor Suozzi had recommended staying away from.

"This is something we would like information on," said DeRiggi, staring down at her from the podium. "Could you tell us the truth, Mrs. Slezak? Tell me what you told me and Mr. Iversen."

"I would prefer not to discuss that publicly," she said.

"I had a conversation with this young lady and various answers came out that I think would be of great interest to this audience," DeRiggi continued. "Tell us what you told me and Mr. Iversen, Mrs. Slezak. Will the record indicate that there is a consultation going on with the attorney and Dr. Vogrin. I would like the truth; tell us what you said to Mr. Iversen and myself."

Linda Slezak was stuck, caught between the Scylla and Charibdis of Glen Cove politics, Suozzi and DeRiggi. Three times the men had run against each other for mayor. The first two elections had gone to Suozzi, the most recent to DeRiggi. Their mutual contempt went far beyond election day and some measly group home. Linda felt no obligation to protect Mayor Suozzi; he had stabbed her in the back by opposing the group home. As for DeRiggi—was there anything on the animal chain lower than a snake and his pro bono private investigator? The least complicated way out was to answer the questions truthfully.

DeRiggi was trying to show that Mayor Suozzi had steered Linda away from several sites but had not privately opposed 9 Highland Road, only delaying its selection until after the election. He elicited from Linda that Mayor Suozzi had asked for delays when it came to Highland Road, but never actually said he opposed the site in their private meetings. By this time Linda had realized that delay was just another way of opposing a group home, that a politician would never support one, but DeRiggi gave her no opening to say this.

Finished with Linda, DeRiggi quickly turned on Mayor Suozzi. No matter how much Mayor Suozzi said he opposed Highland Road, it was not enough for Mayor-elect DeRiggi. "Why didn't you object to the Highland Road project the way you had objected to these others?" asked DeRiggi.

"I did object to this," said Suozzi.

"Did you tell them not to pursue it?" asked DeRiggi.

"It is a bad site because of the traffic and the [residential] area," said Suozzi.

"You interfered with Elwood," said DeRiggi, "You interfered with

Landing and I want to know why you didn't interfere with Highland Road."

"I did, Mr. DeRiggi." Mayor Suozzi was beside himself. What did he have to say to convince the man he hated this group home? "I will say it, I will swear under oath, I did object to Highland Road, back in July and now. Do you want my blood?"

Soon supporters of the incoming—and outgoing—mayors were taking the podium to argue about who was the bigger phony. At 11 P.M., three and a half hours after the meeting started, Mayor Suozzi and his people on the council suddenly marched out. The public hearing for the purpose of discussing a proposed group home at 9 Highland Road was over.

MAYOR SUOZZI went upstairs to his office. He was furious, at DeRiggi for not knowing when to quit, at Speiser for using a group home to turn himself into a hero chiropractor, and at that Slezak woman. Didn't she know when to shut up?

DeRiggi stayed in the council chambers while a large part of the audience remained, milling about. He was basking in his victory. He wasn't even mayor yet and he had already taken control of things. The meeting had ended so abruptly, people lingered, gathering in small groups.

Seth Stein felt the meeting had been a little more hostile than average, but not disastrous. A few times he had had that feeling of being in a crowd when people are on the verge of losing control. Linda and Dan, the novices, were clearly shaken. She was afraid to go out into the parking lot alone. Seth felt bad for them. Working with the mentally ill wasn't an easy way to make a living. There were no big bucks in it, lots of aggravation, the rewards weren't great, and the disappointments enormous. He'd seen very few miracles when it came to mental illness. You deal with the public mental-health system, and if you're lucky it's indifferent to what you're trying. Then you go to a meeting like this, and it's bam, "You should be ashamed, you're a disgrace, who's paying you under the table? Who's the broker? Who's the banker? Why are you really doing this?" You spend a career with little positive feedback and then you're suddenly tossed into the public ring and treated like a criminal. He could keep telling them the public meeting didn't matter, and legally it didn't, but he knew psychologically it did. If they lost their fire to fight, they could lose the group home.

Dan and Gil McGill walked Linda to her Toyota. She'd hated every minute of the meeting, all that anger turned her way. She'd felt so outnumbered. Dan wasn't the confrontational type and had spoken mainly when called on. Karen Mankin from the state had barely opened her mouth. Apparently she had decided against using the meeting to educate the public. It was terrifying, the way it could shake your confidence. Linda wasn't the scared type. She had worked on some of the toughest men's locked wards at Creedmoor state hospital and never felt frightened. Yet tonight she was. When she finally reached home and locked the front door behind her, she was relieved. She was exhausted and yet wired from the meeting. She wanted to sleep. There was no bourbon in the house, so she poured herself a scotch. It didn't make her sleepy, though, just fuzzy and wide awake.

ON THE WAY to his car Seth bumped into Mayor-elect De-Riggi. The two had worked together once years before as co-counsels on some case.

"It's not a good site," DeRiggi said.

"You do what you have to do and I'll do what I have to do," Seth said. "I think we know what the outcome will be." DeRiggi nodded. Seth didn't see him as the evil opposition. He saw him as a typical Nassau Republican, a member of a political machine whose primary job was getting reelected. It made him think of an attorney in another Republican-dominated Nassau town he'd faced in several group-home cases. Even as the attorney was filing legal motions to block a group home, he told Seth, "I know what you're doing, keep doing it. We need them." Who knew what was going on in these politicians' heart of hearts? They were politicians.

AFTER THE MEETING, Dr. Edward Woodman climbed into his Porsche and drove up the hill to his home at 11 Highland, right across from this planned group home. He pulled in beside his wife's Mercedes. Dr. Woodman also had his dental office there. He was hopeful they'd be able to stop this thing. Who welcomes a group home right across the street? Maybe Mother Teresa. Like most of his neighbors, he'd given the civic association a couple of hundred dollars to pay for hiring an attorney. He'd gone to all the strategy meetings. He'd heard about the Padavan law and felt frustrated that he had no control over this house that was going to affect his life so dramatically.

He had not spoken at city hall that night. He'd sat and listened and left with some uneasiness. He had a bad feeling about the men on his side leading the opposition. The stuff between Suozzi and DeRiggi was embarrassing to watch. He had no illusions about why DeRiggi was bashing the house; you just had to look at Highland Road, "Pill Hill" —doctors, dentists, chiropractors, professionals with money and influence. He also couldn't stomach Roy Speiser. Granted, the chiropractor had done much work organizing the civic association against the house, but Dr. Woodman felt a lot of his comments were unfair. Dr. Woodman was sure this agency was intelligent enough not to stick a knife-wielding schizoid in the neighborhood; it was in the agency's self-interest to be cautious. Dr. Woodman saw Speiser as an instigator, someone who was "leaching out all the innuendos": the steep hill, the traffic, the little children. He felt the chiropractor was playing neighborhood golden boy to boost his practice.

Dr. Woodman still opposed the group home for one simple reason: You just don't put these things in this kind of neighborhood. He believed they should put it elsewhere on Long Island, in Long Beach or Freeport where there were more poor people and a group home would seem less out of place.

He didn't like admitting it, but in that entire three and a half hours he hadn't heard one compelling reason to oppose the house.

chapter 3

"No," said The Mayor

P R O S P E R O U S , highly educated, sophisticated Nassau County was the most fiercely resistant enclave in New York State to group homes. By the late 1980s, 75 percent of group homes for the mentally ill and retarded that had been planned in Nassau had been opposed by the municipalities in administrative hearings. Nassau's mayors and supervisors did not stop there; they went on to file lawsuits against 57 percent of these homes. Across the state, lawsuits were brought in only 5 to 10 percent of cases.

Why did Nassau offer such resistance? A significant part of the county's population had moved from neighboring New York City. These people were primarily single-family homeowners, whose biggest investment was the house. The last thing they wanted was having a little piece of New York City re-created in Nassau County.

Social services were not a high priority in Nassau. Press releases from the county welfare office announced antifraud measures, not innovative programs. As late as 1987 the director of social services, Joseph D'Elia, was denying that there were homeless people in Nassau.

When the county finally funded a few homeless shelters—after being sued—officials would not make their location public for fear of alienating neighbors.

Nassau is primarily a white suburb, but feelings about group homes transcended race, religion, ethnicity, class, political affiliation, and educational background. A principal at a Hebrew school in Woodmere, Long Island, spoke against one, saying it would scare away people, reducing school attendance. Black and white residents of Freeport, one of the few mixed sections of the county, argued that a group home would undermine the "renaissance" going on there. Democratic leaders in North Hempstead and their Republican counterparts in Hempstead agreed on practically nothing except their contempt for a proposed group home in New Hyde Park.

Three weeks after the Glen Cove hearing, on December 30, 1987, Linda Slezak called her friend Marge Vezer, who ran a group home program for a nonprofit agency on the South Shore of Long Island. The two women had a lot in common. Marge Vezer had started as a social worker assisting former state-hospital patients dumped in Long Beach, Long Island's welfare hotels. She switched to the group home field a little sooner than Linda; she'd already opened one home, and expected to open a second in early 1988. Her experience had toughened her to the opposition. Neighbors had been picketing her new house, planned for Hewlett, Long Island, carrying signs that read "No More Mental Motels." From time to time, Linda would call Marge to discuss strategy. That Wednesday morning, when Linda heard Marge's voice, she knew something was wrong. "I can't talk right now," Marge said. "I'm running to the Hewlett house. It's been burned down." That day investigators from the county fire marshall's office ruled the blaze arson. Damage was one hundred thousand dollars. Fortunately, nobody was living in the house yet; staff was to have moved in later that week.

Linda was frightened again. She spoke with state officials, who agreed she should hire security to guard 9 Highland—assuming the purchase went through.

GLEN COVE leaders had decided to challenge the house on the grounds there were better alternate sites. The other legal avenue permitted by the Padavan law—arguing that the city was oversaturated with such facilities—was not very promising. This was the first group home for the mentally ill in a city of twenty-five thousand; the only existing group home was for retarded adults.

Yet the city's alternate-site strategy had a built-in problem for the politicians. The law required them to find another house somewhere *in Glen Cove*. If they won, the Highland Road neighbors would be off their backs, but they risked upsetting another section of town. As a result, this tack was rarely taken by municipalities. Linda, Dan, and Seth couldn't figure why the city was going this route. They assumed Glen Cove was simply trying to delay, then pressure and batter the agency into giving up. Melillo board members were receiving as many as a dozen letters a day asking that they abandon the Highland site. Many had friends on Highland Road. A few were close with Mayor DeRiggi.

In early January, DeRiggi made it clear that stopping this group home was a key priority. His first emergency resolution introduced as the new mayor was to hire outside counsel to fight the home. For $125 an hour, Glen Cove signed up Rivkin, Radler, Dunne and Bayh.

Rivkin Radler, located right in Nassau County, was one of the nation's ten fastest-growing law firms, with two hundred lawyers. Business was so good the firm couldn't find office space fast enough. Some junior lawyers were tripled-up on phones. It was mainly a corporate firm that specialized in representing companies charged in toxic pollution or product liability cases—insurance and real estate companies. Among the senior partners was Edward J. Hart, "Mr. Nassau Republican Lawyer," counsel to the party that had dominated county politics for seventy-five years, former president of the county bar association —a very well-connected individual. (In Nassau, getting the Republican endorsement for judge was tantamount to being elected. Hart himself would later become a judge.) Mayor DeRiggi's selection of Rivkin

Radler was a message that he was playing political hardball. The firm used at least four attorneys on the case.

ON JANUARY 7, 1988, legal papers were served on Melillo, notifying Dan and Linda that a temporary restraining order had been issued by Nassau supreme court justice Albert Oppido, preventing Melillo from taking ownership of 9 Highland. It was a clever bit of strategy by Rivkin Radler—sneaky, though perfectly legal. Linda and Dan didn't know what it meant, and called Seth. They had watched Seth stand tall as bombs landed all around him at the public hearing and were in awe of his composure, but now, for the first time, they heard worry in his voice. He was talking even faster than usual. Evidently, this did matter. He told them he needed the legal papers immediately. He explained that he would fight it in court, but there were no guarantees and the order could affect the house purchase date. Linda herself drove the half hour to his office in Garden City to deliver the legal papers.

The request for a temporary restraining order had been heard without a representative from Melillo present. The laws of procedure in New York permitted a judge to issue such an order based on the testimony of just one party, an ex parte ruling. Still, such orders were not routine. Seth had rarely been able to get one in his years of practicing and knew it was a commentary on the Rivkin Radler firm's reputation in this county that the request had been granted. Seth feared this might be just the delay that could kill the 9 Highland site. Melillo was scheduled to take possession of the house at a closing January 13. Seth had always counseled his clients to be aggressive about buying a house as early as practical. The longer you waited, the more you risked the homeowner's backing out of the deal in the face of community hostility. If, after buying the house, the agency lost the Padavan hearing— which rarely happened—it could always resell the place as a single-family home. Also, buying a house early on sent a powerful political message to opponents.

Losing a house sent just as powerful a message. The receiver for the divorced couple that owned 9 Highland was growing impatient. The deal had been delayed twice already. In court papers the receiver stressed that his clients were five months behind on mortgage payments, and the bank was threatening action. If they didn't go through with the sale this time, Seth feared the bank would foreclose, complicating and delaying the purchase for months, perhaps for good. Finding a new site and going through the process all over could add a year's delay, and who knew what might happen to the state grant in the meantime?

If Seth was unsuccessful in getting the temporary restraining order lifted, it could stay in effect for months while a judge decided whether a preliminary injunction was merited. All the fine principles in the world didn't matter if he was outmaneuvered on this. He put in a call to Bob Schonfeld in the New York State attorney general's office. Group homes had been Schonfeld's specialty for almost a decade. Advocates from around the state relied on him for guidance. Any time a municipality filed a lawsuit challenging a group home (and the state mental-health commissioner's administrative ruling) it was Bob's job to defend the group home (and the state commissioner's ruling). In nearly a decade of this work, he had defended 150 group homes and won every case. The body of case law that had cemented the Padavan law as a progressive force for opening group homes had to a large degree been Bob's doing. He had been around long enough to create the legal precedents and then cite his precedents to uphold the next wave of challenges.

He laid out the two ways to undo the temporary restraining order. Seth could ask to have it lifted by going back to the same judge, Judge Oppido. This is what most lawyers would do. Bob recommended against it. No judge likes to overturn his own order. The other alternative was to request a hearing before an appellate judge for the second department. Most of those judges were based in Brooklyn, and most were Democrats removed from the day-to-day politics of Nassau County. Bob had used the strategy successfully in many group-home cases. That afternoon, he sent a sample copy of relevant legal papers to Seth by Federal Express.

Seth did his own research and typed his legal motions on a computer system he'd assembled and programmed himself. On Thursday night he stayed until midnight drafting papers. He wanted to move on this as fast as possible. The longer the restraining order was in place, the more force it would have and the harder it would be to overturn.

On Friday morning, the eighth, he was back at work at 7 A.M. The weather was awful, heavy snow and windy. The forecast was for blizzard conditions all day. Schools were closed all over the region. At eleven o'clock, Seth called the appellate division in Brooklyn. He feared he'd never make it in because of the road conditions. He did not want to wait until Monday, the eleventh. If something went wrong, he'd have just two days to the closing on 9 Highland. No room to maneuver. He asked the clerk in Brooklyn if there was an appellate judge sitting in Nassau that week. Judge Harwood, the clerk said.

This was immense good fortune. Stanley Harwood was the former Democratic party chairman in Nassau, a very liberal man. Seth described the case briefly to Judge Harwood's clerk. The courts were closing in Nassau at noon because of the storm. The clerk checked with the judge, then came back on. "If you're coming over, we'll be here," said the clerk. Seth notified Rivkin Radler of the hearing set for one o'clock. He needed every minute to prepare the exhibits. His secretary had not come in, and he had to finish all the copying.

He was the last to arrive in Judge Harwood's office. At a glance, Seth is easy to underestimate. He is five feet, eight inches tall, 140 pounds, and though forty at the time, he looked ten years younger. Ed Hart, sixty-one, a round, ruddy-faced man, was there with two younger associates. No pleasantries were exchanged. The waiting area was uncomfortably quiet. As Seth handed out copies of his legal papers, he heard Hart complaining about how ridiculous it was to be called out in this kind of weather. Hart had plenty of reason to be in a foul mood. In Judge Harwood's courtroom, being Mr. Republican was no asset.

The judge's law clerk called the lawyers into chambers, wh⟋ ⟍⟍⟍hey sat in stuffed leather chairs around his desk. Hart sat in the center facing the judge, his two younger associates beside him. Seth was on the judge's right. Through the windows they could see the snow swirling fiercely in the parking lot four stories below. The hearing took a half hour. Hart argued that if Melillo was allowed to buy the house it would prejudice the whole Padavan hearing procedure. How could the agency be objective about alternative sites if it already owned a house?

Seth countered that it was the state hearing officer who decided on the alternate sites, not the agency. He pointed out that the courts had upheld an agency's right to buy a house before the process was finished and that it was the agency's risk. At a later date, a court might stop the agency from using this house to operate a group home, but that was a different issue.

Hart wondered what Melillo was doing acquiring a house that it might not be able to use.

"That's their risk," said Judge Harwood. The words sent a rush through Seth. It was one of those rare moments in law or life when you know you are going to win cleanly. "I don't see any harm to the city" if the sale goes through, said the Judge. And "irreparable harm" was the only reason for a restraining order.

Judge Harwood took Seth's copy of the order. In pen, he marked a bracket beside the key paragraph, wrote "Denied," signed his name and the date.

Ed Hart looked furious. He had been outmaneuvered in his home court. As they put on their coats, Seth heard him complaining under his breath. Before leaving, he turned to Seth and warned that Rivkin Radler was going to pull out all the stops on this one. His face was a bright red. Then he stormed out of the room, his associates trailing behind.

FIVE DAYS LATER, Melillo bought 9 Highland Road. Seth, Dan, and Linda all attended the closing. It was a great relief.

But the Rivkin Radler attorneys marched right back to court a few days later in another attempt at delay, seeking a preliminary injunction to halt the administrative hearing. Citing a 1979 Queens case, they contended that Melillo had asked for a Padavan hearing too soon, before the city's period to suggest alternate sites had elapsed. The lower court in the 1979 Queens case had sided with the community opponents. When Bob Schonfeld in the attorney general's office saw the latest Rivkin Radler brief on Glen Cove, he was surprised and delighted. He knew the 1979 Queens case well. He had litigated it and succeeded in having it overturned in the appellate division. He wondered why such a prestigious law firm would base a motion on a case that was reversed. It was one of the cardinal sins of litigation, a rookie mistake. Were they that desperate for delay? The judge was also unimpressed. Again Rivkin Radler lost. The Padavan hearing would begin as scheduled.

MOST ADMINISTRATIVE hearings take half a day, some a day. The 9 Highland hearing went on for three days. Seth Stein felt that Donald McMillan, the Rivkin Radler attorney representing Glen Cove, did the best job of any lawyer he'd been up against in a Padavan hearing. Bob Schonfeld called it a toss-up as to who won. Unfortunately, McMillan made one major oversight, and though Seth missed it too, it cost McMillan dearly.

His strategy was to show that 9 Highland had been picked not because it was best, but for political expediency; that the site had too many shortcomings; that the alternate selected by the city was better; and that Melillo and Linda Slezak had never seriously considered the alternate site. (The city had suggested a half dozen alternates, but it was clear that only one, 8 Crow Lane, was comparable to 9 Highland, and McMillan devoted most of his time to it.)

Stein argued that under the Padavan law, it made no difference why 9 Highland was picked; it mattered only that the house was as good as or better than the alternates.

McMillan embarrassed Melillo early on by calling two of its board members—the two anthropology professors, Jean Wagner and Ruth Shaffer, who testified they did not support 9 Highland. Wagner was upset about traffic, proximity to neighbors, backyard size; Shaffer preferred a site that gave "the least resistance."

Linda Slezak had seen Wagner and Shaffer enter the hearing room, but assumed they came in support. It never occurred to her that they were testifying against the house until McMillan called them. Linda felt like she'd been kicked by just about everybody. She wondered if the good professors had any clue about how much work went into finding a decent place that someone was willing to sell, if they had any sense of how much prejudice there was out there. These two were supposed to be among the handful of human beings on her side. What the hell were they doing on the Melillo board?

Afterward Seth Stein took Dan Vogrin aside and suggested he get control of the board. Seth preferred not meeting anybody else from the agency on cross-examination.

LINDA WAS ON the stand two days. McMillan cross-examined her four hours. The hearing officer kept complaining that the questioning was "way off the beam" but let it go on, until finally he grew so exasperated he called a halt: "I have never, never done this before but . . . I'm going to permit you to go on for one hour more and that's it."

A key advantage 9 Highland had over the alternate sites was being so close to downtown—a block away—important for a house full of people who don't drive. Some alternate sites were over a mile away. McMillan tried to minimize this advantage by challenging Linda's assertions about what was "easy walking distance."

"What is walking distance," McMillan asked, "a mile, two miles?"

"No," said Linda, "Walking distance is under a half mile."

"How do you determine that? What standard or criteria, or is that just your personal opinion?"

"My personal opinion."

"Is there a reason why your opinion of walking distance could not be as much as a mile?"

"I would think a mile would be excessive."

"Why?"

"It's my opinion."

"What's your opinion based on?"

"It's based on what I consider a reasonable distance to walk."

The hearing officer interrupted. "She said, 'in her opinion.' She thinks a mile would be excessive, in her opinion."

"I want to know the basis of an opinion," said McMillan.

The hearing officer asked Linda, "Do you have any scientific reasoning?"

"No."

The hearing officer said, "She just feels a half a mile is all right to walk but a mile is too much."

McMillan was just warming up. "Mrs. Slezak, am I correct that based upon the fact you don't have any scientific studies as to form the basis of your opinion on that distance, that there is no scientific basis for any of the distance criteria that you put in the summaries which are part of the exhibit, whatever the last exhibit is in evidence? I believe it's 16. Is that correct?"

"I don't understand the question," said Linda.

This went on and on. Had she done studies on how far schizophrenics could walk, on how far depressed people could walk?

The city's attorneys argued that the selection of the site was tainted because the chairman of the Melillo board, Gil McGill, was an owner of Gil Realty, the company that had represented the 9 Highland owner. But this argument went nowhere after McGill filed an affidavit stating that, while he once was a partner in Gil Realty, he had severed his ties many years before the acquisition.

In the end McMillan and the assisting Rivkin Radler attorneys generated 666 pages of hearing transcript. It boiled down to this: 9 Highland and 8 Crow cost about the same to buy and renovate and could each house twelve residents. While 9 Highland was considerably closer to downtown, in a prettier neighborhood, with a better driveway, 8 Crow had a bigger backyard and was in better structural shape (it was two years old; 9 Highland was twenty years old).

Privately, Linda felt if she had been shown Crow Lane before Highland, she would have considered it. Because of location, she didn't like it as much, but 8 Crow had possibilities; it could have been a group home. Yet supposing she gave the opponents the benefit of the doubt and called the two houses equal, what purpose would had been served by all this? Months of delays already, months of delays ahead, tens of thousands of dollars in legal fees wasted, because politicians weren't willing to stand up to a small group of neighbors.

MAYOR DERIGGI WAS the last witness called. After testifying that 9 Highland was "the bottom of the barrel," with "major, major traffic," Seth cross-examined him. The mayor had been quite outraged that Melillo hadn't immediately informed the neighbors about the proposed group home at 9 Highland. Seth was curious: had Mayor DeRiggi met yet with any of the neighbors of the alternate site he was proposing, 8 Crow Lane?

"No," said the mayor.

Before writing the official letter recommending 8 Crow Lane, did he speak to the neighbors? Seth asked.

"No," said the mayor.

Did he know if there was any civic association in that neighborhood? Seth asked.

"No," said the mayor.

And did he send any letters to the neighbors and say, "We're going to suggest this site?"

"No," said the mayor.

Did he endeavor to ascertain whether there would be any community opposition to 8 Crow Lane?

"No," said the mayor.

A FEW DAYS after the hearing, Daisy Miller, who lives near 8 Crow Lane, saw in the Glen Cove newspaper that the mayor was trying to switch the group home to her neighborhood. She called her friend Juanita Burnett. The two black women were angry. They had a pretty good idea of why city hall was trying to dump a group home on Crow. "We're predominantly black," said Burnett. "Who cares about us?" Republican DeRiggi got a lot more votes from all those fancy-pants white doctors on Highland than he did on Crow, said Burnett, a computer operator. She was the president of the Glen Cove NAACP chapter, Miller the vice president. The two women sat down and composed a letter to Mayor DeRiggi on NAACP stationery listing reasons for not putting a group home at 8 Crow. They came up with five: too small a backyard for recreation, proximity to a day care center at 2 Crow Lane, influx of traffic, poor landscaping of the site, and failure to consider the community residents affected.

THE NAACP leaders were not the only ones surprised to read about 8 Crow. Diane Kutner was, too. She lived at 8 Crow with her daughter. She rented half the house and had a lease for nine more months, through October 14, 1988. How could the mayor be planning a group home there? She called the Melillo agency. Linda was stunned to hear from her, stunned-ecstatic. They had all failed to check something so basic. The state doesn't permit agencies to purchase a house unless it's vacant. And the state certainly wasn't going to want to wait until October when there was a fine vacant house on Highland now. Linda called Seth.

"Ha-ha," said Seth. "Let's get an affidavit." He hung up the phone and thought, God smiles on you.

THE MENTAL HEALTH commissioner's decision was expected in early March. Melillo's main concern was not letting politics interfere, just allowing the Padavan law to run its course. Mayor De-Riggi began aggressively courting board members, trying to get them to back down on 9 Highland. Suddenly, he was sounding like a warm, fuzzy teddy bear. He wanted to bury the hatchet and start over. Both sides had made mistakes, he said in letters to board members. Why not get together and form a special committee to pick a site that would be acceptable to everyone in Glen Cove? Linda could imagine such a site—it would probably be in Connecticut.

Dan and board president Gil McGill reined in the board. Besides the two who had testified, two others had written the hearing officer saying they opposed the site. Gil strongly suspected the two had been feeding Mayor DeRiggi details of the board's inner workings. He made it clear they weren't welcome anymore. He instructed the secretary at Melillo to stop notifying those two of monthly meetings. He wrote letters to board members setting out strict guidelines for any meeting with the mayor.

When the mayor didn't have any further success cracking the board from outside, he requested to come in to Melillo for a visit, to speak at the next board meeting. On February 23, the all-new friendly Mayor DeRiggi suggested a blue-ribbon site selection committee, and on February 25 Dan Vogrin wrote him what a great idea it was for the *next* group home in Glen Cove. However, for 9 Highland, Dan wrote, the case was closed.

The irrepressible Mayor DeRiggi apparently had a different interpretation. A few days later he wrote the state mental-health commissioner asking for a delay in the decision on 9 Highland, since he and the Melillo board were "in the process of discussing an alternative to the contested selection method."

Linda could not believe the man's audacity. Discussing an alternative! With whom? He must have been discussing it with his pro bono private investigator. But she was even more startled when she heard that the state mental-health commissioner was seriously considering granting a delay.

DR. RICHARD SURLES had been New York's mental health commissioner just a few months. He was a handsome, sharply dressed, charismatic type who spoke eloquently of the need to move people out of state hospitals and into community programs. He was Governor Cuomo's man, and the governor was the rare politician in America who still spoke with compassion for the poor and disadvantaged. The group home advocates assumed this was all good news for them. But the longer Commissioner Surles was around, the more they wondered.

Several years before, the group home agencies for the mentally ill in New York had banded together to form an association representing their interests, the Association of Community Living Agencies in Mental Health (ACLAIMH). It was a low-key group, run by social workers like Linda Slezak in their spare time, that lobbied state officials on group home issues. (Not until mid-1988 did ACLAIMH hire its own full-time executive director.)

In the past, ACLAIMH, which represents 90 percent of the group homes for the mentally ill in the state, always had access to the state commissioner when necessary. In the early months of Dr. Surles's tenure, leaders were surprised by how hard it was to arrange a meeting with him. (Later, Surles would write a letter to ACLAIMH's president saying he was "unwilling to meet," suggesting they deal through his aides.)

ACLAIMH sent two members down to Philadelphia, where Surles had just served five years as director of the city's department for the mentally ill and retarded. The ACLAIMH officials heard stories of a hands-on administrator who'd improved the Philadelphia community-care system there. But they also heard things that worried them. He cared about his popularity. No one would ever be popular supporting group homes. Dr. Surles also liked making his imprint on a system. He was most interested in creating new programs, *his* new programs. Group homes were well established by the time he arrived in New York. They were the backbone of a growing community mental-health system. But they were no longer the sexy new thing in community care. And they were not *Dr. Surles's* group homes.

In February, Concern for Mental Health, an agency in neighboring Suffolk County, Long Island, was planning to open a group home in a middle-class section of Shoreham. A few weeks before Melillo's hearing on Glen Cove, the Suffolk agency had its Padavan hearing. On February 16, Dr. Surles wrote that the Shoreham site was fine and the agency should be allowed to proceed, BUT he was going to consider community concerns and give opponents thirty more days to come up with another site. This was the first time a commissioner had ever intervened to circumvent the Padavan process, as far as assistant attorney general Bob Schonfeld could recall. Dr. Surles's predecessors had been strictly hands-off. So had the commissioners for mental retardation. Group home advocates warned that he was opening a Pandora's box, that once he meddled in the process, all the politicians in the state would be asking him to do it for their constituents, too. Commissioner Surles told them they were overreacting.

The Suffolk agency had planned to open the group home in the middle of a quiet residential block. The neighbors and state assemblyman now began pushing hard for an isolated alternate site, near a shopping center on Route 25A, one of the busiest highways on Long Island. Charles Russo, the attorney for the agency, was heartsick. The official legislative history of the Padavan law called for putting homes "within the mainstream of community life," not on the side of a four-lane highway with eighteen-wheelers buzzing by at sixty miles per hour. But the agency's board of directors felt that since the commissioner was not behind them and the community and politicians were banging away, they were obliged to take the Route 25A site. Charles Russo called it "a sophisticated form of burning the house down."

LINDA DIDN'T THINK it possible, but it appeared that the same was about to happen to Melillo. Commissioner Surles had told his deputies he was going to give the Glen Cove opposition thirty more days and asked that a letter be drafted to Melillo saying so.

Linda was not going down without a fight. She and other members of ACLAIMH sent an angry letter to Commissioner Surles calling his action "dangerous" and warning that until he clarified his position, they would open no new group homes on Long Island. Bob Schonfeld told state officials he felt that the commissioner's thirty-day delay action was a violation of the law.

In early March, Sarah Rose, one of the commissioner's top assistants, sent her boss an internal memo explaining why she had not yet drafted his letter calling for a thirty-day delay in the Glen Cove case. She clearly felt he was making a mistake, although she wasn't that direct in the memo. She described the fury over the Suffolk County case, the attorney general's opinion, ACLAIMH's threat. She also included the expanding list of local politicians who were taking an interest in the Glen Cove house, including the two state legislators from the area: Democratic assemblyman Lew Yevoli, famed for his support of Not in My Backyard issues; and Ralph Marino, the Republican senate majority leader and no friend of social service programs. The commissioner's deputy just stated the facts in her memo, but she picked all the pertinent ones and the conclusion to be drawn was obvious: the sharks were circling, and with thirty more days there'd be blood in Glen Cove too.

Commissioner Surles backed down. Why he changed his mind is not clear, but it plainly angered him to have to do so. In a letter to ACLAIMH he called the group home agency's aggressive stance "violative of any behavior to which I subscribe . . . To issue a threat and ultimatum without an opportunity for discussion is not the way I do business."

On March 15 the commissioner released his decision, picking 9 Highland as the best site. His opinion said 8 Crow was eliminated because of the tenants. Dan Vogrin was quoted in *Newsday* promising that the house would be an "asset" and "never an eyesore." He hoped people would see that the mentally ill could make good neighbors. Mayor DeRiggi told the newspaper the city would fight on. In April, the city filed a notice of petition challenging the commissioner's ruling. Seth wasn't worried. Since the Padavan law, a group home had never been defeated in the courts. He told Linda it was safe to begin work on the house. The courts had also upheld an agency's right to open a group home while the legal appeal was continuing.

LINDA PUT OUT bids and hired a construction firm to renovate 9 Highland. She was anxious to move quickly. While they waited for the building permit, workers gutted the house's insides. Then, on May 5, Linda received a letter from Steven Misiakiewicz, head of the Glen Cove Building Department, denying a permit. A house for more than five unrelated people living together violated Glen Cove zoning, he wrote. Neither Linda or Seth had expected this. It was the kind of stuff towns pulled *before* the Padavan law. All work on the house stopped. Back to court they went.

At the end of May, Seth and the New York State attorney general's office filed motions seeking to have the building permit issued. The attorney general called the city's denial "a bald attempt to delay and impede" the group home. On July 7 state supreme court justice George A. Murphy ordered the city to issue the building permit. He based his decision on a case that Bob Schonfeld had won in 1982. Dan Vogrin told the local papers: "I'm thrilled. We've been waiting much too long." Still no building permit, and on July 19 the city appealed. Under the laws of procedure in New York, the city didn't have to issue the permit until the appeal was resolved. This was a disaster in the making. It could drag things out another year. On July 22 Seth filed a motion in the appellate division seeking to have the automatic stay lifted. He argued the delay was doing irreparable harm to the dozen people waiting in institutions for a group home bed.

Then assistant attorney general Bob Schonfeld came up with one last procedural magic trick. He'd noticed that Glen Cove had slipped up in its appeal of the commissioner's ruling. The city was supposed to have filed its complete case record with the appeals court by July 17. Glen Cove missed the filing deadline. On July 25, Bob entered a motion with the appellate division asking that Glen Cove's Padavan appeal be dismissed. Normally he would not stoop to relying on such a technicality. Bob routinely won these appeals on their merits and was sure Glen Cove would be the same. Despite the adversarial relationship, he tried to keep on as good terms as possible with local municipalities. He knew the group home residents were going to be living in these towns, and he wanted to minimize animosity. But Glen Cove was fighting dirty. He'd succeeded at getting an equally dirty case dismissed in Hempstead, Long Island, a few months before, using this technicality. Bob attached a copy of the Hempstead court order to his motion and sent the papers to Glen Cove officials. If there was one thing being an assistant attorney general had taught him, it was this: Much of law is intimidation. He had Mayor DeRiggi in a rather bad spot. By this time, the mayor had dropped Rivkin Radler and was relying on the city attorney, John V. Terrana, to handle the case. How would it look if it became public that the DeRiggi administration had taken charge and immediately bungled it, to the point that Glen Cove was about to be booted out of court for missing a filing date? It might raise many embarrassing questions. Mayor DeRiggi had decided to have the city take over after getting Rivkin Radler's bill—$36,000 and not a thing to show for it. (DeRiggi was so upset by the bill, he launched into a shouting match with a Rivkin Radler lawyer, ultimately succeeding in having the fee cut in half, to $18,000.)

So Glen Cove quietly made a deal with Bob Schonfeld and Seth Stein. The city would issue the building permit for 9 Highland, and in return, the attorney general would withdraw his technical motion to block the city's Padavan hearing appeal.

Not a word of the deal, or the city's screwup reached the local papers. It was kept so quiet, even the deputy mayor, Anna Iversen, didn't know. The size of the Rivkin Radler fees never became public either.

On August 12, Glen Cove agreed to issue a building permit for 9 Highland.

All fall, workmen renovated the house. Things went slowly at first. The construction firm had taken other jobs because of the building permit delay, and didn't get back to full manpower for weeks. By December the house was nearly ready. The state notified Linda that it wanted to move at least a few people in before the end of the year, for funding purposes. After so much waiting, she suddenly was rushing to pull things together. Several residents moved in right after Christmas.

SOME CAME ALONE, some with parents, some with social workers they barely knew, and one drove up in a red Cadillac. They were anxious to get on with it. Their lives had been on hold for months while they waited for the group home to open.

Stan Gunter brought his guitar and was delighted when he learned the house was getting a piano donated, so he could continue work on his music composition.

Julie Callahan, the twenty-year-old homeless runaway and ward of the state, did not own a suitcase. She arrived from the borderline unit with six large cardboard boxes, one filled with stuffed animals. A few days later her most recent foster mother dropped off another half dozen boxes and quickly drove away without waiting to say good-bye to Julie. Julie never saw the woman again.

About half of the twelve new residents had close relatives who cared, none more than Charlotte and Gary Grasso. Linda Slezak had suggested that they drop off their thirty-three-year-old son Fred at about 10:30, and at exactly 10:30 they pulled up in their Bronco. One of Linda Slezak's assistants, Laurie Nardo, met the Grassos at the front door. She was all smiles and good cheer as she took the parents' coats. Fred would not give up his leather jacket. For the last six years he had lived at a run-down, two-hundred-bed psychiatric facility in Brooklyn where his clothes had been stolen several times. It had taught Fred to be very cautious about his clothes. Only after his mother said, "Fred, this is your home now," did he agree to let the counselor hang his jacket in the closet.

"OK, Fred," said Laurie Nardo, "since this is your day, we'll see what you want to do. Would you like to have a tour of the house?"

"Yeah," Fred said. Right away Mrs. Grasso remarked on the new parquet floor, the handsome wooden coffee table, the brick fireplace. "Look at this, absolutely gorgeous," said Mrs. Grasso. "What a beautiful home, a beautiful home."

"Yeah, Ma," said Fred. She noticed the translucent blinds. "Gorgeous," said Mrs. Grasso. "Isn't this gorgeous, Fred?"

"Nice, Mom."

"Fred's a little nervous," Mrs. Grasso said. The three Grassos weaved through the downstairs and upstairs rooms, peeking into all four bathrooms. In the dining room there was a long oak table and chairs. "Nice," said Fred.

"I count ten chairs," Mrs. Grasso said to the counselor. "I thought twelve people are going to live here."

The counselor just stared at Mrs. Grasso for a moment. More chairs were on order.

Mrs. Grasso is a fabulous baker and cook, and it was the tour of the kitchen that touched her most—the garbage disposal, the cupboards, the Whirlpool dishwasher, the Westinghouse FrostFree refrigerator. "Fred," she said, "look at here." Mrs. Grasso blew her nose. The Sharp Carousel II microwave was making her cry.

"Unbelievable," said Mr. Grasso. "Who'd think the state would have something like this for people like Fred?"

For the first time in years they weren't ashamed of where their son was going to live. When Fred had been diagnosed with schizophrenia in the early 1980s, there wasn't a group home on suburban Long Island. They had tried to keep him at their home in nearby Oyster Bay, but as they approached retirement age they found the illness too much for them. That awful two-hundred-bed Brooklyn institution was all they could find.

The counselor put on water for coffee and the Grassos took seats in the living room to talk about Fred's new routine at the home. Fred said little. His schizophrenia, or the medication, or the drugs he'd once done, or maybe all of those things made him mostly quiet now. Fred didn't seem to know how to explain it himself. "There are times my head doesn't work right," was how he expressed it if asked. Or he'd point to his head and say, "There's something wrong in here. I'm a degenerate." While Mrs. Grasso and Laurie Nardo spoke of Fred's medication, Fred's preferences, Fred's old life, Fred's new life, Fred ran his hand over the sofa and said, "This is nice, Ma."

The kettle whistled and Fred said, "Mom, the water's boiling."

"Fred, you can get it," said Mrs. Grasso. Getting up, Fred almost knocked over an ashtray. "See!" he said to his mother, but then he went in and turned it off.

Laurie Nardo asked which bedroom Fred wanted. He was one of the first to move in and had plenty of choice. Maybe too much. "I don't know," he said.

So the three Grassos filed back upstairs and Mr. Grasso paced off each room, measuring which was biggest. Upstairs is best, the father said, more privacy. Fred nodded. He said nothing while his parents debated rooms. Mr. Grasso told Fred, "Take the one upstairs in front." The three filed back down, where Ms. Nardo was waiting for them. She asked Fred which room he wanted and he remembered. "The one upstairs in front," he said.

The Grassos wanted to know if someone on the staff would supervise what Fred did with his pocket money. They wanted Fred restricted to a small weekly allowance. "He doesn't know the value of money," said Mrs. Grasso. "If you give Fred all his money at once, he'll give it away. I'm telling you, I know."

"In Brooklyn he used to give everyone his cigarettes," said Mr. Grasso. "People like Fred are so timid, they are so vulnerable, it's a sin. In Brooklyn they took his jewelry, they took his clothes. Fred would have given it to them if they just asked."

Ms. Nardo was noncommittal about the allowance money. She felt Fred might be more capable than the Grassos believed. She wanted to stress this point from the start. Fred was here to learn independence. This was what a group home was all about. "We'll see what Fred says about an allowance," Ms. Nardo said. "He might have his own ideas. After all, he picked out his own room."

Mrs. Grasso just smiled at Ms. Nardo. She didn't want to do anything to dampen youthful enthusiasm.

Fred's mother and father took a long time leaving the group home that first day. They were trying to drink everything in, trying to make the best impression possible on Ms. Nardo. Practically every minute they thanked her again. "You don't know what this means to me," Mrs. Grasso said, her eyes filling with tears once more. "You don't know." She looked out the sliding-glass patio doors to the backyard. There were blackbirds sitting in the high hedge. A light rain had started falling. The house was so quiet, the street so quiet, the pattering of rain actually sounded noisy on the window air conditioner. "Listen to the rain," Mrs. Grasso said. "I'm blowing my nose again."

The parents collected their coats. Mrs. Grasso kissed Fred good-bye. Mr. Grasso patted him on the shoulder. They headed up the driveway to their Bronco. Fred peeked in the closet to make sure his leather jacket was still there.

IN THOSE FIRST few weeks, the counselors were on the phone constantly, trying to ensure that the residents' transition to 9 Highland would be smooth. The group home looked fancy, but it was a basic, public mental-health program, funded from the same fiscal pots as the worst state mental hospitals. There were tons of government bureaucracy to move. For Julie Callahan alone, the staff was in frequent contact with her discharging hospital, her foster-care social worker, her most recent foster-care mother, her new therapist at her new day-treatment program, the Social Security Administration to make sure Julie was signed up for her disability check and would receive the group home rate (aggregate care level II, rather than the hospital rate), and the county welfare department to make sure Julie would get a welfare check until her first Social Security disability check arrived. (Social Security was backed up about a year.) Every agency had to be notified of her change of address, usually many times.

The day-to-day business of running a group home is never routine. Staff and residents got used to living with a normal amount of surprise. There was a rhythm to daily life at the house: the hectic rush in the morning to get out to day program, counselors making sure people were up, residents coming to the office for their meds, twelve people vying for four bathrooms, the cup of coffee, the first smoke, the pop tart, then the mad dash out the door.

During the day, the house was quiet. A couple of counselors caught up on paperwork and used the phone to untangle red tape for residents, making all those follow-up calls that hardly anyone else in the mental health system had time to make. Starting at four, residents trickled back. There was time for a smoke, a little MTV, some quiet in your bedroom, and then a couple of them had to get dinner going. Dinner was usually at six. Everyone had a chore to do afterward, then they went their own way. Every Tuesday night, they all gathered in the living room for the weekly community meeting.

It took some of the residents a while to learn the rules of behavior in Glen Cove. Jason Smith was having a cup of coffee downtown in front of a deli when one cop eyed him, then another. Later, back at the house, he said, "One thing I noticed in wealthy towns, the police are around. In Hempstead where my dad lived, they don't mind if you stand outside and have a cup of coffee." He wasn't going back to that particular deli anyway. He had taken too long to order, and the man behind the counter said, "What do you want, the psycho special?" On the other hand, Jason liked going to Uncle Dai's to get Chinese. "For $4.60 you get soup, egg roll, a meal, rice and soda. I give the waitress a dollar. Fifty cents looks miserly."

THE GLEN COVE RECORD-PILOT is normally the sort of weekly newspaper that tries to stress the good. If there's bad news, it's usually played down. In the January 19, 1989, issue there was just one paragraph about a Glen Cove man charged with attempted murder. The story did not name the man or his victim. Maggie Polk, the editor of the paper, felt that in sensitive matters it was best not to. She thought of herself as being very civic minded, had spent decades in Girl Scouting. An assistant publisher once told her, "We don't want to embarrass a guy's family."

Yet in that same January 19, 1989, edition there was a much longer story about a man reported temporarily missing from 9 Highland. The story noted that he was soon located (the next day) at his brother's house in Iowa. There were extensive comments from Roy Speiser of the Highland civic association about the need to "protect ourselves" against such "escapes." An accompanying letter by Speiser called residents "inmates" who "roamed the streets."

The *Record-Pilot* story used the group home resident's name, Jason Smith.

Linda Slezak could not figure why a newspaper would withhold the name in an attempted murder case, but use the name of a recovering mentally ill man accused of no crime.

"It's true we don't want to embarrass residents," editor Polk explained. "And this probably would embarrass Jason Smith. But in terms of Glen Cove he's not a resident, he's a temporary resident."

After that attack the group home was largely forgotten by the Glen Cove paper.

THE ACTUAL FACTS of Jason Smith's disappearance were less sensational. On Saturday, January 14, Jason, who has schizophrenia, told the group home staff he was going for the $4.60 lunch special at Uncle Dai's, then rode the Long Island Rail Road into Manhattan to the Port Authority bus terminal. He had withdrawn $200 in savings and used $140 of it to buy a bus ticket to his brother's in Des Moines. He had not told his brother. The trip took a day and a half. Jason enjoyed it. He favors bus travel; as he often says, "No one bothers you on a bus. No one knows who you are. No one looks at you too much." At the Chicago bus terminal, during a layover, he called his father in Florida to explain his travel plans. The father immediately called Linda Slezak. Jason Smith had no specific idea of how long he would stay with his older brother, a married father of two who owns a building maintenance business. When Jason arrived he said, "If you're upset with me, take me to the hospital and they'll kick me out in the street. Then in two weeks Dad will have to deal with it." After a week the brother suggested it would be best to return to the group home so Jason wouldn't lose his bed. Later, Jason Smith would say, "I would have liked a little longer vacation."

He felt embarrassed coming back and apologized to everyone for having run away. Linda Slezak asked him why he'd left the house after waiting so long in the hospital for a group home bed. "I got caught smoking in my room," Smith answered. The cigarette burned a mark on the dresser. Having broken the group home rules, he feared he would be sent back to Pilgrim State. "Last time I was at Pilgrim, I had to stay six extra months waiting for a group home bed," he told Linda. "I didn't want to go through another six months, so I split."

Linda said, "Jason, don't you know we don't hospitalize someone who's not sick? Breaking a rule is not the same as being sick."

"I've been hospitalized so many times when I didn't know I was sick," he replied.

He was pleased it had not turned out worse. "I thought they'd kick me out," he told a friend. "They told me a million times, 'no smoking in the room.' I'm not smoking anymore. I learned my lesson."

When he heard of the news report in the Glen Cove *Record-Pilot*, his face darkened. He hadn't seen the article. Gazing down at the dining room floor, he asked, "It didn't say I was doing crazy things, did it?"

THE CITY OF Glen Cove continued its legal appeal. There was still one more wild card it could play. Glen Cove could try to get an injunction preventing the house from operating while the appeal continued. It did not. Assistant attorney general Bob Schonfeld had seen the pattern many times. At some point, bashing a group home loses its political luster. Mayors get weary of being defeated in court. While their local newspapers praise them, the larger newspapers— *Newsday* and *The New York Times*, in this case—are supportive of group homes. Glen Cove officials realized there were only a small number of neighborhood people who remained interested. The final ruling on the city appeal didn't come until January 1990, but by then, Glen Cove was just going through the motions.

MAYOR DERIGGI actually agreed to come visit the home after it had been open a few months. The residents and staff met and planned for it. The first thing Julie Callahan thought when he walked in was: He's scared. Julie watched the way he shook their hands—he seemed afraid he might catch something. He made attempts to joke around, but looked stiff. At one point Julie turned to Linda Slezak and whispered, "He's really an uptight man, isn't he?" Linda Slezak almost fell over. She'd been thinking the same. The mayor talked to them about what a great place Glen Cove was and raved on and on about Zanghi, a local three-star gourmet restaurant. They listened politely to the mayor. They each received a ninety-dollar monthly allowance from Social Security, not enough for one person to eat and drink at Zanghi. They had bought a cake and expected the mayor to join them, but he said he had to be running. Afterward, they ate the mayor's cake without him. Julie Callahan was mad. "You could tell it was a token appearance," she said. "It really made me feel insulted, because I'm not here to be looked at like a fucking zoo animal." She said it seemed like it was all public relations and had nothing to do with welcoming them to the neighborhood. "It was obvious," said Julie, "he wanted to get out. 'Oh no, I can't stay.' He didn't want our cake or coffee. He must think we're contagious."

NOT LONG AFTER that, Linda Slezak got a call from the Glen Cove deputy mayor, Anna Iversen. Mrs. Iversen was Mayor DeRiggi's appointee; she was also married to Jim Iversen, the Highland civic association's very own pro bono private investigator. "We have a favor to ask," said the deputy mayor. A longtime City of Glen Cove worker had a grown daughter suffering from manic depression and drug dependency. The troubled woman was on the psychiatric wing at Glen Cove Hospital. The deputy mayor explained that the woman's father was not capable of taking care of her at his home. Since the daughter was a Glen Cove resident, it seemed like she'd be a good candidate for the group home. "We really want this favor," the deputy mayor told Linda.

Linda Slezak promised she'd arrange a screening and then make a decision. She hung up the phone and sat there in her little windowless office at Melillo, amazed. Here were the very people who had done everything in their power to kill the group home, now pleading for a bed for one of their own. Linda had to smile. Did they really want a drug-addicted, chemically controlled, delusional manic-depressive living so close to a school bus stop?

The Melillo staff screened the woman and concluded that she could benefit from a group home. Several weeks later she moved in. Linda Slezak certainly wasn't going to penalize the woman just because she'd been referred by Mayor Snake.

chapter 4

JASPER SANTIAGO:
"YOU DON'T SEE GAMBINOS?"

JANUARY 1991. Two years had passed. Linda Slezak was now overseeing three group homes for Melillo. In addition to 9 Highland, she'd opened houses in the nearby suburbs of Glen Head and East Hills.

The daily routine at 9 Highland took on a larger rhythm, of people leaving and new ones arriving. When retarded adults move into a group home, it is expected they will reside there for life. At a group home for the mentally ill, the stay was meant to be short-term. Two years was the goal in New York. With each departure, Linda and her staff took a measure of how they'd done. She'd come to see how hard it was to predict someone's prospects. People she thought were on the verge of going on to a more independent life suddenly collapsed. People she felt might be too ill to even be accepted into the group home flourished. In her three group homes, she counted small, medium, and large successes, and one that was truly extraordinary.

She'd had her disappointments, too. Three months after his high-profile Iowa bus-capade, Jason Smith moved out, to a large adult home, where he could sit around and do nothing all day. A few others had relapses within weeks of arriving at 9 Highland and were sent off for long-term hospitalizations.

As the house moved into its third year of operation that winter of 1991, Linda's biggest headache was Jasper Santiago.

"WHAT'S GOING TO happen to Jasper?" she asked at the staff meeting Monday, February 25, 1991. She had doubts about Jasper's future at the group home. On the last Saturday in January, Jasper had been sitting on the couch closest to the TV having a smoke, when he picked up a scissors from the coffee table and winged it at the kitchen door. "Jasper, what are you doing!" shouted Jodie Schwartz, a counselor sitting beside him.

"Saw a demon," said Jasper. He was taken to Central General in Plainview, the closest hospital with an available bed. Linda Slezak knew what that would amount to. Stays on the psychiatric wings of these small suburban general hospitals went like clockwork. They'd fiddle with his medication and he'd be returned to the group home within a month—even if he was still psychotic. The incident and the hospitalization itself didn't bother Linda so much—these things happened. Saving a bed for him at the house was a routine matter. More serious for Linda was that the group home really wasn't helping the twenty-seven-year-old Jasper. He'd been there almost two years and hadn't made any progress. The stretches when he was hallucinating, laughing, and talking to himself were lengthening. And he didn't seem to be picking up any of the day-to-day skills they tried to teach. Two years later they were still lecturing him on his hygiene. When it got warm, Jasper's odor was all over the house. Passing his bedroom some days was like living downwind from a pig farm. The eating problem was worse than ever—he was up to 350 pounds. He'd awaken three or four times at night and gorge himself. The overnight counselor would get up to check on the noise in the darkened house and there was Jasper in the kitchen, lit only by the opened refrigerator door, his head stuffed inside, using his fingers to scoop leftovers from a plate to his mouth. Jasper went to his treatment program, did his chores, but had little interest in much beside listening to the stereo.

The State of New York's Office of Mental Health program model gave a person two years to get healthier, acquire independent living skills, and learn to cope with the illness, and then expected him to be ready to move on. The problem was, the illnesses weren't familiar with the state model. Schizophrenia is usually a lifetime cyclical disorder. Should a group home push a schizophrenic out during a good period, knowing from his case history that a bad period was likely to follow? At the same time, Linda Slezak knew that if she kept too many people beyond the two-year mark, she would get pressure from state auditors. As long as she felt someone was getting something from the home, she was willing to take that heat. She had started thinking about Jasper while doing the year-end state-mandated utilization review on 9 Highland. The evaluation sheets the group home counselors filled out twice a year indicated that Jasper's living skills—hygiene, shopping, cooking, impulse control, thirteen in all—were actually deteriorating. Linda had asked the group home manager at 9 Highland, Maureen Coley, to work up transfer papers on him. Jasper might be better off in a less demanding program.

As house manager, Maureen Coley would normally act on a request from her boss immediately, but this time she stalled. She and her 9 Highland staff didn't want to give up on Jasper, had a real fondness for him, felt there was more there than met the eye. He had grown up hanging out on Glen Cove's tougher streets, was powerfully strong, and yet if another resident made a cruel crack about him, he'd let it go. Jasper was gentle. His father had done prison time. His brother had died from a drug overdose. Jasper had lived the drug life for a while and had the strength to quit. There was still a lot of little boy in Jasper. Despite his weight, he could dance and would often rocket out of the chair beside the stereo, earphones on, and sashay around the room. Sometimes when he got home from program at the end of the day, he'd come into the office and give Maureen or Jodie Schwartz a kiss hello on the hand. Maureen thought it said something for Jasper that his hallucinations were usually happy ones. He'd frequently surprise the staff and fellow residents. Maureen would think he was lost in one of his fogs, and then out of nowhere he'd say something that touched her. Jasper felt things that caught them off guard. Maureen was impressed by his performance at a Tuesday community meeting in early 1991 when several of his fellow residents complained about people with body odor. Everyone understood this was a thinly veiled attack on Jasper.

"I'm not singling anybody out," said Sherry, one of the younger residents, "But the personal hygiene is getting disgusting."

"Anyone else agree?" said JoAnn Mendrina, the senior counselor.

"Some people have a bad odor," said Sherry, "and drag it around with themselves. It gets in the couch and all over the stuff. It doesn't bother anyone else?"

A few mumbled yes.

Maureen, who as house manager moderated these meetings, suggested they take the person aside and be honest. Sherry was peeved. She'd talked to Jasper before; he'd be good for a few days, then smell awful again.

"Does anyone have anything else they want to say?" Maureen asked.

"Just take more showers and watch your personal hygiene," said Jasper.

Jasper! Maureen didn't know whether to laugh or cry.

"Are you going to take your own advice?" someone asked.

"Sometimes people might be on medication," said Jasper. "It slows you up."

"Jasper, if someone brought it up, how would you handle it?" asked Maureen.

"If they told me, I'd take a shower," said Jasper.

"I told him last night," said Sherry quietly. "He did."

"How about just looking out for each other?" said Jasper. The place went dead. Maureen was amazed—delighted. Everyone knew he'd stink tomorrow, but somehow, from deep inside his hallucinatory swirl, Jasper had found the words and feelings to disarm them when he needed to.

IN MOST MATTERS related to the house, Maureen and Linda Slezak agreed. Both are politically liberal, feminist, anti-authoritarian, and sweet-tempered. Both have lots of energy and a deceptively quiet style, usually persevering until they've outlasted opponents and won their point. At twenty-seven, Maureen Coley was twenty years Linda Slezak's junior and usually deferred to her. But there were subtle differences between the two women that shaped the way they thought about Jasper. Linda was a professional social worker—and a good one. She cared, she was brave when she needed to challenge authority, and she always managed to put a good face on things (she'd been a high school cheerleader). This was her second career. As a young woman she'd graduated from the Fashion Institute of Technology in New York City and worked in the garment district, married, moved to the suburbs, and raised three children. She'd gone back to college in her thirties to get degrees in social work, partly because she wanted to do something more meaningful, but also for a practical reason: she was getting divorced and needed to support her three kids. Linda was remarried now, and though more liberal than most of her Glen Cove neighbors, she was very much the Long Island suburbanite.

Maureen was more the idealist, a crusader and outsider. She'd grown up in a large, wealthy Catholic family on the Island, but it was not Maureen's destiny to be the high school cheerleader. (She used to travel into Manhattan for No Nuke demonstrations.) Maureen is gay and open about it, though discreet and professional. None of the residents at the house knew, and straight friends would generally figure it out gradually, from the casual comments she'd make about Kate, another social worker who was her partner. After college at the state university in Oswego, New York, Maureen joined the Jesuit Volunteer Corps, relocated in Seattle, and worked in a homeless women's shelter. She'd moved back to Long Island and taken a job as a counselor at the group home to pay the bills. She stayed because the group home had more to do with the homeless problem than she'd understood at first. Maureen was from the suburbs, but never the suburbanite.

As program director, Linda was aware of the people who'd been on the waiting list six months and could make better use of the group home than Jasper. She had sympathy for Jasper, but, supervising three homes, ran into him only occasionally. When she stepped back and reviewed Jasper's record, it did not look good. Maureen, on the other hand, saw Jasper daily and worried about how alone he was. She saw too clearly where he could land if he was moved out of 9 Highland: a homeless shelter like the one she'd worked at; or, just as bad, locked away long-term at Pilgrim State. He had no other advocate. Jasper's mother lived in Glen Cove but rarely was in touch. Mrs. Santiago didn't tell him when she changed her unlisted phone number. She missed his birthdays, didn't invite him home for the holidays. Shortly after his most recent hospitalization began, Mrs. Santiago left for vacation in her native Puerto Rico. Jasper's therapist did not go to see him during his stay at Central General. Nor did his county caseworker. His only visitors were Maureen and the group home counselors. If the group home really was a home and not some mini-institution, if it really was community mental-health care, Jasper ought to be able to stay there, Maureen felt. Glen Cove was Jasper's hometown. She didn't care what the state regs said, or if Jasper made the turnover rate at the house look bad. She hoped she wouldn't have to go to war with Linda Slezak over this.

"Jasper did seem better when we visited," Maureen told the others at that February 25 staff meeting. "He insisted on kissing me and Jodie. He's been attending group therapy and said he wanted to come back to the house. He hasn't been smoking—it's a no-smoking unit—and he's actually lost some weight, which is good news. His clothes are even fitting him better." They'd modified the dosage of his antipsychotic medication, Haldol, and he'd be out soon.

"What do we do with him, then?" said Heidi Kaminsky, Linda's assistant. "I have the referrals ready. They're the only two options I can think of." One was a program at Pilgrim State. "I think the next step should be—"

"—So I said to Jasper," Maureen interrupted, "maybe when you come home, when you're still in this mood, maybe you might join Weight Watchers, watch what you eat, be more involved with things. He seemed to think it was a good idea."

Linda Slezak asked if Maureen had had any luck finding him a specialized therapy program for his eating problem. The answer was no. The only one around that would take Medicaid was geared toward young women who were anorexic or bulimic. Maureen could just imagine poor Jasper sitting around in a circle with a group of painfully thin suburban teenage girls talking about their mothers. "It's for people that Jasper wouldn't fit in with," said Maureen.

Linda nodded, then moved on to something else. She wasn't going to back Maureen into a corner yet.

AFTER JASPER WAS at Central General thirty-one days, Maureen went to bring him back to the house. Waiting for her in room 331, he looked like an overgrown child. He was sitting on the edge of the bed, staring straight at the door, a blank expression on his face, a shopping bag of clothes on the floor beside each leg. When she walked in, his face lit up and he stood to go. "I'm all ready, Maureen," he said. As they waited for an attendant with keys on his belt to unlock the steel door leading off the ward, a female patient gave Jasper a big hug, touseled his curly hair, and said, "You're so cute, Jasper, I'm going to miss you." She told Maureen she bought her clothes at Bergdorf Goodman and worked exclusively for Vice President Quayle. "That's good," said Maureen.

"See you around," said Jasper. Downstairs he had some difficulty, but squeezed into the front seat of Maureen's Dodge Shadow. She complimented him on going so long without a cigarette. Like most people at the group home, Jasper was a chain smoker. "I'm dying," he said.

"We'll stop by the pharmacy to fill your prescriptions and you can get cigarettes."

"I'm not really desperate for a cigarette, but I have no deodorant, no nothing. I stink like a dog. I'll quit one day. You could save a lot of money by not smoking, you know?" Jasper told Maureen he didn't ever want to go back to the hospital, though he didn't go as far as saying he felt all better. "I think I still need treatment, but you know, maybe another facility like a farm. Something outdoors. Locked up, you feel like a kook in there."

Maureen asked if he was interested in bowling Saturday with other residents. Jasper said yes. "I feel better. Maybe I had too much gook in my brain—in my blood from the cigarettes. Maybe it slowed me down."

"Gook in your brain?" Maureen asked.

Jasper got quiet. "Nothing," he said. Maureen suggested he continue the hospital's fourteen-hundred-calorie regimen. Jasper nodded. On the car radio the announcer said the estimate of Iraqis killed in the war was now over eighty thousand. They were driving north on Route 107, past some of the richest horse farms on Long Island's North Shore.

"Surprised the war was over so fast, Jasper?"

"It's over?" he said. "Who won? I read it in the papers but I didn't understand they said it was all over."

"The papers can be kind of vague if you don't read them carefully," said Maureen. Jasper had noticed the same thing.

There was a yellow ribbon tied around Glen Cove City Hall. "Looks like four more years of George Bush," Maureen said.

"I don't mind," said Jasper.

"Did you vote in the last election?"

"I don't know," said Jasper. "I can't remember." At the pharmacy Jasper bought a pack of Marlboro 100s. "They look different," he said, studying the gold and white box carefully. Maureen wasn't going to let him smoke in her car. "I'll just smoke on the way to the car," he said, dragging deep and finishing nearly half the cigarette in the fifty feet from the pharmacy. Then he put it out, saving the butt.

· · · ·

JASPER DID NOT go bowling Saturday. He said he felt "slouchy." His shadow, lit by the refrigerator door, was spotted that first night home. Maureen decided that one way to keep his mind on the external world more was to have him take notes at the Tuesday evening community meetings—to turn Jasper into a recording secretary. She was going to try to compete with his hallucinatory world. "Let's turn off the TV," she said, handing Jasper a legal pad and pencil. President Bush had just finished saying, "Just look what we did in the sands of the Gulf. America is a can-do nation." Jasper wrote something on the top of the pad and looked at Maureen. "What month is it?" he said.

It was the first week of March. The weather would be getting warm soon. For a while they discussed weekend outings, then the conversation shifted to how quickly the food was disappearing.

A counselor and a resident shopped together once a week, spending about three hundred dollars, and within hours much of the snack food was eaten. This week they'd shopped Friday. "All three boxes of cookies were gone Saturday night," said Grace Wallace, the woman the mayor had helped get into the house. "I'm on a diet, but I wanted one cookie and one glass of skim milk and it was gone."

Jasper had stopped taking notes and was leaning forward in his chair. "And there's not one drop of soda left," said JoAnn, the senior counselor. Maureen tapped Jasper on the back gently. The crack of his butt was showing halfway out of his pants. "You relating to this, Jasper?" Jasper laughed. "No matter how much soda," said JoAnn, "if we bought sixty bottles, it'd be gone."

"And I didn't get one cookie," said Grace. Jasper rose from his chair beside Maureen and took a seat on the couch. He had put down the notepad and was laughing to himself and fiddling with the venetian blinds.

"Jasper, don't do that. You're going to break that."

Jasper said, "Do I . . . Can I go to the . . ."

"Do you think you'll need the hospital again?" asked Maureen.

"I'll let you know if I'm going to snap and start saying things like Fred had a big head," said Jasper. He leaned back on the couch and his shirt rode up, exposing his huge stomach.

"Jasper, pull down your shirt," Maureen said quietly. There was an edge to her voice. *What was going to happen to Jasper?*

After the meeting she took him aside. She asked about the hospital, but he said he was just joking. He didn't like Central General. "But if there's an opening at Glen Cove Hospital, would you let me know?" said Jasper. "That's a nice place." Maureen told him being hospitalized is serious, it wasn't like picking out a restaurant for lunch. "They let you smoke at Glen Cove Hospital," Jasper said.

On March 12, Jasper went into the hospital again. The hallucinating and laughing were worse. A counselor had found him in a corner of the living room sitting by himself, chatting with members of the Gambino crime family. She'd asked Jasper what was up, and he said, "You don't see Gambinos?"

Maureen arranged for him to go to Glen Cove Hospital, but not for Jasper's reasons. She respected the chief psychiatrist there, Dr. Michael Melamed, and wanted him to do a complete review of Jasper's medications. Sometimes a switch to a different antipsychotic medicine could have an impact on the schizophrenia. She spent a good deal of time preparing a chronology of Jasper's meds in recent years, as well as the dosages. At least the psychiatrist would know what antipsychotics had not helped.

Jasper was pleased. Maureen had come through again—a hospital where he could smoke.

She told the others about Jasper that evening. "That's funny," said one resident, "he didn't seem to be doing any worse." It was a scary moment for Maureen. Laughing, talking to himself, hallucinating were beginning to be perceived as normal Jasper.

COUNSELORS WHO VISITED at Glen Cove Hospital reported that he seemed pretty out of it. At the March 19 group home staff meeting, Jasper occupied a good deal of the conversation. "He's been switched onto Stelazine," said JoAnn.

"He's not doing well," said Maureen. "He wants to just continually sit and masturbate by the fish tank in the lounge. It's causing a little bit of a problem. They asked me if he did this at the group home. I told them never in a public part of the house . . . He didn't used to be like this."

"So what will they do?" asked Jodie Schwartz. "Ship him out to Pilgrim?"

"We've got to see," said Maureen. "Glen Cove Hospital's pretty good. They're trying to do something for him. There might not be a lot they can do."

On March 25, Maureen went to see him on 3-West, the hospital's psychiatric wing, during afternoon visiting hours. She was surprised. He was sitting with his mother, a small, nervous-looking, birdy little thing, one-third Jasper's size. Mother and son spoke in a mix of English and Spanish. "Mrs. Santiago, how you doing?" Maureen asked.

"Fifty-fifty," said Mrs. Santiago. How was she doing? She has a nineteen-year-old daughter who just won a big accident settlement and blew twenty thousand dollars in two months. Her husband had left her after thirty-five years of marriage and was living with another woman. And Jasper was in the nuthouse again. She said she was going to family court next month to try to get some money from Jasper's father.

Maureen felt Jasper looked tired.

"Must be the meds," said Jasper.

A middle-aged woman sat down and interrupted their conversation, asking Jasper to fetch her some juice. It took Maureen a few moments to realize the woman was a patient. "I get him juice, so it's his turn to get me juice," the woman said. "I'm a special education teacher. I'm doing what's called behavior modification on Jasper. If he sits up, I give him a kiss. It's improved his posture." Everyone glanced at Jasper. He looked slouchy. Kissing therapy apparently wasn't working on Jasper either. "You can't tell on these chairs," said the woman, wandering off.

Maureen questioned Jasper about his new medication. "Strazine," said Jasper.

"Stelazine," said Maureen.

"Something like that," said Jasper. "I feel anxious." A side effect. Jasper was flapping his big legs back and forth. His fingers were intertwined and were picked around the nails. Mrs. Santiago complained about his sister. Jasper said, "Her brain has yucky stuff up top." He told his mother to be tough with her.

"I try," said Mrs. Santiago, "but girls won't listen. They're only good to others. I fought with her and she told me to get out of the house. It's my house."

"I used to be like that," said Jasper, "but I got out of it." Maureen asked Jasper if he'd heard from his county caseworker. He hadn't. Visiting hours were ending. She told him she'd be back soon. An aide pressed a button behind the counter at the main nurse's station, releasing the lock on the door, and Maureen walked out of 3-West. She was worried. Linda Slezak had been asking again if the transfer papers on Jasper were ready yet.

chapter 5

THE SPHINX'S RIDDLES

A FEW DAYS later, on Wednesday, April 3, Fred Grasso did not get off the little yellow social service bus at 4 P.M. when it pulled up at the corner of Highland near the group home. "No Freddy?" said senior counselor JoAnn Mendrina. "That's funny, no Freddy. We have something that's very out of character for Freddy—no Freddy." She immediately went into the office and began making phone calls. For anyone else it would be no big deal, she'd probably wait until the 11 P.M. curfew. Though residents usually returned straight from their day programs, they didn't have to. As a courtesy they were supposed to tell staff, but sometimes they forgot and sometimes they didn't feel like it. Fred, however, was not one to deviate from routine, even a little bit. He got up in the morning when he was supposed to, went to program when he was supposed to, came home at four, smoked Camels, watched TV, ate dinner, took his meds, did his chore without being asked, watched more TV, and went to bed at 9:30. He rarely said anything unless spoken to, never had outbursts, may have been the most amiable person on the planet, and definitely was the quietest resident of the group home. Every weekend the thirty-five-year-old

Fred visited his parents. A lot of initiative for Fred at the group home was slapping Jasper five as he headed into the kitchen for a cookie.

JoAnn called a counselor at Fred's program, Micrographics. The most capable people there learned how to produce microfilm and then graduated to jobs in industry. Fred was mired in a training phase of the program, learning typing. All day he sat quietly in a corner copying business letters from a manual. Fred had gone to lunch and did not return. He was an easy person to overlook, and no one noticed him missing until the buses were loading at the end of the afternoon. On Wednesdays Fred picked up his week's supply of meds at Micrographics—twenty-eight tabs of clozapine to control his schizophrenia. He was last seen at noontime, walking with a young woman who lived in a MICA group home, a residence for Mentally Ill Chemical Abusers, former drug addicts and alcoholics. Fred himself had been a drug abuser as a younger man.

It was warm and sunny, one of the first spectacular spring days of the year, and JoAnn was worried about what Fred's fancy might have turned to.

She made a few more calls, without any luck. "Fred knows the number of our pay phone and should have his ID on him," she said. "I'll give him a little longer." She walked around the house, keeping busy, checking the chore schedule, taking a friendly peek at Snuffy, the house's new pet rabbit.

In ten minutes, she phoned the Melillo supervisor on twenty-four-hour call that week, Antoinette Storey. "I don't have any problem with Fred in and of himself," said JoAnn, "but there's this young lady . . ."

Antoinette reminded JoAnn that there was no need to call the police. Ever since Jason Smith's widely publicized bus-capade two years earlier, the Melillo policy had been not to call police unless it was a definite emergency. The police didn't run out looking for missing people, but they did file reports that found their way into the local paper.

JoAnn reached the MICA house. "Has your resident Debbie arrived at home? Did she bring a friend with her, by any chance? One of our gentlemen is missing . . . Could you ask Debbie if perchance Fred mentioned to her if he had any other plans for the day?" JoAnn had a gift for making the whole thing sound like an ice-cream social. "No? I see. Very good. Thank you so much."

She was getting worried. JoAnn was the senior staffer, a somewhat old-fashioned forty-nine-year-old disciplinarian, who had maternal feelings about most of the residents, including Fred. "This isn't like our Freddy," she kept saying. She checked his progress notes. A recent entry indicated that Fred was feeling unhappy about his program lately. When counselor Charles Winslow came in at six, JoAnn sent him to cruise the streets in his van. It was a long shot; the program was in Hicksville, ten miles away. Fred had a six-hour lead. He could be anywhere. More than anything, JoAnn was worried about someone taking advantage of Fred, harming Fred. She couldn't envision it the other way around. The counselors did not tell the group home residents. "Don't want to alarm anyone," JoAnn said. She did notify the Grassos, though she hated to. They were the nicest people and didn't need more grief.

WHEN MRS. GRASSO got the call from the group home, she was worried, but amazed that this place paid enough attention to know her schizophrenic son was a couple hours late getting home. Fred had been in programs where he could have fallen off the planet and no one would have commented. This is why Charlotte Grasso had wanted the group home so badly. Because of her persistence, Fred was one of the original residents to get into 9 Highland. She had called every week for months to find out when they'd be interviewing. During his screening he'd said he didn't care if he was accepted or not; Mrs. Grasso insisted to the Melillo people that this was the illness talking and a sure sign that Fred needed the group home to recapture his enthusiasm. Because she pushed, Fred had been one of the first schizophrenic people in America to be treated with clozapine—the most hopeful medication to come along in the field in twenty years. She got him into a national test program in 1985, years before most psychiatrists had heard of clozapine. He hadn't been hospitalized since. The Grassos joined the National Alliance for the Mentally Ill, the main family advocacy group in the field, and traveled to Washington and Albany to lobby the politicians for more research aid.

Charlotte and Gary Grasso had been active, involved, caring parents for their four children, and they did not stop when their pride, their older boy, the brightest and most athletic, developed severe schizophrenia.

They had been slow to see it. He'd been a warm, energetic kid, always working, delivering *Newsday* at age twelve, mowing lawns, caddying, busing tables at a restaurant after school. Mrs. Grasso never regarded Fred as a hard child, certainly no harder than her other three, all of whom had gone to college, built their own lives and families. If anything, Fred had seemed more sensitive and thoughtful than the others. At the end of their street was a pond. Kids caught small fish there and kept them in jars. Young Fred was always letting the fish go. He was kind about playing with his younger brother, at an age when older brothers don't want to be caught dead with some shrimp. He'd walk his older sister, a cheerleader, to the high school games at night —the protective Fred.

They grew up in a large, immaculate ranch house in Oyster Bay, an upper-middle-class suburb that is a fifteen-minute ride from Glen Cove. Mrs. Grasso, an insurance agent, worked at home to be with the kids. She is a gifted amateur artist. Her sophisticated watercolor landscapes line their walls. Mr. Grasso, a truck driver, did years of overtime shifts so his family could afford this house on the North Shore. He'd made much of their furniture in his basement workshop. At Oyster Bay High, where 90 percent of the kids go on to college, Fred had a B-plus average while playing soccer, basketball, and baseball. A tall, lean, good-looking Italian American boy, he never had trouble getting dates. The girl next door, Patty Rogers, one of the smartest kids in school, Ivy League material, was crazy about Fred and disappointed when he took someone else to the prom.

Looking back, there were suspicious signs as he hit his late teens, but they certainly didn't seem so extraordinary at the time. The Grassos were surprised when Fred wanted to take a year off to kick around before going away to Buffalo for college. But it was 1974, and a lot of kids were doing the same. They compromised. Fred attended Nassau Community College and did well. They suspected he was smoking marijuana, but a lot of kids were then. Although the Grassos never supported such things and are conservative people (Mrs. Grasso used to warn her daughter Rebecca, "Remember, young lady, no boy will pay for the cow if he can get the milk free"), they understood that pot was supposed to be like beer in these modern times. At any rate, Fred wouldn't talk about it, not even with his sisters and brother. He seemed to be getting quieter, more withdrawn—but he was a teenager, riddled with hormones, and the males in the Grasso family were never chatty anyway.

This the parents knew: he went off to Buffalo in January 1977 and came back changed forever. Academically, he did fine: A in European literature; B in personality studies; B in economics; B in creative writing; C in twentieth-century Europe. But now he was moody, surly, angry, completely uncommunicative. They tried to piece together what had happened in Buffalo. It was getting harder. Fred was saying less and less, and when he did say something it was hard to know if he was kidding or serious. The crucial junctures in Fred's life were like unfinished puzzles, because Fred wouldn't provide all the pieces, or couldn't. That was the winter of the big blizzard in the Northeast, and he talked about how hard it was to be cooped up for weeks, of walking to class through campus tunnels. Maybe he'd had a breakdown. They suspected he did a lot of drugs—more serious than marijuana, maybe LSD, maybe PCP—but just what, they were not sure. There was trouble with a roommate. "He had a colored roommate, they had a fistfight," said Mr. Grasso. "He threw the colored guy out. That seemed to be a big thing."

"Buffalo ruined him," said Mrs. Grasso.

Much later, Fred would tell his sister Rebecca that the cause of his Buffalo trouble was drugs. "Fred told a story about being tied down by these guys and having drugs shot into his veins and the room swirling around." The sister didn't know how much of it to believe. "I don't know if he'd done it willingly and made up the story because he felt guilty. I don't know if these were the ravings of a madman. I don't know." She believed Fred had abused drugs, but nowhere near as much as he implied. It was Rebecca's feeling that Fred found it easier, cooler, more acceptable to blame drugs than admit he was losing his mind.

Fred wasn't returning to college, but didn't want a job either. He'd been working all his life and needed to relax, he told them. He started doing things that weren't Fred, going to a party and stealing an album, getting into a fistfight with his father on the lawn in front of the whole neighborhood. The father had tried to never let it show, but Fred had always been his favorite child. The other kids recognized it. Rebecca, who would go on to get a graduate degree in public health policy, considered Fred the brightest of the four kids, a prodigious son. The high school teachers would tell her, "I have your brother Freddy in class, I love him." Fred was soft-spoken, he had polish, he'd grown up on the North Shore, was six feet one, handsome, and he *had* been kind. Mr. Grasso was five feet six, a high school dropout from Queens who looked like a working guy and talked like one. He didn't know the young man in his house anymore. The real Fred was slipping away from them. "He used to be such a surefooted boy," the father said.

It would be a few years before they'd learn that late teens to early twenties was the most common period for schizophrenia to emerge. Instead, they kept attacking symptoms. One counselor said Fred needed discipline. They got him a job with American Airlines as a bill collector. He failed. "I always said that was bad for Fred," Mr. Grasso said. "Fred is basically a nice person. Bill collecting made him do things against his grain." Mr. Grasso took Fred along on his delivery route, but Fred coudn't handle that, either. Maybe it was a mistake working with his father.

They got him drug treatment and therapy. They figured, dry him out and Fred would come home a new man. Mr. Grasso said to his wife, "Fred has friends who did a lot more drugs and they're lawyers today." He was drug free, but still not better. Maybe they'd been too hard on Fred; maybe they'd been mistaken to pressure him to go to college when he'd wanted that year off. They let him use a family car and he took a nine-thousand-mile cross-country trip. As best they could tell, he'd spent almost the whole trip in the car. Twice he was jailed after routine traffic violations escalated into fights with police. The second time, Mr. Grasso had to go to Delaware to bail him out.

Years later, when asked about the trip, Fred said, "I wish I'd taken someone. It was lonely."

Fred worked menial jobs, took his savings, bought a plane ticket, and announced he was moving to San Francisco to start over. His parents were skeptical, but weren't going to stop him. It was January 12, 1979, United flight 94805, 11 P.M. departure. He'd reserved a seat, 34 H. The Grassos drove Fred to the airport. Maybe this would be it, though they doubted it.

An hour after departure the phone rang. It was Fred. He'd fallen asleep and missed the plane.

"He really didn't want to go," said Mrs. Grasso.

"He was scared to death," said Mr. Grasso. They still have the ticket.

THOUGH FRED'S SISTER Rebecca was a nurse and had done part of her training in New York City on Bellevue's psychiatric ward, she herself did not recognize what was wrong with Fred for a long time—or wouldn't see it. She was angry with her younger brother. She kept thinking he was being an obstinate SOB and wondered when he was going to grow up and pull his life together.

One night when he was really behaving oddly—he kept saying "Charlotte's Web, Charlotte's Web," and making whistling sounds like a bomb dropping—Mrs. Grasso asked her daughter to take Fred. "He can't be here," the mother said, "You bring him home."

Rebecca got him back to her apartment and put him to bed in her room, but he kept calling to her, "Rebecca, hold me, please."

"There was a trundle bed, he wanted me to sleep in it," she recalled. "He pulled out the trundle and his leg came out [from his bath robe] and he didn't have anything on. He kept calling, 'Rebecca hold me. I want you to lie with me and hold me.' I couldn't. I was too scared. We'd always been so close, but I don't know what he meant, what he wanted.

"My roommate wasn't there. I didn't sleep one wink that night. He kept calling, 'Rebecca, hold me.' I sat on the couch waiting for the sun. I wanted quick access in case I had to get out of there.

"That night was the first time the word 'schizophrenia' came into my head. We're all good at denial in my family. This was my brother, and I knew from my training, once it's schizophrenia, you're finished. It's not like a broken leg.

"As soon as the sun came up, I put him in my car and drove him to my parents' and said, 'He has to go to the hospital.' " She didn't tell them her suspicion.

FRED FILED HIS last income tax return in 1979. He had earned two thousand dollars. For the next three years he was in and out of private hospitals. The parents' first hint of what was in store came from a hospital counselor. The Grassos were sitting in a pretty courtyard and the counselor said, "What would you do if I was to tell you Fred was going to be like this forever?" The counselor's expression is frozen in Mr. Grasso's mind. They had been expecting to find out when they could look for some progress. The most anyone had said until then was "thought disorder." The Grassos hadn't recognized the code words. So this counselor said it out loud. Afterward, talking it over, Mr. Grasso said to his wife, "I don't think the doctors have the heart to say, 'You have a schizo son.' "

Rebecca and her husband, a doctor, broke the news to Fred's younger brother Gary, Jr., who was nineteen at the time. As a boy Gary had followed Fred everywhere. They'd ride bikes, swim, and because there was a four-year difference and Fred had such a sweet disposition, there was little of the normal rivalry. Gary idolized Fred.

"Fred is very, very sick," Rebecca's husband explained. "He has schizophrenia."

"You're full of shit," said Gary. "There's nothing wrong with my brother. You're the one who's sick." And he walked out of the house and has never talked to Rebecca or her husband since. And if he talks about them, he doesn't use their names.

FRED LIVED AT home between hospitalizations. The Grassos were lost. One Saturday night while watching TV he lit a cigarette, flicking ashes on the floor. Mr. Grasso told him to get an ashtray. Fred punched his father. The father got him in a bear hug, trying to ride out the storm. They were rolling on the floor when Fred looked into Mr. Grasso's face and said, "Dad, your nose is bleeding." He didn't remember why. The Grassos called the police on their son. Fred ran upstairs and locked himself in his bedroom. The police stood outside his door, asking him to come out. They had guns. Suddenly Fred threw open the door and shouted, "You can't come in, you don't have a search warrant." Then he went off quietly with them. That night the Grassos knew they were too old to care for Fred themselves.

IN 1982 THERE wasn't a single group home for the mentally ill in suburban Nassau County. The best the Grassos could do was Boerum Hill Psychosocial Rehabilitation Institute in Brooklyn, a fancy name for a shabby two-hundred-bed single-room-occupancy hotel in a poor neighborhood. State officials had licensed it in 1979 as a mental health facility, in one of their earlier, more feeble attempts to do something about the homeless mentally ill. When Fred first saw Boerum Hill in June of 1982, he could not believe this was where they meant him to live. It was eight stories high, with small, dirty rooms. There was no bell to call the elevator; you yelled your floor and hoped the elevator attendant, usually another mentally ill resident, heard. "I want to come home," Fred pleaded with his parents. "I want to go with you. Don't leave me, please." Once he actually started walking the twenty-five miles from Brooklyn to Oyster Bay, but turned back after several miles, discouraged. Another failed idea.

The Grassos were ashamed of where he lived. They brought him home each weekend. They joined a small group of family members meeting monthly in a room on the eighth floor, off the Boerum Hill cafeteria, and tried to make the place a little nicer. Mrs. Grasso became the group's fund-raiser. She ran a raffle each year, buying 250 tickets herself. She went to cosmetics companies and got them to donate samples for Christmas presents for the two hundred residents. She collected old clothes.

At Boerum Hill one patient stole all Fred's clothes. Another nearly threw him out of an upper-story window. For several years he did not receive a personal allowance he was entitled to.

In October of 1985, a dozen inspectors from the State Commission on Quality Care for the Mentally Disabled descended unannounced on Boerum Hill. They found filth everywhere, rooms caked with soot, rolls of dust, moldy food, linens soiled by week-old dried vomit, windows so dirty they were difficult to see through, a pervasive stench. Inspectors noted that the owners cut every corner. The state mandated a minimum of two towels to a room; there was one. Each room had one light, a twelve-inch fluorescent lamp. Many did not work. The place wasn't air conditioned; the windows opened only a crack. The solution to preventing people like Fred from being thrown out or jumping out was blocking window latches so they'd barely open—it was cheaper than hiring enough supervisory staff. The inspectors found an unshaven twenty-five-year-old man in filthy clothes who hadn't been to program or seen a therapist for weeks, smoking and pacing endlessly in his bedroom.

A state inspector wrote: "Not a single mirror offered a clear reflection."

The owner, a psychologist, Dr. Karl Easton, was charged by the state attorney general with fraudulently billing Medicaid and diverting public funds to himself. A state appeals court eventually ordered him to pay $7.5 million in penalties and fines. (Because Dr. Easton attempted to appeal all the way to the U.S. Supreme Court, it took the state seven years to close out the case.)

This was the choice before group homes.

Two and a half years later, the same Commission on Quality Care made surprise inspections at thirty-two group homes for the mentally ill throughout the state. These same inspectors found group homes to be "safe, nurturing and rehabilitative." Where deficiencies were found, they were quickly corrected, the report noted. Eighty-nine percent of group home residents questioned by inspectors found the group homes a good place to live; 96 percent of the staff found them a good place to work.

FRED LIVED IN Boerum Hill five years, until his mother got him into 9 Highland. On the day his parents went to move him out of the Brooklyn facility, they were in great spirits. It was hard to read Fred. He wore sunglasses, even indoors. "Fred, take a good look," said Mr. Grasso. "This is your last time."

"Yeah," said Fred, "I won't be able to steal in the stores."

"Come on Fred, you don't steal," said Mrs. Grasso.

"Yeah, I don't," said Fred.

Mrs. Grasso said how excited she was about Fred moving to the group home.

Under his breath, Fred said, "Another jail."

"Fred!" said Mrs. Grasso, who missed nothing. "It's a beautiful house, it's near all these restaurants and stores, it's going to be a nice place, Fred."

"Right," said Fred, "I know it." They went up to the third floor and began moving Fred's things from 329. A young man saw them and gave a funny look. "This is my mom and dad," said Fred.

"I thought you was the inspectors," said the man. Fred's closet was stuffed with clothes, some in such bad shape Mrs. Grasso just threw them into a trash can in the room. On the ride home Fred said he was glad to be going. "There's a lot of violence and gangsters on the street. They always try to mug you."

When the Grassos got back to Oyster Bay, they put Fred's things in the garage until his mother had time to sort through them. She didn't want cockroaches getting in the house.

The Grassos returned to Boerum Hill once more without Fred, to say good-bye to the parents' group. A dozen parents were still meeting monthly in the room off the cafeteria, still trying to make the place a little better. Mrs. Grasso brought four bags of clean used clothes. The group leader said, "I wanted to say how I'm very happy for both of you. Without you and your raffle support I don't know what we'll do."

"You'll have to find a new fund-raiser," said Mrs. Grasso. "My son's in a beautiful home. It was a hard struggle getting him in, but it's worth it."

SEVEN O'CLOCK, April 3, and still no Fred. JoAnn wanted to know if he'd called the Grassos. He hadn't. Charles came back after a couple of hours' driving all over. No Fred. It was dark now. A few residents were watching TV. Most were upstairs in their rooms. About ten, the front screen door opened and there was Fred. He told the overnight counselor he just didn't feel like staying in program that afternoon and had taken a walk. He'd been walking ten hours. The counselor waited for more, but that's all there was. Jasper, just back from his most recent hospital stay, rumbled out of his room by the front door on the way to the kitchen for another evening snack. "Hey Fred, how you doing?" said Jasper.

"Hey, Jas," said Fred. Fred was pooped. Would it be all right if he took his meds and went to bed?

Next morning Maureen casually asked Fred about his absence. "I just wanted to get out of program," Fred said. He was walking to his parents' house, he said, and a cop stopped him but didn't arrest him. Maureen waited, but that's all there was. This was touchy. She didn't want to intrude—Fred had done nothing wrong, hadn't even missed curfew. Her best guess was that Fred had probably been inspired by the lovely weather to get himself a beer or two. The spring before, JoAnn had looked out the window one afternoon and saw Fred out front, sucking a beer, a violation of house rules. She'd approached him, but before she could utter a word, Fred had said, "It's not good to drink beer with your meds." Maureen's guess was that he'd been drinking on a curb in some nice neighborhood, hadn't bothered to put the can in a brown bag, and a cop had spotted him. This was apparently Fred's spring ritual.

She wondered why he hadn't stopped at his parents' and saved himself ten miles of walking. "Didn't want to bother them," said Fred. Maureen made it clear she wasn't upset, just concerned about him. "Yeah," said Fred, "I was really tired." Maureen figured he'd probably walked twenty-five miles.

Maureen spoke to the Grassos and explained that the best she could make of it was spring fever.

"I don't believe that spring fever stuff," Mrs. Grasso said to her husband. She asked Fred herself. Spring fever, said Fred. She still didn't buy it. "I think that's just something they put in his head. He heard them say it." Still, she had no better explanation. This was it with Fred—all theories, all conjecture, no emotion, no anger: a Sphinx.

JoAnn thought he was so quiet and reserved because he heard voices constantly and was covering. His parents didn't think he heard voices at all. Maureen wasn't sure, but didn't think it was often, if at all.

Fred said he didn't hear voices. But was he being truthful? Was it a matter of pride? Years before, when he was first getting sick, he'd asked his sister Rebecca a lot of questions about Van Gogh and people who hear voices. He wanted to know what it meant. Once, before his first hospitalization, he'd told his sister that Jesus Christ was in the bushes in front of their house and wanted Fred to kill somebody.

"He never told me he heard voices," Rebecca said, "and I don't think he does now, with the clozapine. But Fred is well enough to know he's sick and is very embarrassed by it, so it would be hard to say for sure."

The roots of his schizophrenia were just as mysterious. Maureen felt that Fred, like most victims of the illness, probably had a genetic predisposition which in his case was triggered by his heavy drug abuse. She felt he was so quiet and passive because of the damage drugs had done to his brain.

Linda Slezak disagreed. She believed that Fred was this way because his schizophrenia was very severe. She had seen people like Fred at the hospitals with these "negative symptoms"—very apathetic and withdrawn—who had never done drugs. She felt the drugs had been Fred's means of medicating himself as his brain betrayed him in ways he could not understand.

Fred's sister Rebecca, who was there during the onset of his problems, believed the schizophrenia came first. (She felt the root of his illness could be traced to their paternal grandparents, who had married despite being first cousins, laying the foundation for a "genetic weakness." "I know it in my heart that's the reason my brother's sick," Rebecca said.)

Fred's girlfriend at the time, Patty Rogers, who was also there during the onset and went on to be a college professor, was convinced the heavy drug use came first.

By now Mr. and Mrs. Grasso had read everything they could find on schizophrenia, attended dozens of lectures, turned it over in their minds a billion times, but concluded they'd be as likely to solve the chicken-and-egg riddle as the mystery of Fred.

And from Fred you got only more riddles. In the middle of a going-away party for one of his friends at the house, he'd quietly said, "Who's leaving?" But he'd had a smile on his face. Was he serious? Joking?

Did Fred like the group home? "It's nice," he said, "warm in the winter. I hate the cold." Anything else? "It's nice." Was this the only answer Fred could produce? Or did he dislike the house but feel it would be wrong to say so?

Fred had once been a good athlete; now he wouldn't pick up a glove for a catch in front of the house. If he did the minimum, maybe he'd have a minimum number of failures. When he first came, staffer Laurie Nardo had said how independent she was going to make him. But over two years later, he still couldn't manage his allowance, still couldn't take meds by himself without losing track a couple of days a week and messing up.

Stan Gunter, one of the group home's success stories, now living in an apartment, stopped by to see his friends at 9 Highland one day that spring and spotted Fred. "Freddy!" said Stan. "You've been sitting in that chair since I left a year ago."

AND YET THERE were times he'd catch them all off guard. He'd do considerable extra work around the house without being asked, clean Snuffy's rabbit cage on his own. Saturday mornings he'd whip up French toast or pancakes for himself for breakfast. Sometimes they'd all be sitting around watching MTV and Fred would hit their mood right on the nose. In the middle of a song by the Animals, he'd pick out the perfect lyric and sing it out loud: "We got to get out of this place, if it's the last thing we ever do." They'd look at him. Fred was there. He'd smile back in recognition. And then Fred would go silent again.

The counselors discussed his mystery walk at a Tuesday staff meeting.

"There's a lot there inside Fred," said JoAnn.

"I get the sense Fred's a silent recorder," said Maureen.

"You should see Fred with Snuffy," said Paula Marsters. "He sits there, kissing her. Little kisses."

STEPHEN DEROSA'S schizophrenia was different from Fred's and Jasper's. He didn't hallucinate or hear voices, and was quite involved in the world around him. Fridays and Saturdays he put in several hours at the DeRosa family business in town, doing cleaning work. Saturday nights he volunteered at a local charity bingo game, calling numbers. Sunday he attended mass faithfully and went to his elderly mother's for dinner. During his healthy stretches Stephen—who at forty-eight was the group home's oldest resident—was a delight. He laughed easily, was magnanimous about people's shortcomings, flirted shamelessly with female residents and counselors, and was a good sport when teased about his eccentricities. At these times he would attack his house chores with ferocious energy. His bathroom-cleaning skills were legendary at 9 Highland. On an evening when he had bathroom duty, they'd yell, "Stand back, Stephen's going in for the kill," and Stephen would march by, dead serious, like General Patton taking Sicily, carrying mops, sponges, and cleaning fluids, wearing rubber gloves and galoshes. By the time he was through hours later, you could have run a neonatal clinic in the toilet.

When he was feeling well, he looked good. Walking around the house on a Sunday before church in a conservative dark suit, sipping from a mug of coffee, he could have been one of Glen Cove's town fathers. He had a handsome, masculine face and a full head of thick, dark hair that was graying. When Julie Callahan first met him at the house in 1989, she kept trying to figure out—was he resident or staff?

His illness had long since settled into a predictable cycle. When Linda Slezak first read his records, she was angered that he'd been kept ten years at Pilgrim State Psychiatric Hospital in neighboring Suffolk County. Nothing indicated he needed that length of institutionalization. Pilgrim was the worst fear of every 9 Highland resident.

In an era when smaller is considered better for treatment purposes, Pilgrim State held the dubious distinction of being the largest mental hospital in the nation. During the 1940s and '50s, it was a national leader in lobotomizing patients. By 1991, the sixty-year-old mental institution was so badly underfunded, its director was inviting in reporters to do exposés on the conditions.

Stephen might become unhinged occasionally and require a short hospital stay for a rest-and-medication tune-up, but ten years at Pilgrim was a sin. His life would have been so much richer, Linda Slezak felt, if group homes had existed when he came of age. It wasn't until 9 Highland opened that Stephen was able to return to his hometown to live.

Stephen's bad periods rattled the whole house. He grew paranoid, extremely sensitive to noise, intolerant, and angry. One of schizophrenia's symptoms can be a hypersensitivity to the environment. Linda Slezak thought of Stephen as a person whose brain was missing the filters most people have to screen out the extraneous noise of day-to-day life. When he was ill, he couldn't shut out background sound the way most people do. At these times it was awful for Stephen to be living in a house with eleven other people.

Once his paranoia took hold, he was sure a horn honking on Highland was meant for him—even if he was in his bedroom. Residents had a hard enough time living with their own severe illnesses; on top of this they had to tiptoe around Stephen's paranoia. Stephen would periodically be convinced that someone he lived or worked with was his sworn enemy. That spring of 1991, he realized it was Eve, the newest resident at the house. She'd moved into the room across from his on the first floor.

"There's one person in the house, I don't know, she's kind of snobby," he hissed, gritting his teeth fiercely. "She's sending me bad feelings. It's that new black girl. I don't know why she's doing it, but it's really bothering me. I've had problems with blacks at my day program too."

He was convinced Eve was scorning him because she'd found out about the porno magazines under his bed. He'd been tormented by magazines under his bed all his life. "I had a nervous breakdown after high school," he told a friend. "I had a lot of time. I used to think about girls. I used to read *National Geographic* and do something to myself. Something that I shouldn't tell you. I did something to myself, it left a mark on my belly button. I think she can tell," he said, pointing toward Eve's room.

A few days later he was standing in the first-floor hallway screaming, "Eve's out to get me! Eve's out to get me!" She had sneezed when Stephen walked past. "Right when I was going by! She's trying to get me sick."

All he talked about at the community meetings now was noise. "Whose dog is that always out there barking?" he asked one Tuesday. "It was out there two weeks ago Sunday, too." No one had noticed.

Maureen tried keeping his mind on more constructive endeavors. Stephen was supposed to go to a group homes consumer meeting that night. The state was really pushing consumerism lately, encouraging people in the mental health system to speak up about their needs. What kind of housing arrangements did they really want? What kind of job assistance did they need? The state had hired consultants from Boston University to help shape a more consumer-oriented mental health system for New York. "Empowerment" was the new watchword. But as much as she cajoled and pushed, Maureen had trouble getting any of the 9 Highland residents—or "consumers," as the state now officially preferred to call them—interested. She kept asking for volunteers, and Stephen had finally agreed to go to Melillo's consumer meetings because there might be some pretty girls there.

"Would you like to talk a little about what went on at the last meeting?" Maureen asked.

"I don't remember anything," Stephen said. He had more pressing problems. He noticed Fred had used his hands to rub butter on his corn at dinner. "It's uncivilized," Stephen said. "I can't stand living around all these sick people."

Stephen reluctantly got ready for the consumer meeting being held at the East Hills group home that night. He put on his coat, then gargled. Fred walked by whistling.

"Please!" said Stephen.

East Hills is the newest of the three group homes Linda Slezak oversees. It had been open just a few months. Stephen admired how fresh and clean everything looked. Antoinette Storey, the house manager, had designed the house as she'd hoped her own home would look someday, emphasizing pastels. "Very nice," Stephen said, making a short downstairs tour before the meeting, nodding and smiling at the East Hills house residents. During the consumer meeting—about a dozen people Stephen didn't know and didn't care to—he'd peeked around often, eyeballing the East Hills residents in the back of the house who were smoking and reading. As for the meeting, Stephen spoke only if asked a question, and then said as little as possible.

Afterward, walking back in the dark to where the car that was taking him back to Glen Cove was parked, he said, "There was a fat girl in the other room. Did you see her? She was beautiful. I love fat girls; the only problem is the religion thing gets in the way. If I did anything, I'd just be doing it for sex, that's the problem. There were actually two fat girls in there. That's a nice house."

The car started, he settled into the front passenger seat and buckled his seat belt for the ride back to Glen Cove. He didn't get to ride in a car much; just those humiliating yellow county social-service buses. "I get this magazine, it's mostly skinny girls, but it has six pages of this fat girl, a big spread, and six pages of another fat girl. I don't know what I'm going to do. I've been waiting for this magazine *Buff* to come out again, and it hasn't come out for three to four months." He got quiet. This was pleasant. It was dark and late; there weren't many cars on the road making noise. No idiots honking at him or trying to see in his window. "I have to build up my spirit . . . My spirit's not so good right now. I do things in my room, it takes away my spirit, if you know what I mean. But that's up to me to change. I can do something about that."

The car was cruising a stretch where Glen Cove Road turns into a divided highway and you can do seventy. Stephen leaned back, relaxing, a small smile on his face. "I'm forty-eight and I'm a virgin," he said. "Isn't that pathetic? You want to hear a story? I had a fat girlfriend once. In Building 45 at Pilgrim. She'd make a signal to tell me when to kiss her. I really loved her, from the first day we met. She was beautiful. She was sitting on the stairs and I was staring at her. She said, 'Hi.' She said, 'I have to make a phone call. You want to come?' She was so nice. It lasted a week and a half. I got mad at her. I was very mean. I thought she was planning against me. I feel bad about it now. I'd like to apologize but I don't know where she is."

MAUREEN TRIED keeping a cap on Stephen, but she was riding a geyser. She had hoped to prevent a hospitalization by hanging on until this cycle in his schizophrenia passed, but it would not. Every day now, he'd blow. Some boob had cleared away his dinner plate without asking if he'd finished. ("I can't stand being with sick people. No manners!") His roommate Jasper accidentally stepped on the TV remote control. ("The sheerest stupidity!") At the sheltered workshop where he packaged baking kits for supermarkets, his supervisor kept snapping her gum. ("A really snobby colored girl.")

Maureen waited for Glen Cove Hospital to get a bed open.

On April 17, in the afternoon, the call came. Stephen put on a clean white shirt, packed some clothes, walked into the office, gave Jodie and JoAnn good-bye kisses, and thanked them for everything. He saw his roommate Jasper, and said pleasantly, "Now it's your turn to have the room to yourself."

. . .

LATER THAT SAME evening Julie Callahan stopped by the group home, just to say hello. Since leaving 9 Highland the previous fall, she'd returned for visits several times. She looked great. She was wearing a tan fitted skirt that came to her knees, a flowing white blouse, stockings, and medium-height heels in matching tan and white. Her hair fell loose over her shoulders.

Staff was always glad to see Julie. It was like teachers getting a visit from a former star pupil and being reminded that some of those seeds you plant really do flower. Residents were glad to see her, too. It was nice to know one of your own was still hanging on out there. Many from the home who'd gone on to live independently had severed their ties. It was like they were afraid if they stepped back into the group home, they'd be sucked into the system again. Not Julie. "Julie!" said one of the men. "How you doing? This is the only success story the mental health system's ever produced." The long-termers who'd been there during Julie's hard times could never get over it. "How did she get better so fast?" they'd ask. Her illness had been a mystery to them. There was almost something magical about Julie. She was friendly to everyone in the house. If Stan Gunter was playing classical music on the piano, she'd accompany him, or she could dish street jive with Jasper. Julie was one of the few non-hallucinations that could make Jasper smile. "You're looking good, girl," he said. "You doing good?" She *was*. She looked like someone you'd see on the cover of *Glamour* or *Mademoiselle*.

She stayed for dinner, talking a lot with Jodie, one of her favorite counselors from her days as a resident. Julie casually mentioned that she wasn't working part-time any more, that she'd just been hired full-time as a secretary for twenty-seven thousand dollars a year. This was Julie's style, to understate things.

"Julie, that's great!" said Jodie. "You're amazing."

After that, when another counselor asked Julie how she was doing, Jodie waited, then said, "Come on Julie, tell her the best part."

"The best part?" said Julie.

"Tell her you're working."

"That's the best part?" said Julie.

"I think it is," said Jodie. "You're making more money than we are."

This was one of the reasons Julie returned for visits. She felt important. She had a gift for making things look easy, though her life even now was anything but. She still lived in fear of being hospitalized —or worse, becoming homeless again. She needed to come back occasionally to this place where they knew how it had been.

Julie was disappointed Stephen wasn't there. She asked JoAnn if it would be all right for him to have a visitor at the hospital. "I'll check, dear," said JoAnn, going into the office to call one of the pay phones on 3-West. "Stephen DeRosa, please . . . It's JoAnn. How you doing? . . . Not to worry about your program. You're there to have your medication evaluated and relax . . . Would you like a visitor this evening? Sometime before eight for a short visit? Oh, you want to be surprised? Fine . . . But you are up to facing visitors this evening? Good . . . You took communion at the hospital this afternoon? Very nice . . . If you get communion every day, it's going to straighten you out? Good, good . . . How about your medication, did Dr. Melamed make any changes? . . . Yes you're going to have a surprise visitor this evening . . . You want to know? . . . Sure. How about Julie? . . . No, not that Julie. Our Julie."

JULIE RODE the elevator to the third floor. She pressed the bell beside the heavy, locked, windowless door marked 3-West. A little voice came out of the box, "Yes?"

"I'm here to see Stephen DeRosa," Julie said, leaning forward to talk into the box. The door buzzed and she pulled it open. At the front desk she signed in. A couple of staff members on duty recognized her, were surprised, and asked how she was doing. There seemed to be just a touch of nervousness in their smiles, but maybe not. Julie made a joke of it. "Just visiting this time," she smiled back. She walked down the hall to Stephen's room, her heels clicking softly on the shiny white linoleum. Wherever she went, heads turned. Passing room 9, she said, "That used to be my old room here." Julie had spent big chunks of 1989 and 1990 on 3-West.

Stephen was sitting at the edge of his bed in a white shirt, black flannel slacks, and dress shoes. He could have been a businessman who'd just arrived home from work and taken off his tie. He stood when Julie entered, a big smile on his face. Stephen was fond of Julie. She always took an interest in him. He was sorry when she left the group home. He liked classical music and enjoyed it when Julie and Stan Gunter played Mozart together. Stephen's only regret about Julie was that she was too skinny. It limited the feelings he could have for her. "You look fantastic," he said. Stephen was looking fairly trim himself.

"Oh no, I still have my belly," Stephen replied, cradling it for emphasis. He told her about a woman he'd walked by downtown who'd retched when she'd seen it *("Bleh!")* and brought Julie up-to-date on his fat-women magazines. "You should see how *their* bellies hang down," he said.

"I'll bet," said Julie. She asked him, "Do you need change?" Julie knew how important quarters for the pay phone were on a locked ward. They were your only link to the outside world. She still carried plenty, just in case. That was what Stephen liked about Julie. She remembered the bad times. Just because she was doing great now, she didn't go around snubbing people.

chapter 6

JULIE,
SPRING/SUMMER 1989

BACK AT THE start of 1989, when Julie first moved into the group home, there were people who felt she was too well to be there. Mrs. Grasso, Fred's mother, commented, "That girl seems terrific, not like my Fred. I'm wondering if these new homes are taking the better ones to make themselves look good?"

Julie was the one who toured the mayor around when he visited. Julie was the one who volunteered to go door-to-door to hostile neighbors' homes to invite them to an open house at 9 Highland. When a counselor left that first March the house was open, it was Julie who took up a collection, bought a tea set, and decorated the cake. Though Julie didn't say who was behind it, the honoree knew, commenting, "Classic Julie C." She had been at North Shore Day Treatment program four days when fellow patients nominated her to be president of the patient council. She won. Her victory speech was, "This is great, but I just got here, I don't know what to do." Her therapist at the program, Nan Case, used to tease her for being too goody-goody. The therapist told Julie it was OK to be less than perfect, maybe get in late one day.

Not that Julie was a pushover. She'd be the first at the group home to stand up for her rights. After Jason Smith's bus-capade, Julie asked to read the file of newspaper articles the agency kept. The counselor tried to give her only the positive stories written about the group home. "Since the other articles had nothing nice to say, there's no reason to show them" the counselor explained. Julie was teed off. "We're being treated like insignificant mental patients!" she complained. February 2, 1989, the counselor wrote in the daily log: "After . . . awhile Julie became more relaxed. I tried to help her to focus on the good articles because those are the ones that count. However, she claims she can't really appreciate the good articles until she can read the negative ones. I told her I will check into the idea." Julie persisted, and Julie prevailed.

After reading the file, she told the counselor that the bad ones weren't as bad as she was expecting. "They're mostly just stupid," Julie said.

In her early days there, Julie loved the group home and felt better than she ever had. She saw no shame in needing it. She was learning the basic skills she'd never picked up because her family life had been so crazy and brutal. Within a week there, she helped prepare her first meal ever: breaded pork chops, corn, and french fries. She learned how to do comparative price shopping at the supermarket, cash a check, open a savings account. (Years before as a high school student she'd never cashed her paychecks from a part-time job because she didn't know how and was too ashamed to ask.)

The curfews didn't bother her. She liked hanging around the house watching TV with a counselor. Just talking with a normal person about how the day went, a TV show, the news, clothes, made her feel human. After twenty-seven months in hospitals, she felt free.

At the group home she soaked up everything, making up for a lost childhood. Julie's mother had never let her wash her hair or shower and rarely let her take a bath. Julie was always sure she was an ugly girl. As a child she owned just two pairs of pants, neither of which fit, one of them iridescent. Kids called her dirtbag. She was such a proud little kid, it used to humiliate her when a teacher who meant well would suggest she bathe more. She'd have angry conversations in her young mind with the teachers: "Don't you see? Don't you think I'd like to wash, but my mother won't let me? Do you think I want to be this way?" She swore to herself when she grew up, she'd understand girls with dirty hair. As she got older, she'd conceal shampoo packets in her purse, sneak into the ladies' room, and before anyone saw, would quickly wash a section of her hair in the sink, until it was reasonably clean. She couldn't get it too nice—she was scared to death her mother would find out she was shampooing on the sly and beat her. It wasn't until she was in her late teens, living in a foster home, that she first stepped into a shower and then was petrified she wouldn't figure it out. It took months of showers before she started to feel clean. Just by observing female counselors and residents at the group home as well as people in the streets and stores of Glen Cove, Julie learned about hygiene, grooming, makeup. She'd study TV to teach herself how to make a better appearance. All her life, if Julie wanted to learn something, she'd make a study of it. As a girl, she'd taught herself to throw a ball by going to the library and reading a book on it.

Terry Gaylo, a counselor, told her about a beauticians' school, where Julie got her hair cut at a reduced price. They took her to her first 50 percent–off sales.

Julie wasn't bothered by the sickest people at the house. She danced with Jasper at parties; went to Friendly's for ice cream with a man who had such severe schizophrenia, he lasted at 9 Highland only a few weeks before being institutionalized long-term. She was nervous for him, didn't know if the poor guy was together enough to answer the waitress. The moment came and out of nowhere, he said peppermint stick ice cream with marshmallow in a sugar cone. Julie was dumbstruck. This obviously was a priority.

Perhaps Julie's greatest gift was her insight into people. She saw things most missed. Julie didn't have to gossip; she often could sense what would happen before it did, because she read human behavior. If there were seven people in a room, Julie knew how to put each one at ease. She had an ability to learn from each person she met.

Julie practically was a counselor at times. In one of his nutty cycles, Stephen had invited her into his room to explain about the magazines under his bed and how he feared Christ would banish him to Hell for it. Julie didn't feel Stephen was in that kind of danger, but listened sympathetically. "Do you want to see the magazine?" Stephen asked. They studied it together. "Look at that girl's can," Stephen said. Julie agreed it was something. She'd never seen a fat-women magazine before. "No?" said Stephen. He explained this was doing terrible things to his spirit.

"I think you need some help with this," said Julie.

"You're right," said Stephen.

"Would you like me to take this magazine away when I go out?"

"Would you?" said Stephen. Julie would.

Later, as she'd put on her coat, she heard her name. "Julie," whispered Stephen, peeking out of his room. "Don't forget this." He handed her a brown bag with the magazine inside.

A FEW TIMES in these early months, the group home staff picked up behavior that didn't seem to fit. Julie would normally swear once in a while, but on a couple of occasions every other word out of her mouth was "fuck." Not like Julie. Something else odd. One evening during her first months, she approached counselor Joy Curran and asked, "Is there a baby in the house?" Joy was surprised. A baby?

"I don't hear it now," Julie said, "but I could hear it really clearly up in my room."

SHE WAS DOING so well that, when she'd been at 9 Highland only two months, her day treatment therapist tried to get her to move out. The therapist persuaded Julie to attend an orientation session about an apartment program that provided more independence; the only supervision would be brief daily visits from a caseworker. Julie was resistant. At the group home she felt stability for the first time.

But Julie was also an achiever. Within the mental health system there was a pecking order. Private hospital patients looked down on state hospital patients. Apartment people looked down on group home people. Julie was soon asking to be referred to an apartment. She wanted to return to college in the fall and felt it was time to make the move so she'd be well established in a new routine when school started. The group home staff and Julie's therapist argued over it. The therapist said it had been a mistake to send Julie to a group home in the first place, she was too well. The Melillo staff contended a longer stay was necessary to ensure she was stabilized. Julie and staff members fought, too. A counselor wrote in the daily notes that Julie was "obsessing" on this. Finally a truce was reached. If Julie continued doing well, she'd be referred to an apartment after six months at the house, in June.

May 25, 1989, she fell apart.

AT STAFF meetings you'd rarely hear a counselor describe someone as a "classic schizophrenic" or a "typical obsessive-compulsive." Staff knew the residents too well and the unique form the illnesses took in each. However, group home workers were still well aware of everyone's diagnosis. And it affected their thinking. In Julie's case they were looking for signs of borderline behavior—her diagnosis at the two prestigious private hospitals where she'd been treated. There weren't many. The other two borderline women at the house had eating disorders: one was anorexic, the other bulimic (staff suspected the resident was forcing herself to throw up in the shower after dinner each night). Julie had no eating problem.

A borderline personality often latches onto one other person to the exclusion of everyone else; Julie was friendly with almost everyone at the house. Narcissism is another common trait; Julie was giving. There was no evidence she was defacing herself, no scars on her arms, no razor blade wounds. Nowhere in the daily log is there a mention of the mercurial mood swings so common to the borderline disorder.

In just one respect she conformed to the borderline pattern: Julie was socially active. If she wanted, Julie could have had a date every night. Counselors were on the lookout for evidence of the promiscuity mentioned in her hospital records. It can be a symptom of a borderline problem. A person can have poor sense of self, little idea how to form balanced relationships, and so use sex as a shortcut to intimacy. But if this was Julie, she wasn't advertising it. They'd have to keep a close watch. The other two at the house dressed hot; their breasts always seemed on the verge of popping out of their halter tops. Julie's clothes were tasteful.

She was well aware that she was suspected of being a sex fiend. When Don Berlin had given her that big, wet good-bye smooch during her trial visit to the house, Julie wasn't sure she should tell the staff. She didn't think anyone would believe her, given her reputation. A therapist on the borderline unit had once said Julie was so highly seductive it was unlikely that even the most esteemed male therapists could resist her, and to be safe she should always seek out female therapists. She was flattered but it scared the hell out of her, like she was equipped with a mysterious sex force that she didn't feel, but others sensed.

She took a chance and, her first week at the house, told counselor Terry Gaylo about Don. Terry jumped to Julie's defense and Don apologized next day. They did not have a problem again, and became friends. It grew into a joke. Don would be cooking Chinese for dinner and if Julie said, "Looks delicious," Don would say, *"Now* can I have a kiss?"

Every few weeks there was something suspicious with men. Julie went for Sunday brunch with a guy in his forties. He picked her up looking neat, and when they returned he looked disheveled. She explained that he was just a sloppy guy with a messy car, but counselors wondered. At the open house, a strange man was noticed sitting beside her in a close, suggestive way. A few times she went out on dates without telling anyone, returning late, with red glassy eyes. "We were worried something might've happened," said Jodie. "We just want to know when to expect you back." Julie said the date had treated her decently and she found that hard to deal with. She said she felt disgusting and stupid and not worthy of anyone's attention.

On the yellow bus to program, a man with severe schizophrenia sitting beside her tried kissing her out of the clear blue. She ducked him. For days, he'd ask if he could ride beside her. He wanted to date. She kept refusing. The 9 Highland staff offered to handle it—they knew this man had been obsessive about other women—but Julie said she needed to learn to deal with these problems herself. This apparently was what life was all about—fending off men, starting with your father and foster father.

The counselors suggested she cultivate more women friends. They conferred with her therapist, Dr. Robert Blank. Julie was struggling with impulse controls and sexual acting out, he said, showing "very disturbing thought patterns in therapy." At the house, they were noticing the same. In mid-April of 1989, she started laughing so hysterically one evening, she was nearly crying. When a counselor offered help, Julie said, "I feel like I'm losing my mind." She went up to rest. A counselor checked on her, but Julie didn't want to talk, saying that the group home staff and Dr. Blank "are trying to take everything away from me . . . You're trying to change me and eventually I'll be left alone . . . You're trying to take my sister away." Voices in her head warned her not to say what was on her mind.

Next day she left program early, arriving home at midday. She did not say her usual hello, but wandered the house aimlessly, keeping her coat on, making no eye contact. Her hair was down over her face. She seemed to be avoiding well-lit parts of the house.

"Sweetie, is anything bothering you?" asked counselor JoAnn Mendrina.

"I'm scared they're going to get me," Julie said. "I feel separated from everything and everybody." Her hair still down, she asked JoAnn, "Where are we going with this conversation?" Julie lay down on the sofa and watched TV. JoAnn sat nearby at the dining room table, finishing med log paperwork. "Don't you write about me," said Julie.

The house staff consulted the psychiatrist again. Julie's always been psychotic off and on, Dr. Blank said, with impulses to hurt herself. He suggested being supportive and monitoring suicide potential. Julie at first was furious that they had spoken with Dr. Blank, but a few days later apologized. She said she hadn't known what she was saying, it was like she was drugged.

She was having trouble sleeping. She'd do her chore at 1 A.M., cleaning the refrigerator and laundry room, then be up at 6, before the overnight counselor. In late-night talks with staff, she'd tell them little snatches of her life. When she was still a girl a younger sister had died of an illness, and Julie was ashamed for having laughed hysterically at the funeral.

About this time, April 1989, the first group home manager left because her husband was being transferred. A new manager, Tim Cook, was hired. He would stay only eight months, but would play a crucial role in Julie's life.

THE FIRST TIME Tim Cook toured 9 Highland, he was struck by Julie's room. A ton of stuffed animals covered the bed, but the one that made an impression was a little dog placed on the floor, at the foot of the bed, pointed at an angle toward the door, like a guard dog.

"Sexually abused?" Tim said to the counselor touring him.

"Whoa!" said the counselor. "You'll do just fine here."

Tim, who was in his early thirties, did not have a traditional background for running a group home. While he had worked in a half dozen community mental-health programs—apartments, homes, shelters—his master's degree from St. John's University was in the philosophy of religion, not social work. He saw people with a fresh eye and had a nontraditional view of these disorders. He believed the medical model of treatment was badly flawed, that medically trained psychiatrists had too much power and relied too heavily on prescribing medications often of questionable value to patients they hardly knew. Today schizophrenia is generally viewed as a biochemical breakdown in the brain to be treated with medications. To this Tim says, "If it's an illness, how come there's no chemical means of identifying schizophrenia in the brain the way you'd identify other illnesses?'' In Tim's view, the psychiatrists didn't treat individuals; they medicated a diagnosis. Tim is a voracious reader and saw worth in writers no longer popular in the eighties, like R. D. Laing and Thomas Szasz. He liked their questioning of the medical model of treatment and their emphasis on how little was known of the disorders' biological nature. Tim didn't go so far as embracing Laing's and Szasz's conclusion that there is no mental illness, but he admired their skepticism about the mainstream approach. He had a far more radical outlook than 99 percent of the people working in the system. To Tim the group home was like a laboratory, where all sorts of creative approaches could come into play.

Linda Slezak didn't agree with a lot of Tim's ideas, but she hired him because he was bright, hardworking, humane, charismatic, insightful, had a terrific belly laugh—and ultimately was a pragmatist. If Tim was radical, it was always from within traditional organizations. He'd been an Eagle Scout. His interest in social issues came through the Catholic church. At one point he'd thought of being a priest, and attended a seminary preparatory school.

As a condition of living in a group home, residents must take medications, if prescribed, and in accepting the job Tim agreed to enforce these rules. Linda Slezak welcomed his skepticism. She herself had seen how disappointing the psychiatrists and their medications could be.

TIM IS A striking presence, a former high school athlete with a handsome, round, boyish face; about five feet, eight inches tall; weighing well over 250 pounds. He looks a little like the Pillsbury Dough Boy, and has a freshness and enthusiasm that would have made him a perfect sidekick to Mickey Rooney in *Boys Town*. "Jasper!" Tim said one day. "We're going to take you to a big man's shop, get you some new clothes. Don't feel bad about it. The clothes will fit you, you'll look great and feel great."

"You wear them, Tim?"

"You bet, Jasper!" said Tim. "You're looking at a twenty-inch neck." Jasper hugged him, and Tim said, "It's OK to be big, feller."

During his first weeks at the house, watching Julie, a couple of things struck Tim. He loved the way she listened to the other residents, advising and helping them. She touched his heart. The other thing Tim was sure of: No one had a clue what was wrong with her. He didn't buy the borderline stuff. And while he didn't have an answer yet, he was noticing things. When her hair was over her face, something major was up. She wouldn't talk to you, just grunt, pacing the house like a caged fawn, trying to find a comfortable spot. She'd sometimes disappear into a bathroom, later emerging composed. Tim had a guess on this: Growing up, the bathroom was probably one of the few places she could hide from her abusive father.

Tim would visit her room, trying to draw her out. She was guarded about discussing herself. He sat on a corner of the bed, and Julie would be as far away as possible, knees up, pillows clenched in front of her legs. Slowly, he picked up leads. Counselors reported that Julie took solitary walks, and when they'd ask where, she'd say Saint Patrick's Church. She said she was praying for her dead younger sister. But when she described her visits to Tim there was almost a surrealistic quality to them. She'd speak about going to be with her dead sister. Tim had a hunch that Julie was having a bizarre fantasy or hallucination, maybe those post-traumatic stress episodes mentioned in her records. He wasn't even sure she was actually visiting the church, and went himself to see what Saint Pat's looked like. It was as Julie described. So she was going inside. But something didn't seem right.

One evening she missed dinner. Tim drove around looking for her. She wasn't at Saint Patrick's. He checked Saint Paul's Episcopal—just up the street from the group home. Saint Paul's has a cemetery. In the past Julie had mentioned visiting her sister's grave. He saw Julie walking among the headstones. "Julie," called Tim, "Julie!" It was like she couldn't hear him. He figured maybe she was having some kind of psychotic episode. She came out of the cemetery and Tim joined her on the curb in front of the church. Her hair was over her face and she was rocking back and forth, crying. After a few minutes, she pulled her hair back and gave Tim a startled look.

"What are you doing here?" she asked.

Tim explained that she'd missed dinner and he was concerned. No one knew where she'd gone.

"I went to pray for my sister," said Julie. "I like going to Saint Pat's."

"But you didn't go," said Tim.

Julie paused for just an instant. "Well, I just needed to walk around," she said. After a while she agreed to go back to the house. As she walked up the stairs, Tim asked if she would like some dinner. They'd saved a dish for her.

"No," said Julie. "I need to rest."

As the weeks passed, she grew more and more depressed.

JULIE WAS TRYING to hide as much as possible. She assumed she was going crazy. She could make no sense of what was happening and it terrified her.

She kept blacking out and figured maybe she had a sleep disorder. A half dozen nights that spring, well past curfew, she would wake and find herself on the stairs of Saint Patrick's Church, looking up at the sky as birds circled overhead. She did not remember dressing, leaving the group home, or arriving at the church. She figured it might be some form of sleepwalking. It was spooky. What happened during the lost time? Had anyone noticed her behaving peculiarly? Waking and realizing it had happened again was the worst. She'd walk back to the house as fast as possible, quietly sneak upstairs, and go to bed, hoping nothing would be said next day.

No one caught on. Julie got used to thinking of this as something queer that happened to her at night, but if she went home and went to sleep everything would be all right in the morning.

A few times at Tuesday meetings counselors asked if anyone was leaving the side door to the house open at night. There was no response. Residents guessed it was Jasper, in his typical sloppy fashion stepping out for a smoke, then forgetting to close up. Tim Cook thought so too. Julie never remembered using the side door. Though she had a vague sense of guilt, she kept quiet.

Tim found bowls of leftover cereal in the sink in the middle of the night and figured it was Jasper.

Julie was losing more and more time to the blackouts. She'd feel light-headed, dizzy, on the verge of fainting, and at times, when she came to, many hours had passed. She had a gynecological exam at a clinic and when she learned it was being done by two male doctors, she felt frantic and blacked out. When it was over, she ran the whole way to her therapist's office, chanting to herself, "Help me, help me, help me." If she didn't talk to herself, she felt she'd lose control, disappear. Keeping her mind racing, she could hold off the blackouts some.

The only person she confided even a little of this to was Dr. Blank. During her regular session on May 22, he told her he was prescribing something for a thought disorder, Trilafon, an antipsychotic. Julie tried not to let him see how devastated she was. She was enormously fond of Dr. Blank. He had been her doctor the first time she was hospitalized, at seventeen. He'd always gone out of his way, taking her for walks around the hospital when no one visited her, leaving her sweet, encouraging notes to help her get through lonely weekends on a locked ward, even coming in a few times on his day off to make sure she was all right. Dr. Blank was very protective and fatherly, the first person in her life she'd ever had the confidence to trust. Now it didn't matter how many nice words he used; he was thinking "schizophrenic." Lifetime sentence.

Julie told no one at the group home. God knows, she didn't have much in life, but one thing that gave her standing at the house was not needing medication. Most residents had to visit the office morning, noon, and night, taking their pills in front of a counselor. They used to call the place Club Med. It was humiliating. She didn't want anyone waking her at nine on Saturday morning telling her to take her meds.

The more people watched her, the worse she got. She couldn't stand losing the little freedom she had.

If she did decide to take the medication, she would do it on her own, telling no one. She filled the prescription, but during a blackout it disappeared.

AT 5:15 ON THURSDAY, May 25, Mike Long, director of North Shore Day Treatment, called the house to speak with Tim. Julie had come to his office extremely upset after her regular session with Dr. Blank. She didn't want to return to the group home. She wasn't making sense. Mike was going to have a counselor drive her back.

Tim called her psychiatrist. Dr. Blank explained that he was seeing more delusional symptoms, was considering changing her diagnosis to schizophrenia, and mentioned the meds. "I told Julie at our Monday session," said Dr. Blank. "She didn't say anything?"

Tim suggested to Dr. Blank that the decision to place her on medication might explain why Julie was so upset. "Is it really essential?" Tim asked. Dr. Blank was quite certain. He assured Tim that Julie was open to it.

Julie had an awful headache. Everything was spinning and dizzy. The blackouts were spreading. It was like she was watching a movie. She'd see a few frames of a person speaking to her, have the screen go black, then suddenly the person would reappear in the middle of a new conversation. She knew she was sitting with Mike Long, waiting to be driven home. She'd see Mike, black out, see him again for a few moments doing something new, black out again. And the craziest thing was, she must have looked somewhat normal from the outside, because Mike was right in the middle of talking to her when she came out of a blackout. She clearly wasn't falling on the floor or flailing about. But she couldn't remember what she'd been saying. She listened intently to him, trying to pick up hints of what they were talking about.

The ride back to the house was like being in a thick dream. She knew the counselor was talking to her, but felt far off and incapable of getting any closer to the action.

JULIE CAME into the house disheveled, her hair in front of her face, her shoulders hunched forward. She paced the rooms. Tim suggested she get herself some dinner, then rest. He went into the office to take care of a few matters and when he came back out, couldn't find her. "Have you seen Julie?" he asked a counselor.

"Yeah, she just left for a walk."

"Aw, shit," said Tim.

About an hour later Julie came to, in Glen Head, the next town over. She could not remember how she got there. She called a friend on the house pay phone. "Everything OK at the house?" Julie asked. It was her way of trying to pick up a hint of whether she'd created a disturbance while she'd been blacked out, without giving away too much. If they said something like, 'Are you joking?' Julie would know it was bad.

"Everything's OK," said the other resident, "except they're worried about you."

The woman drove to pick Julie up and was startled. To the rest of the house, Julie was the rock. They weren't used to seeing her falling apart.

She went right up to her room. Tim could see she was having trouble staying in touch with reality. She repeatedly said, "I'm losing myself, I'm afraid I'm going to disappear." She feared she wouldn't make it through the night and would cut off her face. "You people are trying to make me disappear," she said. She told Tim she'd blacked out on the way to Glen Head—the first time she gave him any indication of that. She wavered about going to the hospital, saying she needed it—"I'm going crazy"—then saying it would be too big a setback. She was terrified of losing control of her life. She was supposed to be done with the hospitals. She didn't want to be one of those people going back over and over again. At times, Tim noticed, she seemed to be struggling with another person. She'd become inaudible, mumble, then later would have bizarre conversations with someone else.

"What's going on inside?" Tim asked. "Are you hearing voices? Seeing things?" Julie was sitting on the bed, her hair down in front of her face, hunched over. She looked like a petrified child. Then, in an instant, she lifted her head, tossed her hair back in a confident, casual way, looked directly at Tim, and said, "No, I'm fine. I'm not hearing voices. I don't want to talk. Leave me alone now, OK? I just want to be left alone. I AM NOT GOING TO THE HOSPITAL!"

A chill went through Tim. Her voice was like a different person's. She looked different—her facial muscles had changed. It was like she was possessed. "OK," said Tim. "I'm going downstairs. You get some rest." He went down to speak to staff and call Dr. Blank. For the first time, he was pretty sure what was wrong with Julie.

"JULIE'S NOT doing well," he told the staff. "We may have a hospitalization on our hands." He didn't want to say more. He closed the office door and consulted the Diagnostic and Statistical Manual of Mental Disorders III, the standard physicians' desk reference that lists all psychiatric disorders and their symptoms. "Holy shit, this is it," he said. The sexual abuse, blackouts, the sudden change in appearance and voice—it all fit. Tim called Dr. Blank to explain how bad Julie was. Dr. Blank recommended hospitalization and Tim agreed, but asked for time so he could talk to Julie and get her to agree to go in voluntarily.

Then Tim said, "This will sound crazy, but have you ever seen a drastic personality shift in Julie?"

"What do you mean?" asked Dr. Blank. Tim could tell immediately, from his voice, that the psychiatrist had seen it too, but he wanted Tim to go first.

"This will sound crazy," said Tim, "but I just had a conversation with Julie and in the middle of it, I had a conversation with someone who wasn't Julie, who was a totally different personality."

"What do you mean, a totally different personality?" asked Dr. Blank.

"The quality of the voice was different," said Tim. "Muscles in her face tightened in a different way. The contours of her expressions were different. The person was belligerent, cocky. Before, she'd sat with hair down, meek. Have you ever seen it?"

There was a pause on the other end, and then Dr. Blank said he thought he'd seen it, too. "To be honest, I've never said anything to anybody else, but I've had my suspicions that something else might be going on," said the doctor. "But now someone else is telling me the same thing."

Tim said he'd met one other person with the same behavior, at a program where he'd once worked. "Maybe it's crazy, but I seemed to see it," Tim said. "It was very bizarre, but may be very real."

"No, there's something there we have to follow up on," said Dr. Blank. "I never said anything before because I thought people would think I was crazy." Tim asked if he'd consider a diagnosis of multiple personality disorder and Dr. Blank said he would.

After their talk, Tim made a note in the group home log: "Dr. Blank feels schizophrenia or personality disorder (multiple personality), may be indicated. Expressed interest in consulting with expert in multiple personality disorders . . . and to see if antipsychotic [medication] reduces delusional symptoms." It appeared to Tim that Julie had more than one personality, like in those books *Sybil* and *Three Faces of Eve*.

IT TOOK A while, but after speaking several times with Tim and with Dr. Blank on the phone, Julie agreed to go to the hospital. Tim arranged with Dr. Blank to make it a voluntary commitment. "Don't worry, they won't 2PC you," he assured Julie. A 2PC is an involuntary hospitalization, ordered by two physicians, that would involve a longer stay. Tim drove them in his 1981 Toyota and Julie was her lively, witty self again. "You're going to be in hot water with the little woman," Julie teased. Tim had missed a dinner date with his fiancée to make the hospital trip. Several times Julie said she felt better and asked if Tim really thought this necessary.

"It'll help us figure out what's going on," Tim said. "Let's check this out."

"You have no idea how confusing this is," said Julie. Tim did not tell her his suspicion—she'd had enough that night. At the hospital, there was a foul-up and they insisted on 2PC-ing her. Tim threatened to write a letter of complaint, but it did no good. At 11:45 P.M. Julie was committed. An emergency room psychiatric intern, reviewing the paperwork, noticed that for diagnosis, Tim had written multiple personality disorder. "Are you a psychiatrist?" she asked.

Julie woke the next morning with an overwhelming sadness. She was back in the same hospital where she'd first been committed as a teenager. It was like she hadn't made a stitch of progress. She did not remember what happened the evening before at the house, the ride to the hospital with Tim, or the admission.

. . .

DR. BLANK MAY have told Tim he saw signs of a multiple personality disorder, but in the hospital he treated Julie as if she were schizophrenic. There is an enormous difference in the way you'd respond to each diagnosis. A personality disorder would rely on long-term, intensive therapy, taking Julie back—often through hypnosis to the childhood brutalities that were the root of her problem. Medication would be unlikely.

On the other hand, for schizophrenics, therapy becomes secondary and centers mainly on ways to cope with the illness. Powerful medication is the primary treatment. Dr. Blank prescribed Julie Trilafon, an antipsychotic, and Tegretol, a medication used to calm people in a manic state.

For four days, Julie refused to take anything. But they had her. She was involuntary, and if she continued to say no she'd never get out. She feared they'd ship her to Pilgrim State.

So she gave in. Finally, she looked like a mental patient. Her hair was scraggly, and she walked around with her head down, shoulders drooping. The meds made her move in slow motion and there wasn't anything she could do about it. All she wanted was sleep. She had no desire to get up, get dressed, eat, or shower. When she was awake, she fantasized about going back to bed. They'd try to get her to do things, rousting her from bed to shoot baskets at a toy hoop they had on the ward. But even in the middle of the day, she felt like it was 3 A.M. and someone was shaking her from a dense sleep.

She was jittery and restless. Dr. Blank prescribed a third drug, Artane, to control the side effects of the other two drugs. Then he went on vacation the first two weeks of June, leaving instructions for an intern to continue the medication. There was no way she could talk her way out of the meds then.

Every few days one of the staff from 9 Highland visited. She complained about the meds to them all. Since being on the medication, she had never been so depressed in her life, she told them. At least before the medication there were days when she felt like she was improving. JoAnn compared taking meds to a diabetic's needing insulin and asked if Julie felt there was anything wrong with that. Another counselor reminded her about the group home rules on meds. Tim told her to just try to hang on. He suggested she give some thought to what was going on with the switching personalities, so she could better explain it to Dr. Blank, but Julie seemed resentful and preoccupied. He didn't push—he didn't know that much about it himself and needed to do more research. Julie had more immediate fears. She was scared the hospitalization would hurt her chances of getting into an apartment.

When house staff visited on June 6, Julie mentioned that she'd been switched to a private room because she was "too crazy to be with other people." She'd told the hospital staff she felt she had killed her dead sister. She received a visit from a priest, which she said helped. Julie believed God was punishing her, but the priest explained otherwise. Julie said she was trying to get something useful out of the hospitalization; in occupational therapy she was making a stool for her stuffed dog. She was worried about being able to come back to the group home. She'd seen other residents hospitalized who didn't return. JoAnn Mendrina assured her that they were saving her bed and that everyone was pulling for her to come home soon. JoAnn had a card for her signed by everyone. Julie hugged the counselors when they left.

The days dragged on in stupefying boredom. She found the bed she'd slept in when she'd been hospitalized the first time, three years before. On the crossbar, an inscription she'd scratched with another patient was still there: *Julie and Janey, bff* (best friends forever). She was seventeen then and everything was an adventure.

They kept her five weeks this time and then discharged her to the group home. She knew she'd be back. She felt like hell.

NOW AT LEAST Tim knew what to look for. His plan was to try to get Julie to manage these crises better, get her to let staff know when an episode was coming on. During one of their talks upstairs in Julie's room, Tim suggested she keep a journal. Julie didn't want to. She'd kept one at the hospital on the borderline unit and it scared her. She felt like she was losing control. She'd find entries she couldn't remember writing. Julie didn't tell Tim, but there were pages filled with nothing but "Di Di Di Di Di" in the large, unsteady letters of a young child.

On July 3, in the middle of the night she got dressed and sneaked out of the group home, walking to Saint Pat's in her slippers. Staff did not catch her, but next day, she at least told her counselor where she'd been. Julie said she'd wanted to light a candle for her dead sister. She woke on the church stairs with an intense fear, rang the church doorbell, but no one answered. The counselor asked if it was possible to warn staff before leaving the house. "I don't know when I'm leaving," said Julie.

Another evening, Julie was missing and Tim drove around looking for her. He found her hanging out at the Glen Head train station. When she spotted Tim she ran. She was fast. Tim followed in his car. She was heading back toward Highland. He found her a block from the house, sitting on the steps at Saint Paul's. He sat beside her. She was quiet, her head down, then started making cooing noises. She sounded just like a baby.

He waited for her to lift her head. "Hi, Julie," he said. "OK, you had another one of your spells."

"How'd I get here?" she asked.

Tim explained. "You seem OK now."

"This is so bizarre," she said. "I can't believe I'm going through this." Tim suggested if she was about to disassociate—switch personalities—she alert staff instead of going into the bathroom. "So we can get control over it," he said. He was worried about strangers taking advantage of her.

She said she'd try, but the next day Julie didn't remember the conversation.

JULIE'S LIFE in these weeks revolved around trying to get off the meds. She complained to everyone she knew in the mental health system, but it didn't make much impression. Everyone in the system hates their meds. The worst thing about it was that the more she complained, the more medication they put her on. She complained to Dr. Blank that the antipsychotic Trilafon made her feel restless, so he prescribed five milligrams daily of Ativan, an antianxiety medication. At another session Julie tried to convince Dr. Blank that the medication was causing her to be more depressed than she's ever been. But he said, "That's a good sign. I think you're getting better." Before, the depression was masked, Dr. Blank explained to Julie; now, thanks to the medication, her true underlying feelings were emerging. It was healthy being depressed, the psychiatrist said; she was supposed to be depressed, her life had been depressing. To improve her mood, he prescribed an antidepressant.

When Dr. Blank spoke in consultations with group home staff, he was adamant about her need to continue the medication. He said the side effects Julie was feeling—constant drowsiness and depression— were short-term until he found a comfortable regimen for her. Since Julie was being so resistant and manipulative, group home counselors needed to remind her this was her best bet for staying out of the hospital. Tim tried pleading Julie's case with the psychiatrist. After speaking with Tim at one point, Dr. Blank did agree to reduce the antipsychotic Trilafon, from thirty-two milligrams a day to twenty-four. Later, Tim learned this was just lip service; they were going to reduce the Trilafon anyway because it wasn't working, then try her on another antipsychotic.

People at day program were startled by how tired and drawn she looked now. Julie had always been so perfectly dressed, so stylishly groomed. Her regular routine had been to rise at 6:30 in order to be on the day program bus at 8:10. She'd shower, blow-dry her hair, do her makeup, fuss over the right clothes; her morning prep was so elaborate there wasn't time for breakfast. Now, on the meds, she barely had the energy to get out of bed fifteen minutes before the bus pulled up. Through enormous willpower, she forced herself to take a shower every other day, though sometimes she was too tired even for that. Her hair was soaking wet, she never had time to blow-dry it or do her makeup. She threw on whatever clothes she saw first. Brushing her teeth seemed like an enormous project. Summing up this period, Julie said, "I looked and felt like shit."

All she wanted to do at her day program was put two chairs together and lie down. Julie Callahan—day treatment president, adviser to fellow group-home residents—was now dozing off in group therapy. "You have to see the medication's making me worse," Julie pleaded with Nan Case, her day treatment therapist. "Have you ever seen me look this bad?" Nan sent her to the day treatment psychiatrist, Dr. Anthony Donatelli, who said Julie was experiencing a rare side effect and it would pass. He prescribed more medication, more Artane, two milligrams daily to control the shaking from the antipsychotic. For a couple of hours she'd believe these guys knew what they were doing. The worst thing was, she knew these were all decent people who cared about her, but they were destroying her.

Only the other patients listened. Day treatment members rallied behind her at a community meeting. A male patient said, "You've got to stand up to them!" Julie felt the guy needed medication more than anybody there. She didn't want to be a cause célèbre. She wanted off the friggin' meds. One evening she was supposed to go to a party with a couple of other women at the house, but all she could do was lie on the couch. At times she'd scream silently into a pillow. Tim stayed late to watch her.

She couldn't tell if Tim was doing anything to help. If he was her friend, how could he watch while they medicated her to death?

TIM HATED what was going on, but had to enforce Dr. Blank's game plan. Tim didn't believe for a moment Julie was schizophrenic, and neither did his boss Linda Slezak. Julie was too quick, too coherent, too verbal for days and weeks at a time. The group home staff saw Julie day in and day out; Dr. Blank saw her at two forty-five-minute sessions a week. Tim had tried talking to Dr. Blank about the multiple personalities several more times, and the psychiatrist would say, "Yeah, I know what you mean." But Tim could see that Blank was taking the safe, conservative approach: Assume the more traditional diagnosis of schizophrenia until shown wrong and medicate accordingly. Tim felt Blank was afraid of going out on a limb with his colleagues at the hospital. While multiple personality disorder had been recognized and described in the medical journals for years, it was still believed to be quite rare. Schizophrenia might be the wrong diagnosis, but it was safer.

Tim realized he was going to have to take the initiative. He spoke to Linda Slezak and she was supportive. He began making calls, starting with Dr. Richard P. Kluft, the Philadelphia psychiatrist who'd written the entry on the disorder in the standard physicians' desk manual. A specialist in Phoenix led Tim to one in California, who led him to another in Seattle. Slowly he gathered academic papers and a list of a dozen experts nationally. In the meantime, Tim monitored Julie carefully. The only other person at the group home he told his suspicions to was his number-two person at the time, Maureen Coley. To those who don't understand, there is a sensational, freakish quality to multiple personalities, and Tim wanted to protect Julie's privacy as much as possible.

The best Tim could say to Julie was, "We've got to give Dr. Blank's plan a chance to work."

Julie grew more withdrawn at the house. One of her goals was to organize recreational activities for other residents, but that was dropped now. On July 13, she reported hearing voices again. Tim talked with her about ways to push the voices out of her head. Julie agreed that if the voices told her to harm herself, she'd let counselors know. Next day she said she felt like running into the street in front of a car.

On Saturday the 15th, counselor Heidi Friedman went up to check on Julie at 1:45 in the afternoon. She was still in bed. "You OK?" asked Heidi.

"No," said Julie.

"Want to talk about it?"

"No," said Julie. "I'll just rest it off."

She spent the entire weekend in bed, not getting dressed. Counselors were speaking to Dr. Blank daily. She was hearing voices telling her not to take her meds and not to comply with treatment. To Tim it was a sign that after nearly two months, the medication was a failure. To Dr. Blank it was a sign she needed it all the more.

On July 18, Dr. Blank called and changed her antidepressant to fifty milligrams of Pamelor at bedtime. He continued the antipsychotic. "Pamelor should work nicely with Trilafon," he said. He told the group home counselor that Julie's thinking had always been psychotic, but now it was really starting to blossom and she had to learn to handle it. "You must remember that this has been going on for years and has recently begun to surface."

Dr. Blank warned the group home that in therapy Julie was speaking about killing herself with a kitchen knife. He recommended keeping her busy and making sure she wasn't alone, so she wouldn't focus on the delusions as much. He was hoping they could avert a hospitalization, but if she needed it again, he said it would most likely be long-term care at Pilgrim State.

When Tim heard that Blank was thinking Pilgrim, he was furious.

Not only was this guy botching the case, he was ready to dump Julie in the shittiest state hospital around, where they'd warehouse her and medicate her into oblivion. Tim checked with Linda Slezak, and she was furious, too. Leave it to the ivory-tower psychiatrists to refer to what went on at Pilgrim State as "long-term *care.*" He called back Blank and argued for referring Julie to their local hospital if necessary. Then he called Glen Cove Hospital and arranged for an emergency bed just in case.

Tim's legwork came none too soon. The next night, at 1:45 A.M. Terry Gaylo heard someone come downstairs. She went into the kitchen and there was Julie, standing with her back to Terry.

"Julie, are you all right?"

Julie turned around and was holding a large kitchen knife. Terry went to her, took it out of her hands, and placed it on the countertop. Julie appeared to be in a trancelike state. Terry asked her to sit down on the living room couch and Julie did. The counselor asked Julie what she had intended to do with the knife. Julie did not respond. She held her head in her hands, gazing downward. Terry asked if she was hearing voices. She was. And? "They are telling me to do things to myself," said Julie.

Hurt yourself? Kill yourself? Terry asked. Yes, both, said Julie. She asked Julie to lie down on the couch. Julie wanted to go back upstairs to her bedroom. Terry persisted, and sat with Julie. She beeped the Melillo supervisor on call. They tried to get the county mobile crisis team to transport Julie to the hospital, but it didn't work nights.

A second counselor was called and arrived at 2:30. They told Julie she would have to go to the hospital immediately.

"Is this a dream?" asked Julie. Terry wanted to know if she remembered what happened in the kitchen. "It was a dream," said Julie. "My hands were numb and the voices told me to cut off my hands and hair."

Terry had Julie get her belongings together and drove her to Glen Cove Hospital.

JULIE WOKE the next day on 3-West with no recollection of the kitchen incident. For the first time, she talked to hospital staff members about what was happening in terms of multiple personalities. This was due partly to Tim's prodding; partly to the work of the group home staff, which had been telling her how different she seemed at times; partly to the realization that whatever she had, it wouldn't just go away; and, partly to the fact that she was beginning to get a little insight and it made more sense—or at least as much sense as anything else. At the entrance screening by Glen Cove Hospital's chief psychiatrist, Dr. Melamed, Julie said she felt like two people and sometimes three, one telling the other to cut her hands off. She explained she had not been able to "control her personalities" and "they have not been nice to me." She said the night before she was two people and felt in a dream.

Dr. Blank responded to a call from the group home and was brought up-to-date. He was still talking schizophrenia. He kept describing her as delusional, the lingo of schizophrenia. Even if Julie was a multiple personality, it didn't mean she wasn't schizophrenic too, Dr. Blank told Tim. One of the personalities must be schizophrenic, he said. Tim had never seen anything about that in the literature. Dr. Blank said that the antipsychotic medication probably hadn't taken effect yet, but should be continued, and Julie would most likely need it long-term.

Tim knew his best hope was Glen Cove Hospital. He arranged a meeting with the hospital staff and gave the 3-West social worker, Howard Rothenberg, the scholarly papers and list of multiple personality experts. Tim made it sound like Dr. Blank was more receptive to a multiple personality diagnosis than he was. The Glen Cove Hospital staff listened without saying much. Tim felt like a visitor from Mars. Hospital people tend to look down on group home staff; treat them like well-intentioned camp counselors. Tim could tell that the Glen Cove chief of psychiatry wasn't convinced yet, but at least he seemed more open-minded. And almost immediately, he read the papers Tim had brought. Dr. Melamed struck Tim as an objective, caring man.

Tim was well ahead of the psychiatrists. He was now trying to help Julie identify personalities. She spoke of hearing three distinct voices.

As best as Tim could piece it together, they were Didi, a young child; Patricia, the dead sister; and Marlena, a cocky, provocative teenager who talked in profanities. It fit with what he had seen at the house. He felt he'd met all three. As it turned out, he didn't have it quite right, but he was on the right track.

That first day Julie called the group home collect from the locked ward's pay phone. She was frightened and had been staying in her hospital bed, except for meals. "I want to come back," she said. She felt trapped and didn't even have change for a phone call. A counselor from the house came during the evening visiting hours, assuring Julie the hospitalization would be short-term and the group home would stick by her. The counselor handed Julie a plain white envelope full of quarters before leaving.

NOW, LESS THAN two years later, Julie was the visitor offering quarters. Stephen DeRosa reached into his pocket and pulled out a fistful. "I have lots, but thank you Julie," he said. They smiled at each other, two veterans of the mental health system who'd learned too many things the hard way.

She told him a little about her new secretary's job. Stephen said she was dressed very professionally. Julie worried she'd worn the wrong shoes to work that day. Maybe her other pair of heels, the black ones, would have looked better. "You think so?" said Stephen. "I'm not sure."

Julie asked how he and Jasper were getting along. "I don't like him for a roommate," said Stephen. "He's quiet, but he smells."

They walked over to the ward's small recreation area, passing room 9 again. "It was my room so long," said Julie, "they were going to name it after me when I left." Julie played Ping-Pong with another visitor while Stephen watched. Even in heels and stockings, she raced around the table, tossing her hair over her shoulder, smashing and slicing the ball, putting spin on shots. She looked like someone in a movie.

Several patients gathered to watch. "She's good," said one.

"Ping-Pong is a mental institution game," said Stephen. Julie had spent months on end sharpening her game during 1989 and 1990. She knew every inch of the Glen Cove Hospital table.

Stephen admired her grace. "I wish I could love Julie," he said, "but she's so skinny." Julie was going out for dessert with a friend afterward. She wanted to know if Stephen could suggest a place. "I don't go out to eat in Glen Cove very much," Stephen said. "I don't like people looking at me." But he did know a new restaurant, Pastas Cafe near Saint Pat's Church. "The desserts are out of this world," said Stephen. "They have marble tables and coffee is $1.50 a cup."

Julie put her arm around him and they walked together to the door. He was old enough to be her father. In her heels she was a head taller. "You'll be out soon," Julie said. Stephen hugged her good-bye. "Take care of yourself, little girl," he said. The aide behind the counter pressed the button, the door buzzed, and Julie walked out. It felt good to be the one leaving.

She ordered two scoops of the gelato at the restaurant, chocolate and pistachio. It was out of this world, smooth and creamy. She knew the place would be great. When it came to the finer things in life, Stephen's judgment was always excellent.

chapter 7

THE MATTER OF
HEATHER MARTINO VERSUS
GLEN COVE HOSPITAL

THAT SPRING of 1991, Maureen Coley felt like she was spending half her time ferrying between the group home and Glen Cove Hospital. In addition to Stephen and Jasper, Heather Martino was up on 3-West. She had been gone from the group home the longest, and at Tuesday meetings, residents asked, "When's Heather coming back?"

Maureen was evasive. She didn't see any hope. Heather had lived at 9 Highland that previous fall, but was so suicidal she kept landing back in the hospital. She'd be released a few days, become suicidal, and get put in again. "She's not doing great," Maureen said, discouraging visits. The group home wasn't planning to hold a bed for her much longer; the hospital staff had informed Melillo that Heather would require long-term institutionalization. Maureen knew what that meant.

Glen Cove Hospital's psychiatrists felt they'd done what they could. They planned to transfer Heather from 3-West to the only long-term facility that would take her, Pilgrim State. "I won't go back to Pilgrim," the thirty-two-year-old Heather kept telling them. "I'll kill myself before I go back." Once before, she had consented to being placed at Pilgrim voluntarily, for five terrible weeks, in the fall of 1990. This time she would fight. To block the transfer, Heather requested a hearing challenging Glen Cove Hospital's decision.

Maureen didn't give her much chance of winning. Nobody did.

Technically, this hearing was about whether Heather should continue to be committed or be released. If Glen Cove Hospital won, Heather would remain under a commitment order and could be transferred to Pilgrim against her will. The screening had already been done; Pilgrim had agreed to accept her.

If Heather won, she could walk out of the hospital, free to live wherever she pleased. In reality, Heather knew she still needed help and would have preferred staying at Glen Cove Hospital, if they'd have her. Or she would be willing to go to a long-term psychiatric hospital where she could get help, and had applied to two private institutions —Columbia Presbyterian and New York Hospital. But she was on Medicaid. Both rejected her. She had no choice but to fight.

ON A MONDAY they informed Heather that the commitment hearing would be that Friday. She found the card of the legal aid attorney assigned to Glen Cove Hospital tacked to the patients' bulletin board and spoke with him a few minutes, then called Dr. Robert Barris. Dr. Barris had been her therapist during the first half of 1990, when she'd been at North Shore University Hospital. She thought he was terrific and had not found anyone who helped her as much on Glen Cove Hospital's 3-West. Dr. Barris made an extra effort, going beyond simply medicating her, helping her probe her past. In fact, even after he was no longer her therapist she'd stayed in touch, calling him a few times a week, at first from the group home and now from the pay phones on 3-West. He was generous with his time, always returned her calls. He knew how much the threat of Pilgrim frightened Heather. For a while, he was the only one she'd told her story of being sexually molested during her first stay at Pilgrim.

That Monday, when Heather asked Dr. Barris to testify for her, he balked. She'd had so many self-destructive relapses, he wasn't sure he wanted to be advocating her release. He'd gone to bat for her before and she'd let him down. "I have to think about it," he answered. On Wednesday he said yes, if she would agree to his conditions. She had to promise that if she was released and felt suicidal she would call for help and go into the hospital voluntarily. In Dr. Barris's experience, Heather did many stupid things, but kept her word.

THURSDAY EVENING, Heather and the patient she was friendliest with on 3-West, Teresa, sat smoking and talking in the lounge, near the fish tank. "I don't have anything to wear to my hearing," Heather said.

Teresa offered a pair of black loafers. They were only a half size too big. "That'd be great," said Heather. All she had were sneakers.

A woman in for drug detox overheard and offered a cranberry sweater with a floral pattern. Another patient, a beautician, promised he'd do her hair. A middle-aged woman from an adult home said a rosary for her each day that week.

People liked Heather. She'd been elected president of the ward council three times. Often she was the patient who led the group therapy sessions. She could be kind to a fault. She was always giving away her Marlboro 100s. People on a psych ward tend to be withdrawn and self-absorbed; Heather took an interest in others.

On the outside, she'd been the same. As manager of a Record World store, she scheduled herself for the least popular shifts. On holidays, she ran a barbecue for her staff in the rear parking lot, though it violated Record World policy. She was unusually well read, with a huge book collection. Her bowling average was 179. She'd also lived some pretty wild times, dating a couple of professional hockey players on the Islanders, and spending a year in Hawaii with a boyfriend. Most people didn't know these things about her; it was not Heather's way to brag. There was a depth to her that people sensed, without knowing the details.

All week fellow patients and even a few of the staff had been quietly wishing her luck. If anyone could beat the hospital, they said, it was Heather.

THE HEARING was a few hours away and she still hadn't discussed the case with her legal aid attorney that week. He'd probably be so overworked he wouldn't be able to distinguish hers from a hundred other commitment hearings.

Steve Minerva of Mental Hygiene Legal Services was buzzed onto 3-West at 9:30 that Friday morning. They talked in Heather's room, number 3. He surprised her. He seemed to know what he was doing. She noticed he'd written a list of questions for the hospital's psychiatrist. He'd consulted with Dr. Barris and knew more about her than Heather expected. Nothing she said seemed to shock Minerva; he made her feel normal.

He was reserved and businesslike, reviewing the questions he planned for her, and several times asking if she'd be able to get through her testimony without crying. Minerva had lost cases because of excessive crying. Judges took it as a bad sign. "It's important," he said. "Crying could ruin it."

"I can do it," she said.

He kept stressing that he really wanted to win, but if it didn't work out, there were several things he could do to get her out of Pilgrim. They spoke for an hour and a half, then Minerva said he needed to review the hospital records. Heather asked what her chances were.

"Pretty good with Dr. Barris testifying," said Minerva.

STEVE MINERVA practiced this kind of law because he cared. That was the reason to do it; it certainly didn't pay well compared to private practice—thirty-two thousand dollars to start. When he crossed his legs you could see the beginning of two holes on the soles of his brown tie shoes. Minerva knew a fair amount about the mental health system from his own experiences. His mother was a therapy aide, an entry-level job, on a state hospital ward. She used to talk about how bad off the patients were. In his early twenties one of his best friends had a breakdown; Minerva remained close with the young man.

The work was interesting, but there wasn't any glory in it. Hearings were private and confidential; no one saw or read about your victories in the newspaper. Clients were often too sick to appreciate you and at times were so paranoid they harangued you for reasons you couldn't even figure out. Minerva was thirty-six, doing this five years—a hearing every week or two, maybe two-hundred of these cases so far—and rarely in that time had a client touched him as Heather did. He believed it when she said she'd kill herself if sent to Pilgrim. He felt an obligation to try to save her. The Glen Cove Hospital doctors seemed to take the attitude that Heather wasn't serious, and a stay at Pilgrim was just what she needed to snap her back to her senses. Minerva couldn't believe they could be so cavalier. He appeared phlegmatic, but all you had to do was watch him for a few minutes in the season ticketholder section at a St. John's University basketball game—his alma mater—and you saw this was a guy who could get very worked up. He used to call the all-sports radio talk shows to give his opinions about what was wrong with the St. John's team.

In his own quiet way he was getting worked up about Heather's case.

He'd met Heather for the first time in early December, the week after she was hospitalized. Under New York law, all newly hospitalized patients must be seen by a mental hygiene lawyer who informs them of their rights. Minerva had visited Glen Cove Hospital every week for five years. During the first few months of Heather's stay, he chatted with her a half dozen times to see how she was progressing.

He didn't have to read very far into her hospital records to see that life had been miserable to Heather. She'd been a human punching bag for a screwed-up family—or as the hospital records put it, "dysfunctional family system." When she was four her father began having sexual intercourse with her. This prompted her first suicide attempt, also at age four. Little Heather swallowed two bottles of St. Joseph's Aspirin for Children. The father continued with her until she was fifteen. The mother's idea of appropriate punishment was locking Heather in the closet for hours at a time or holding her hand to a burner on the gas stove. ("Family abounds in pathologic dyads, triads, splittings," the record noted.) At twelve she began using illegal drugs, starting with marijuana, then cocaine, PCP, barbiturates, amphetamines, and alcohol.

Despite this mess, Minerva found signs in the records that she outwardly managed her life quite well, having graduated high school a year early and thereafter held several responsible jobs. Despite getting no support from her family, she'd gone looking for help.

In February 1983, her mother died, prompting the twenty-four-year-old Heather to enter a monthlong drug detoxification program. Three weeks after being released, Heather was back on cocaine. In July 1983 she attempted suicide by taking an overdose of pills. She was hospitalized two months, detoxified, and never used illegal drugs again. She began private therapy with Dr. John Imhof and was still seeing him eight years later. From 1984 to 1990 she worked for Record World, becoming the manager of a suburban Long Island store that did $1.5 million in sales yearly.

Through most of these years she lived at home with her father. In October 1989 he died, and Heather was hospitalized shortly after for depression at North Shore University Hospital. That was where she'd met Dr. Barris. She attempted suicide again in April 1990 and was kept at North Shore until September, when doctors decided long-term care was necessary. Heather was transferred to Pilgrim State Hospital and spent just five weeks there.

Minerva checked the Pilgrim record closely. The sexual abuse incident Heather had confided to Dr. Barris and to him was not mentioned. On October 31, 1990, she was released from Pilgrim and moved to the Glen Cove group home. During the month at the group home she talked increasingly about suicide and was eventually committed to Glen Cove Hospital. At the time of the hearing in the spring of 1991, she'd been at Glen Cove Hospital four months.

It took Minerva a couple of hours to sift through the folders. He was disappointed. From the point in late January when the hospital staff had decided to transfer her to Pilgrim, almost every entry in Heather's record was negative. He'd seen this too often in these cases. It was hard to know whether they were deliberately building a case for a transfer or their own decision blinded them to Heather's positive points. Steve Minerva wasn't there twenty-four hours a day, but he had seen her several times on the ward these months and had found her to be quite engaging.

HEATHER SHOWERED and dressed. She put on thick black cotton socks so her friend's loafers wouldn't be floppy. The beautician in for detox blow-dried her long hair straight back and out, and Heather put on makeup, which she hadn't bothered with in weeks. She refused her noon meds. She worried that they might do something to them to dope her up for the hearing. This was being paranoid, she knew, but it didn't hurt to play it safe. On her way down the hall, two nurses sitting in the TV room said how pretty she looked. "If looks can do it, you'll win, sweetie," one said.

Minerva was standing in front of the nurses' station. He stared at her a moment extra. She'd done something to herself, her hair or something. She looked good.

"Anything helpful in the records?" Heather asked.

"Nothing much."

"All those records and nothing?"

"Every time there's something good it's followed by something self-destructive," he said.

THE HEAD NURSE on 3-West led Heather down to the hospital's boardroom on the first floor. When Heather walked in, state supreme court justice Gabriel Kohn, dressed in a dark blue business suit, was seated at the head of the long rectangular mahogany table. Behind him was a stenographer, to his right a court clerk. By the door stood an armed court officer. Heather saw Dr. Barris in a chair against the wall and went over to shake his hand and say thanks. A pitcher of water and cups had been placed on the table. She noticed they were glass. It had been a while; on 3-West, for safety's sake, they were plastic. She took a seat to the judge's right beside Minerva. Across the table were the hospital attorney and psychiatrist. There were also a couple of nurses and the ward's social worker. She was surprised by all the people on the hospital's side.

Minerva didn't mention it to Heather, but before she'd come down, the judge had called both attorneys and the psychiatrists into a conference and tried for ten minutes to work out a deal to avoid a hearing. Judge Kohn asked if the hospital would agree to keep Heather on 3-West. The Glen Cove psychiatrists would not budge. Each time they had prepared to discharge her, Heather sabotaged it. They were fed up. They had done everything for her and she was ungrateful. Manipulation was a major part of her disorder and she had to be taught that there were limits.

'' T H I S   I S   T H E matter of Glen Cove Hospital against Heather Martino. Counsel, are we ready?'' asked the clerk.

The hospital's attorney called Dr. Michael Guervich, Heather's psychiatrist on 3-West. In a thick foreign accent at times broken by a stammer, the Russian-born psychiatrist testified as to his credentials: associate director of psychiatry at the hospital with a local private practice; licensed seven years; board certified in psychiatry and neurology.

It was Dr. Guervich's job to convince the judge that Heather needed long-term commitment. He reviewed her recent history, how she had been at the group home just a month when she relapsed and was put in Glen Cove Hospital for a week during Thanksgiving of 1990 because of suicidal thoughts. She seemed better, was released again, but the first day back at the group home she had suicidal feelings and was taken to the hospital emergency room. "She was expressing thoughts that she wants to kill herself by penetrating her heart with a scissors," explained the doctor. Dr. Guervich saw Heather in the emergency room. She was involuntarily committed to 3-West on November 29, 1990, and had been there since.

The doctor spoke directly to the judge, across the table, describing the treatment plan they'd followed. Dr. Guervich was wearing his white coat, and it made Minerva wonder if this was to remind them all that he was the doctor; usually they came in suits to hearings. Dr. Guervich explained that Heather was put on Wellbutrin, a new antidepressant; Klonopin, an antianxiety medication; and a tranquilizer. When the depression didn't lift, they had administered twelve electric shock treatments. She seemed to improve, he said, and they considered releasing her, but then she grew suicidal again. Dr. Guervich said that she had now exhausted the care that the acute patient unit at Glen Cove Hospital could provide.

At the end of January 1991, Dr. Guervich said, "Heather had an out-of-unit pass and asked a friend to go into a suicidal pact in which she and he would kill themselves . . ."

"He's lying," Heather said to her attorney in a voice loud enough to make Dr. Guervich turn his head.

"Be quiet," Minerva hissed at her. "You'll have your chance."

"She requested the same patient to bring her pills to overdose herself on the unit," Dr. Guervich continued. "We found a knife in her room that she took from our kitchen and she described that was her security blanket . . . Also, Heather had scratched her wrist on a number of occasions with her nails."

"Was that a plastic knife?" the judge asked.

"No," said Dr. Guervich.

The judge said, "That was a . . ."

"A real knife."

"Metal substance?"

"Made out of metal," Dr. Guervich answered. "Heather expressed that if she would be transferred to a state hospital, she would definitely find a way to kill herself." He pointed out that her condition was so serious, the hospital frequently put her on one-to-one supervision, with "a nurse all the time next to her."

In response to a standard list of questions, Dr. Guervich said that

Heather was not delusional, hallucinating, hearing voices, or psychotic.

"Can you describe the patient's judgment?"

"It's kind of difficult," said Dr. Guervich. "At one point she may present herself as nice as she is now. And in a day or two she may appear completely despondent."

The doctor was asked to discuss Heather's diagnosis. He felt she had three. Borderline personality disorder. Major depression, severe. "She also has a disassociative disorder."

The judge looked confused. "What?"

"Disassociative disorder."

"What?"

"A patient tends to split among different people," Dr. Guervich said. He felt she had multiple personalities, like Sybil, like Three Faces of Eve, like Julie Callahan, who'd been treated at Glen Cove Hospital, too. Heather was amazed to hear this. No one had ever mentioned it to her; there'd never been any indications, none of the classic symptoms like blackouts or losing time. Dr. Barris, who'd later be testifying for Heather, was caught off guard too, and was shaking his head. Multiple personalities? He'd never seen a hint of it, nor had it ever been mentioned by Dr. Imhof, who'd treated Heather for years. This sense of a good and bad self was actually a classic borderline trait. In trying to explain her feelings to Dr. Guervich, Heather had said there were times she felt like she was split in two, between good and evil. Had he taken it literally? She was never quite sure how much English he understood. The mental health system was full of foreign-born psychiatrists. It was easier for a foreigner to get a job working with the sickest patients in the public and community hospitals. A few times during the hearing, the judge had interrupted Dr. Guervich to summarize parts of his testimony that were unclear or contradictory.

"Heather has what I would call a split personality," Dr. Guervich went on. "One that represents a kind of a devil in her that all the time gives her ill advice . . . Heather described herself that it was a bad part of her ego who was giving her all the time ill advices . . . And the other is the Heather who is kind, nice and trying to improve . . . There is a constant fight between these two egos inside of her. And unfortunately, too often she wins and influences Heather to attempt to kill herself."

"Today this patient is requesting her release from the hospital. Is this patient in need of continued hospitalization?" the hospital attorney asked his witness.

"Yes," said Dr. Guervich. "I would feel at this point if she would be released, she may kill herself in the very near future. I don't feel she at this point is in control of her impulses and I feel this struggle in personality still continues."

"Could Heather function in a less structured setting?"

"I wish I could say yes, but I don't feel she could," said Dr. Guervich. And with that, the hospital rested its case against Heather Martino.

IN CROSS-EXAMINING Dr. Guervich, Steve Minerva's goal was to distinguish between suicide ideation—thoughts and fantasies of suicide—and serious attempts. His feeling was that Heather's only true attempts had followed real tragedies in her life—being raped by her father and later, the deaths of her mother and father. He believed fantasizing about suicide was an intimate part of Heather's life, a practice that had started as the understandable response of a little girl regularly being brutalized. He was worried that Dr. Guervich's testimony left the impression that Heather was on the verge of suicide twenty-four hours a day. He also felt Guervich's diagnosis was way off. He knew the psychiatrist would not be receptive to being challenged. Once they make a diagnosis, Minerva had found, it was hell getting them to blink.

The last time Heather was admitted to the hospital, Minerva asked, was her threat to stab herself verbal only?

"Yes," said Dr. Guervich.

She was not seen with scissors or close to doing this?

"No. But she was telling everybody persistently that she wants to kill herself, and that caused significant anxiety to the staff."

Minerva believed that the only accurate piece of this psychiatrist's diagnosis was borderline personality disorder. One symptom of the borderline disorder is to cut or mutilate yourself without any intent to commit suicide. A person might take a razor and instead of slashing her wrists, cut a "safe" place, like her upper arm or thigh, to create a physical release for the emotional pain she is feeling. The pain from the flesh wound provides temporary diversion and relief from the diffuse and pervasive emotional pain of depression. Heather had a history of this sort of self-mutilation that dated back to age twelve, and it was totally apart from her suicide attempts. Minerva didn't intend to advertise this—who knew how a judge would respond to self-mutilation? But he needed to get Guervich to talk a little about borderline illness.

"Do you mean it's a lifelong condition, or it will continue to be?"

"Probably it will continue to be for quite a significant time," Dr. Guervich answered, "unless she will get specific treatment, and actually she has been getting treatment."

"People can function with this disorder?

"Yes."

"As a member of society?"

"Yes."

"Was Heather on one-to-one observation yesterday?"

"Yesterday," said Dr. Guervich, "we put her on a close-up investigation because it looks like she was doing somewhat better . . . Every-ten-minute observation."

"Doctor, could a person kill themselves in less than ten minutes?" asked Heather's attorney.

"Yes. Sure."

Minerva asked the doctor if he felt she was alert; responsive; oriented to time, place and person; coherent; relevant; taking care of all her personal needs. "Yes," the doctor responded each time. Dr. Guervich acknowleged she hadn't been disruptive on 3-West and had taken her medications willingly.

"Does that indicate to you that she has an insight into her illness?"

"Oh yes," said Dr. Guervich. "I never disputed that."

Minerva was concerned about Dr. Guervich's multiple-personality comments. He felt that the psychiatrist was just piling it on to make sure Heather lost. He asked Dr. Guervich whether Heather spoke of having "evil" inside her or the "devil." Having the devil inside sounded hallucinatory. Which was it? Minerva asked.

"Evil, evil or devil," Dr. Guervich answered.

Minerva was angry. This man was supposed to communicate for a living with troubled people, and Minerva couldn't even follow him. Was he being evasive? Was it a language problem?

Was it the devil? repeated Minerva.

"Evil," said Dr. Guervich.

Now Minerva moved to pick apart each of the suicide incidents. He asked the psychiatrist about Heather's keeping the knife in her room at the hospital.

"Yes, she explained it," said Dr. Guervich. "That was her security in case she's transferred to Pilgrim. And I have to point out, at that time we did not even address yet her transfer to Pilgrim. It was several weeks prior to our even talking about that, when she took this knife and she indicated clearly that she would not go alive to Pilgrim State Hospital."

This was trouble. Was Heather this irrational? Paranoid? Hiding a knife to kill herself for no reason based in reality? Dr. Guervich was making her sound crazy. It could be devastating for her chances. Minerva had discussed it with Heather that morning. "Where did she get this idea she was going to be sent to Pilgrim?" he asked.

"It came about in December," said Dr. Guervich, "while the patient was refusing to have electroconvulsive therapy, and at the time she was extremely depressed and constantly very, very gloomy and we talked about it. We exhausted what we can do with medications and you know, that would be one of our options."

Minerva eased back. It made sense now. They'd been talking to Heather about Pilgrim since the electric shock in December; Pilgrim had been an issue for weeks when she secured the knife. It might not be exemplary behavior, but at least it was rooted in reality. "So you did mention to her back in December that there was a possibility of her being sent to Pilgrim if she didn't take shock treatments?"

"In a way, yes," said Dr. Guervich.

"So how could you state that nothing was ever mentioned about Pilgrim before she took the knife?"

The judge was confused. "Is that what you just said?"

Dr. Guervich said, "No you see, Heather came from Pilgrim State Hospital—"

"Doctor," said Minerva, "I didn't ask you where she came from. This is strictly a question of: Had you or anyone else from this hospital discussed the possibility of Heather going to Pilgrim State before the incident with the knife?"

"At the time," said Dr. Guervich, "the issue was not addressed."

Minerva could not get a straight answer. The man was making Heather look a mess and confusing the judge. He wasn't making sense. Minerva asked that the hospital records be checked. Dr. Guervich didn't have the back records in the hearing room and warned that it might take time. "That's all right," said Minerva.

According to the charts, the shock treatments were in December 1990; a nurse observed the knife in Heather's room on January 26, 1991. (On top of this, group home records indicated that Dr. Guervich had again discussed Pilgrim with her on January 24, two days before she took the knife.)

"Didn't you state, Doctor, that one of the ways that you got Heather to accept the shock therapy was to say that if she didn't, she'd be sent to Pilgrim?"

"No," said Dr. Guervich, "what I said to her is that we will have no other choice."

"So the issue was raised that she was possibly going to be transferred to Pilgrim before the incident of January 26 with the knife?"

"No," said Dr. Guervich. Minerva was pissed. His experience in these cases was that the psychiatrists usually testified in a straightforward manner, and left it to the judge to decide the outcome.

Watching them, Heather felt vindicated—they saw what she went through with this doctor all the time. She didn't think she'd win this hearing. She'd never heard of beating a hospital. She realized she'd done enough foolish, harmful things to herself to sink her chances. But it made her furious that this doctor seemed intent on making her sound worse than she was.

"Excuse me," said Minerva. "This is totally unresponsive."

"Let me see if I can help," said the judge, interrupting. And in a few sentences he summed it up, pointing out that Heather clearly had been made aware of the possibility of a transfer to Pilgrim long before hiding the knife, and so she was understandably fearful about the potential switch. "It was real," said the judge. "She was dealing with reality."

"Right," said Dr. Guervich.

MINERVA ASKED Dr. Guervich about Heather's attempt to get another patient to bring her in pills.

"She actually denied that she had asked," said the psychiatrist.

"How about the scratches on her arm?"

"She in a way admitted that it was done to relieve her tensions." Dr. Guervich kept calling them scratches on her "wrist," but when Heather showed the judge, the scratches were several inches above the wrist on the forearm. (Heather had told no one, and they never found out, but she had made the most recent scratches with an earring post, methodically digging the post backward and forward across her forearm.)

"Doctor, do you consider Heather's scratching of her forearms a suicidal gesture?" asked Minerva.

"Yes I do."

"You thought Heather could kill herself by scratching her arms?"

"No. She has a persistent suicidal thought."

"How deep are these scratches?"

"They are superficial."

"Superficial scratches on the forearm indicate an attempted suicide?"

"She wanted to kill herself; however there is no instrument around to do it," said Dr. Guervich. His answer flew in the face of mainstream psychiatry, which would have interpreted the scratches as mild self-mutilation by a borderline personality, rather than suicidal. Heather was fascinated. Did this man who was supposed to be treating her know the difference between self-mutilation and suicide?

Minerva pounced. He'd been on 3-West so often, he knew the ward as well as the psychiatrist, maybe better. "OK," he said. "Does Heather sleep in a bedroom?"

"She does."

"Do those bedrooms have lamps?"

"They have a lamp on the ceiling," said Dr. Guervich.

"And is there a light bulb in those lights?"

"Yes sir."

"Could she not have broken one of those?" asked Minerva. The hospital's attorney objected that the question was hypothetical and Minerva shot back, "He's not being responsive. I asked him if he considered scratching an arm as an indication of someone trying to kill themselves and he said yes."

In a gentle way the judge hinted that he sympathized. "Well," said Judge Kohn, "I think the difficulty is that sometimes when a professional gives an answer or attempts to give an answer, it doesn't come as directly as we might or you might like it . . ."

MINERVA ASKED the professional what sort of long-term care Heather needed now.

"We made an application to several long-term hospitals, but unfortunately, we were unsuccessful," said Dr. Guervich, "and that's why as a last resort we applied for transfer to Pilgrim State."

"And you feel that an institution such as Pilgrim will meet her needs?"

"Well," said Dr. Guervich, "that's the best of what we can do under the circumstances." As much as Dr. Guervich wanted Heather off 3-

West, he could not say Pilgrim was satisfactory. "I'm very skeptical if Heather will be able to really stay alive if she would leave the hospital."

"Doctor, is it true that Heather's suicidal ideations are a chronic condition?"

"Yes."

"And when did they first manifest themselves?"

At the age of four.

"How old is Heather now?"

She was thirty-two. "She's still alive," said Minerva. "Haven't there been long periods of time where Heather has functioned outside of a hospital setting?"

"Yes."

"In fact, seven years, from 1983 to 1990."

"Right."

"And didn't both hospitalizations in 1983 and 1990 follow the death of first her mother and then her father?"

"That's true," said Dr. Guervich.

"She was able to survive on the outside after recovering from the first hospitalization after the death of the first parent?"

"Right."

"She had an opportunity to kill herself all during that time, didn't she?"

"Yes."

The legal aid attorney had one more point to make before he finished with the psychiatrist: Heather and Dr. Guervich did not get along. Heather had felt in their sessions that his primary concern was medicating her or administering electric shock. He seemed to have no interest in probing the sexual and physical abuse that Heather believed were at the core of her problem. At best he would discuss day-to-day coping, and even that was limited. Heather wasn't alone in this perception. Other patients on 3-West believed it was no coincidence that a Russian-born psychiatrist who had some problem communicating would focus on the biological model of mental illness rather than "talk therapy." The Soviet system where Dr. Guervich had first trained relied almost totally on the biological approach. It was a more authoritarian system than the American psychiatric model. The Russian psychiatrist was truly the boss. Minerva figured it must be killing Dr. Guervich to be challenged at a hearing like this based on the testimony of a mental patient with a history of manipulating those around her. Heather, the intelligent, manipulative patient seeking insight, was the worst possible match for an aloof, authoritarian, prescription-toting physician.

In his answers, which were quite candid, Dr. Guervich unwittingly exposed one of the glaring weaknesses of the mental health system. There is no hospital setting where a person like Heather can get the treatment she needs. For long-term care only two options exist: a private, specialized psychiatric hospital which requires private health insurance and is inaccessible to most people; or a state asylum like Pilgrim, which is really a brick warehouse with cockroaches. (One of the most basic complaints about places like Pilgrim was that virtually no one-on-one therapy went on. During her five-week stay there, Heather had to make special requests to see a psychologist, and then got two 15-minute sessions with the man.) With one hospital unattainable, the other undesirable, most people rely on their local private community hospital's psychiatric ward. Because these not-for-profit, community hospitals accepted government aid, the state mental health commissioner, Dr. Surles, had been able to pressure them into taking Medicaid patients beginning in the late 1980's—an important victory.

Still, these community hospital units vary greatly in quality. Glen Cove's is probably above average on Long Island. The group home staff felt it was better than several of the other hospitals their residents were sent to. Minerva felt so, too. Even so, the hospital's goal is to quickly stabilize people through medication and get them out the door.

Dr. Guervich testified that a short-term hospital like Glen Cove couldn't go into any serious psychotherapy. So he focused on the one part of her illness that might benefit from medication. "Major depression is a biological condition and it was treated with medications."

"But treating the biological factors will not enable Heather to overcome her problem, will it?" said Minerva.

"No, I cannot help her," said Dr. Guervich. "As you point out, one of the things that she was suffering from was her childhood sexual and physical abuse."

"So why won't you make that a major topic of your discussion with her?" asked Minerva.

"Well," answered the psychiatrist, "that's not something to consider that I would be able to help her with during her hospitalization."

"Why not?"

"Because it's an issue that has to be addressed in a long-term psychotherapeutic relationship," said Dr. Guervich. "My goal was when Heather was admitted to our short-term psychiatric unit to help her mostly with . . . psychotropic medications."

In a logical world you would think that while she was in a safe environment like Glen Cove Hospital for four months, the staff would permit Heather's therapist—who had known her eight years and *could* address these crucial issues—to provide primary treatment for Heather. Hadn't the hospital psychiatrist said that such therapy was necessary and that he was unable to provide it? Judge Kohn grasped this and asked if something might be worked out. If Heather were to stay at Glen Cove Hospital, would Dr. Guervich see any disadvantage for her to have sessions with either of the two therapists who knew her history best, Dr. Imhof and Dr. Barris?

"Not at all," Dr. Guervich told the judge.

Hospital policy permitted that? asked the judge.

Dr. Guervich quickly retreated. "That is not a usual practice that somebody from another hospital would come see the patient," said Dr. Guervich. "In Heather's case I would be very, very cautious. . . ." The answer was no.

The judge took one more shot at compromise. How about returning her to the group home?

"At this point," said Dr. Guervich, "We feel that she could not function there."

．　　　．　　　．

STEVE MINERVA called Dr. Barris. Heather was pinning everything on him. So was Minerva. Typically, it was hell getting a psychiatrist to cooperate as an expert witness for the patient in one of these hearings. They wouldn't return phone calls, and when you finally reached them, they couldn't wait to get off. Dr. Barris had spoken with Minerva three times, a half hour each call. The doctor had worked hard at making Heather's problems understandable to the lawyer. A lot of these doctors got eight hundred to a thousand dollars to testify at a hearing. Though he never mentioned it to Heather, Dr. Barris had waived any fee—a rarity. Among the mental hygiene lawyers, Dr. Barris was known as a person who was genuinely concerned about patients, which made him stick out.

He explained that he agreed with only one of Dr. Guervich's diagnoses, borderline personality disorder. He made it clear to the judge that neither he nor Heather's longtime therapist, Dr. Imhof, believed the multiple personality disorder Dr. Guervich spoke of had any basis at all. "Because of her history of abuse, she has a very low self-esteem and a self-destructive component that's at odds with a desire to succeed in life," Dr. Barris said. "And there have been unstable periods in her life, but she does not have a split personality disorder."

It frightened Heather listening to them. Here were two psychiatrists with completely different conclusions about her.

Dr. Barris also disputed Dr. Guervich's claim that Heather suffered from major depression. Major depression has a very high response rate to either medication or electric shock. Dr. Guervich's reliance on a biological approach was a mistake in this case, Dr. Barris said. "My focus would have been on the incest and how that contributed to her depression, and I'm quite surprised in his testimony that Dr. Guervich never mentioned that Heather alleged she was sexually abused by other patients at Pilgrim."

The hospital attorney interrupted: "Objection. That's classic hearsay."

The judge wanted to hear it. "It's such a part and parcel of what is going on," Judge Kohn said, "I have to know about it."

"What happened at Pilgrim the last time had devastating psychological consequences," said Dr. Barris, "and I question whether this issue of the sexual abuse at the hands of several female peers at Pilgrim was [addressed sufficiently by Dr. Guervich]. It's no wonder she remains depressed and despondent. I do believe some of the improvement that she has shown of late is because she was able to reveal this information and begin to talk about it with myself and with Dr. Imhof. In fact I did pay a visit to this hospital approximately two weeks ago to meet with Heather in person, where she was able to tell me some of the gory details."

This is what Heather had told Dr. Barris: It was about nine at night, the meds had been distributed, and the Pilgrim aides in Building 22A had called for lights out. She was standing beside her bed undressing in the dark and was down to her bra and panties when a group of women surrounded her. They pulled her to the ground, stripped her, a couple held down her legs, and the rest began touching her all over, fondling her breasts, pinching her lightly, kissing, licking, whispering, "Does that feel good? Do you like that?" She was too shocked to move, too shocked to scream; she just felt numb, like she was hovering above them while they did this to her body. She wasn't terrified, because her father had done worse and she had survived. She lay passively until they stopped. They warned that if she told, she'd be hurt. When they left, she stayed on the floor, lying still in the dark for what seemed like a half hour before getting up.

Dr. Barris had asked Heather if she'd reported the incident. No, she said. She was a week away from getting out of Pilgrim at the time and feared that if she said anything it would only delay her departure. Leaving Pilgrim had been more important.

Dr. Barris noted that Heather had been showing enough improvement at Glen Cove Hospital so that a few weeks before this hearing, Dr. Guervich spoke of discharging her.

"Are you aware of why Dr. Guervich changed his mind on discharging her?" asked Minerva.

"Yes I am. There were some superficial scratches to the forearm that were several days old that were subsequently discovered ... These were clearly not in a dangerous location ... It doesn't take a rocket scientist to know this is not the place where one injures oneself to hurt oneself seriously. Patients know that the risk is the place where the major vessels run, and typically in borderline personality disorder, cutting, scratching, burning themselves with lit cigarettes, etc., are part of the disease, but this is very very different in its nature than suicidality ... The scratches were more of an attempt to put into physical feeling the psychotic pain that she was feeling, and it's completely different than suicidality."

"Is Heather a danger to herself?"

"I believe at this point she is not a serious danger to herself," said Dr. Barris. "She is chronically depressed. There are enormous issues yet to be solved with her being sexually abused at the hands of her father and how the events at Pilgrim impacted upon this."

Were the problems with the knife related to the threat to send her to Pilgrim?

"Yes," said Dr. Barris.

"You characterize Heather as being chronically depressed," said Minerva. "Can someone chronically depressed be treated on an outpatient basis?"

"Certainly," said Dr. Barris. "She did so between 1983 and 1990."

"And what would be the psychological ramifications if Heather were transferred to Pilgrim?"

"Devastating," said Dr. Barris.

Again the Glen Cove hospital attorney moved to have the comments struck. Again the judge overruled him.

"You stated that Heather has expressed to you she was physically and sexually abused at Pilgrim. What effect would that have on her behavior?"

"She told me that it opened up several old wounds of the incest," Dr. Barris said. "I'd like to state that in my conversation with Dr. Guervich I asked his thoughts about the ramifications of the alleged occurrence which I believe to have happened ... Dr. Guervich told me he had great doubt whether it's truthful and whether the patient was fabricating the story, whether she was using that as some manipulative ploy. And I feel that approach would shortchange a patient. It certainly didn't lead to productive dialogue between the two of them to assist her in working through this enormous tragic event."

"Doctor, can you give us your expert opinion, based on a reasonable degree of medical certainty, as to whether Heather can be discharged?"

"I think she can be," Dr. Barris said.

The judge had one psychiatrist telling him that Heather suffered major biological depression, multiple personalities, borderline disorder, and was in danger of killing herself any minute. He had another saying borderline with a less severe, chronic depression, and not suicidal. "Are there tests by which you professionals can determine whether a patient in fact suffers a depression which is biological in nature?" Judge Kohn asked.

"A good question," said Dr. Barris, "but a very complicated question in which there is a lot of research going on." He described some of the scientific efforts.

Are there any tests? repeated the judge.

"Unfortunately, no," said Dr. Barris. "In psychiatry, I guess what makes it so difficult—most of it is by observation."

DURING REBUTTAL, the hospital's attorney asked Dr. Barris how, given Heather's self-destructiveness, she could possibly be discharged.

"Suicidality is not black-and-white, it's a gray zone," Dr. Barris answered. "There are patients who tell you, 'If I leave the hospital I am definitely going to kill myself.' Heather Martino is not in that condition. She is rather chronically depressed and sometimes wishing she were never born."

The hospital's lawyer called Dr. Guervich again, to get his opinion of the Pilgrim incident she had attached such importance to.

"A very controversial issue," said Dr. Guervich. "It came quite late, after we finally began talking about her transfer to Pilgrim State, and only at that time did Heather suddenly come out with this story about Pilgrim State . . . And Heather initially told one story and then she changed. And just now from Dr. Barris I have heard another change of this story, because at this time he indicated that Heather told him she was abused by females on the unit. Before, it was males. At one point it was one male and then it was a group of patients, so that's where my skepticism comes in, because this story keeps changing.

"If this sexual abuse really occurred at Pilgrim State, how come Heather never informed anybody at the hospital?" Dr. Guervich continued. "How come she never mentioned it? That's an enormously important issue. How come she never mentioned it during her five weeks of talking with Dr. Imhof or talking with the staff who are on the treatment program? And how come she never talked about this in the two months of hospitalization? It was something that was developing, OK?" Dr. Guervich believed she was making it up as she went along.

"No further questions," said the hospital attorney. Heather felt rage. Dr. Guervich, she'd say later, had never questioned her directly about it, and now he claimed there were three versions? How would he know? To Heather it showed how little he cared about her, that he was ready to send her to this place without even talking to her about it.

Dr. Barris was asked why he felt Heather had not said anything sooner. "If there's anything that Heather's to be found fault with, it's in delay of sharing this information, but I think it's common, it's classical in people who have been raped or sexually abused to feel humiliated, guilty, worthless. I believe many rape victims never share the information, never go to the police because it's such a devastating and humiliating event. It's unfortunate when she did finally come out with it, it wasn't worked on in a more vigorous way."

Heather had a history of burying these things. The first time she told anyone she'd been sexually abused as a child was in December

1989, when she revealed it to her therapist, Dr. Imhof. That was two months after her father's death and twenty-six years after it first happened.

THREE HOURS into the hearing Heather was called by Minerva. She stood up at her seat briefly to be sworn in. Asked her address, she gave 9 Highland. Her attorney led her through a number of routine questions which she handled easily. She was aware of the judge watching her.

"Tell us what your education background is."

"I finished high school in three years."

"Your employment background?"

"I worked in retail—with the exception of the past year—for the last twelve years, including five years at Record World as assistant manager and managing million-dollar stores."

"Will you tell us why we are here in court today?"

"To determine whether or not I should be released from the hospital."

She told them that if released, she'd live with her older brother and his wife, continue seeing her therapists, take her medication, and live off Social Security disability until she got a job—which she hoped would be soon.

Minerva asked if she'd benefited from Glen Cove Hospital.

"Somewhat. Yes."

In what way?

"Through my interaction with several staff members as well as other patients," Heather said. "I have felt more confidence in myself, particularly in the last month or so. My self-esteem has improved somewhat and I believe that I'm a good person, and that has altered from the fact that I thought I was a totally bad person before."

"Have you benefited from therapy with Dr. Guervich?"

"No," said Heather.

"No?"

"No."

"How about with Dr. Barris and Dr. Imhof?"

"I've benefited from therapy with both."

"Would you tell us what happened that you didn't get discharged?"

"I went up to one of the nurses," Heather said, "and expressed that I was having suicidal ideations, which is definitely different from being actively suicidal."

"Do you have any present desire or plans to physically harm yourself?"

"No, I don't," said Heather.

Her attorney questioned Heather about the knife found in her room, the friend she'd asked to get her pills, and the scratches on her arms.

"I'd like to straighten out something," Heather said. "The incident where I took the knife occurred, I believe, three or four days . . . after the discussion of long-term hospitalization was first broached . . . I was informed that they would be trying Westchester as well as the Psychiatric Institute, then Pilgrim was going to be the last resort. So I took the knife as insurance. If I had to go back to Pilgrim, I would have rather killed myself.

"I did ask another patient to buy me pills for the same reason. I denied asking this patient that because I thought that would only help them send me to Pilgrim.

"As far as the scratches on my arms, I scratched myself once in the presence of some nurses, which left absolutely no marks. And this past occasion, which left several superficial marks on my arm and to me indicated more of a self-sabotage routine than any suicidal gesture."

"Is there anything else you'd like to tell the judge?" asked Minerva.

"The type of therapy I benefit most from is psychotherapy. We discuss issues of relevance about your past and your present, and that's the type of therapy that I receive from both Dr. Imhof and Dr. Barris. That's particularly why I have made many strides . . . I think it would be most beneficial for me to continue that therapy rather than go back to a place like Pilgrim where no therapy is offered, and where you're just handled as an animal and you either get better on your own or you don't get better at all. They don't particularly care what happens.

"Dr. Guervich said there were three versions of the incident at Pilgrim. There was, in fact, only one. I always stated it was by females. I never said it was by males, and that's really all I have to say."

JUDGE KOHN went out of his way to say something kindly to Heather. "I want the record to indicate that as far as her appearance here today is concerned, she impresses the Court as an alert individual who is in control of herself and the surroundings to the extent that any person is in control. Maybe to say it another way: I detect nothing about her to indicate that she has the problems to which the doctors have testified. If I would have walked into this room not knowing what the purpose of my visit was, and she was here, I would never know."

The judge had a few final questions. Clearly, he had no intention of letting Heather go live with her brother, as she'd suggested. This was the same brother who Heather said she'd never gotten along with in the past and had rarely visited while she was hospitalized. Both the brother and his second wife worked during the day and would not be on hand if Heather had a crisis.

Heather knew her brother's wasn't a great place for her. She didn't really plan to stay there long. They always argued—he could be such a bully. She'd met his second wife once, for a half hour. It was just an address to give so she could get out of the hospital. Then she'd find a place, fast.

The judge saw through it.

Judge Kohn wondered whether Heather would call for help if she became suicidal. He got two opinions.

"She answered that in her testimony, and I agree with her," said Dr. Barris. "I think that she would have the capacity to pick up the phone and call myself or Dr. Imhof before acting in any impulsive, self-injurious way." He talked about the trust Heather had for him and

Dr. Imhof. "At this time she has lack of trust in Dr. Guervich. She has poor communication with Dr. Guervich."

Dr. Guervich reminded the judge that while Heather was at North Shore Hospital under Dr. Barris's sensitive, expert care in the spring of 1990, she'd gone home on a pass, collected her dead father's heart medication, brought it back to the hospital, and swallowed two fist-fuls. "Dr. Barris of course can remember quite well that while staying at the North Shore University Hospital . . . she has been feeling much better and has a therapeutic session with Dr. Barris five times a week for forty-five minutes, talking about all the issues of sexual abuse." To a psychiatrist like Dr. Guervich, Dr. Barris had caved in to the manipulative ways of a borderline patient, giving Heather far too much attention. "And she still took all these pills and had a little suicidal overdose which required about a week's treatment in the intensive care unit . . . All their treatment . . . all their psychotherapy had failed."

THE JUDGE was set. "Anybody else?"

Heather whispered to her attorney. "OK," Minerva said. "She would like to be heard."

"Sure," said Judge Kohn.

"I made four suicide attempts in the past. The last two were quite serious. The one that Dr. Guervich is talking about resulted in a day's stay in intensive care, not a week's stay.

"I also would like to point out that each attempt I made, I contacted someone about it, so therefore I sought help in terms of seeking to preserve my life, as well as—"

"Did you contact somebody before or after?" asked the judge.

"Immediately after I had done it," said Heather, "and also this hospital does not intend to retain me here, they intend to transfer me to Pilgrim, in which case I cannot see either one of my therapists, and where I will receive no therapy." She wanted to say so much, she wanted to jump up and tell the judge that this whole thing was an outrage, but she held on.

There was silence. "Anybody else?" the judge asked. "Everybody rests? I just need a couple of minutes. I wish everybody would stay put."

THEY STOOD and stretched, waiting for his return. Heather was dying to smoke, but didn't. No one else lit up. She asked Minerva what he thought.

"We'll see," he said.

Judge Kohn took his seat and began, occasionally glancing down at a standard form on the table. "This is a civil hearing to determine the need for involuntary hospitalization of the patient, Heather Martino, pursuant to section 9.12, 9.31, 9.33, and other pertinent sections of the mental hygiene law of this state . . . In this case the Court finds that the petitioner hospital has proved the following by clear and convincing evidence:

"That the patient Heather Martino has a mental illness; that the care and treatment for the mental illness in a hospital is essential for the patient's welfare; that the hospitalization provides treatment in the least restrictive setting possible; that the relatives of the patient are not able to properly care for the patient . . . "

So that was it. She was screwed. It felt terrible, but she would not react. She remembered what Minerva had said about crying. She'd get through it; she'd been through much worse with her father.

". . . I further find, and it has been proved by clear and convincing evidence, that the patient's judgment is so impaired that she is unable to understand a need for continued care. She believes that she is ready to be released . . ."

A four-and-a-half-hour hearing, and she clearly hadn't made a dent in this judge. He'd believed Guervich. What a world. That numb feeling was settling over her.

". . . And further that the patient does pose a substantial threat of harm to herself. On that basis the Court grants the hospital's petition to retain the patient for up to sixty days and denies the patient's petition for immediate release . . ."

In his mind, Minerva was preparing one last argument to sway the judge.

"... And I thank all of you for cooperating and I do wish for the patient a speedy recovery and wish to say that these are not easy decisions to be made by Courts or anyone."

Judge Kohn seemed done, but wasn't. He was opening his mouth again. She couldn't imagine what else they could do to her.

"I want to add to the decision that I also find that there is proof in this case which comes from both the hospital and the patient's attorney that it would be in the best interest of the patient to remain at this hospital."

It took a moment for Heather to absorb. And then she smiled. To remain at THIS hospital? Glen Cove Hospital?

"And so," continued Judge Kohn, "I am going to direct that she remain here during the period of up to sixty days. And what that means to her is: she will not be transferred without another hearing or without another court order."

My God, she felt like Solomon had spoken. She wasn't going to Pilgrim. It was what she'd wanted from the beginning, to stay at Glen Cove, get more help, and get out when she was stronger. She could not believe it. She'd won. "Thank you," said Heather, "thank you, thank you."

The hospital attorney was caught off guard. The judge had conceded him every last legal point, but had given this Heather Martino person the victory. "Your honor, can I make a statement for the record?" said the attorney. He told the judge this contradicted the case law precedents; he held a five-minute off-the-record discussion with the judge; he said he would appeal.

But Judge Kohn was firm. "In explaining the incident involving her obtaining of a knife, she said herself under oath, very clearly that she did that ... so that she could kill herself if she was transferred to Pilgrim State because she would rather not live than be there, and I think that's quite an accurate statement ... It leaves the court in a very difficult position but with a very, very definite feeling from the proof in this case.

"What I want is for the patient to have every opportunity as a human being to prove to herself and those around her and to the Court that absent the fear of transfer to Pilgrim looming over her head, she can return to a quality of life and behavior which will satisfy the professionals in this case that she's competent to go out and live in a . . . less restrictive setting."

"Thank you very much," Heather kept saying. She would take his words to heart.

"That is the decision of the Court and the reason for it and I thank everybody for cooperating."

Heather could not stop smiling. Minerva shook her hand—effusive for him. The nurse led her upstairs to 3-West and the patients crowded around, hugging and kissing and slapping her on the back of her borrowed sweater. She was shaking so much, she asked for her 6 P.M. Thorazine.

HEADING HOME to Commack, Long Island, in his 1986 Buick, Minerva felt great. Alone, finally he tasted the victory. The hearing had seemed like a matter of life and death and it was a relief to have it off his shoulders. It reminded him of a Jets game in 1982, when Richard Todd led the New York team to a last-minute upset win over the Miami Dolphins.

Rush-hour traffic Friday evening eastbound on the Northern State Parkway was bumper-to-bumper, but he barely noticed. Never had a case given him so much satisfaction. When he got home he told his mother that he'd won his hearing, and when his girlfriend came over later he told her, but he didn't go into detail. It was too hard to explain why it had seemed so important.

A FEW WEEKS later Heather left Glen Cove Hospital and moved back to 9 Highland. She seemed so much better. Maureen regarded the commitment hearing as a turning point. It forced Heather to fight for herself. It made Heather admit that she did care about living. "I have a good feeling about Heather this time," Maureen said at the weekly Tuesday staff meeting. "I used to just dread dealing with her. She's motivated now."

Heather wasn't pleased about returning. She didn't like living with all these people with serious problems—Jasper alone spooked the hell out of her and grossed her out—or submitting to all the rules, often enforced by counselors ten years her junior. The only reason she'd come back was that the hospital had insisted on a supervised setting and she had no alternative yet. But she did have a secret plan.

ONE WEEK LATER Heather moved out. A guy she had met at Glen Cove Hospital who worked at a deli, Larry, had a basement apartment in East Meadow.

While they were together on 3-West they'd quietly agreed to share it. She'd only known him two weeks, but she liked Larry. He seemed sweet and quiet and was nice looking.

Linda Slezak was handling the emergency beeper for Melillo that Friday night. She hurried over to 9 Highland and tried to convince Heather this wasn't the right way to leave the group home. Heather would not be swayed. As a last resort, Linda reminded Heather that they would hold her bed at least two weeks, in case she changed her mind. She didn't want Heather feeling stuck if it didn't work out. She wanted her to have a way back, to understand that leaving was not burning a bridge, that the group home was a safe haven. They had a month's worth of Heather's medication at the house, but Linda would give her enough for only a few days; she was concerned about Heather becoming suicidal, plus the meds would give Heather an incentive to stay in touch.

A little after six Larry was released from 3-West, and by seven he'd arrived at the group home in a taxi, to take Heather away. He hoisted her two large suitcases in the trunk and they were gone.

On Saturday evening, while Larry went out to a deli to get them supper, Heather repacked her suitcases and sat on the couch in the basement apartment waiting for his return. "I don't think I'm ready to live with you," she told him when he walked in with the sandwiches. "The temptation to have sex outside of marriage would be really increased, and I can't do that and it isn't fair to our relationship to have you support me. Would you mind taking me back?"

On Sunday afternoon Linda Slezak was beeped by Donna Rubin, the counselor on duty at 9 Highland. "Heather's back," said Donna.

"How is she?" asked Linda.

"She seems in a great mood."

HEATHER SETTLED into the group home routine. She laid out her stuffed bears and dogs in the room, along with her books—history, mysteries, psychology (*The Courage to Heal, Silently Seduced*)—and her dozens of shampoos and conditioners. Her hair was the one area where Heather really spoiled herself. She wore it long, halfway down her back, and loved trying out new products. She had received a small inheritance when her father died and had more pocket money than most at the house. She usually kept a case of her own Coke Classic or Snapple iced tea in her bedroom.

"I guess I'm here for a little while," she told her primary counselor, Paula Marsters. "I really want to put my life back together. It's amazing how hard it is."

She developed a friendship with Richard, a man in his mid-twenties who'd grown up in Glen Cove and moved into the house a few weeks before Heather's return. The weather was getting nice—it would be one of the hottest springs in years—and they liked sitting in the white plastic lawn chairs in front of the house, smoking and talking.

She began speaking up at the Tuesday community meetings, a sure sign of feeling more at home. "Next time we do a shopping," said Heather, "could we get chicken cutlets?"

"From time to time we can," said JoAnn Mendrina. "They're a little expensive, but an occasional splurge is all right."

"How about veal?" asked Richard.

"No, no veal," said JoAnn.

There always seemed to be one person in the house who had the nerve to raise the complaints that everyone else was thinking, and Heather became that person. "Two rooms smell bad," she said one Tuesday meeting in May. "Jasper's, and Fred and Richard's."

"Fred, how often are you showering?" asked Maureen.

"Twice a week."

"Fred!" said Maureen.

"I only have one towel," said Fred. Maureen rolled her eyes; Fred's parents would have given him a thousand towels if he cared.

"I know this isn't pleasant," said Maureen. "But I think Heather has a point here."

"I'm not mad," said Fred.

"That's life," said Jasper.

IT TOOK MOST of the month, but Heather finally got her car back. It had been repossessed during the year and a half she was hospitalized; she'd fallen three payments behind. Her therapist, John Imhof, was a big help with this. He called the car dealer and persuaded him to cut the storage fee from fourteen hundred dollars to seven hundred. Dr. Imhof went to the bank and had all the money orders made out for Heather. He paid for her to take taxis until the car was ready, on the condition that she'd repay him when she was working again. This was hardly the usual role of a therapist, but Dr. Imhof did not draw the line at his office door. In his eight years with Heather he had reached outside the normal bounds several times to help her, taking her calls on weekends and at odd hours, even phoning her from Switzerland while he was on vacation. During stretches that lasted as long as a couple of years, when she was out of work and had little money, he continued seeing her, carrying her until she could pay. Since she'd been discharged from Glen Cove Hospital, he'd been accepting Medicaid for their sessions—far below his normal rate.

By traditional standards, this was highly unusual for a therapist whose patient has a borderline disorder. The conventional wisdom is to be extremely strict about setting patient-therapist boundaries, limiting any contact outside of regular sessions. Dr. Imhof's answer to this was that he did set boundaries with Heather, they just weren't the classic boundaries delineated in textbooks. Maureen Coley didn't know quite what to make of Dr. Imhof's approach—was Heather manipulating him, too?—though she was attracted to his humanity.

Getting the car back gave Heather an enormous sense of freedom. It is torture being without one in Nassau County, a sprawling, post–World War II suburb. Bus service is terrible. A half-hour drive from the Island's North Shore to the South Shore can take half a day on the buses. At the staff meeting, they all understood the import when Maureen announced, "Heather's picking up her car today. So you'll know, it's a Dodge Daytona." Maureen couldn't resist adding, "It's the next model up from mine, the one I couldn't afford."

"Typical," said Paula Marsters. The pay is so bad for working in a group home, residents often are better off than the staff.

STEPHEN DEROSA visited the house on a four-hour pass from Glen Cove Hospital and spent most of his time with Heather. They'd come to know each other while together on 3-West. Heather thought Stephen looked bad. He was usually clean-cut and well dressed. Now, after a month in the hospital, he needed a shave; his hair was matted, greasy, and hanging over his collar; his white dress shirt hung out, with a button missing; and he was drowsy, a sure tipoff the hospital was heavily medicating him. His eyes often closed while he spoke. "They've changed my meds because I've had a couple of flare-ups," he told Heather. "On top of everything else, they have me on Valium, too."

"I'm happy to see you back," said Heather. "We're all happy."

"Who said that beside you? Did Jasper?" Stephen liked Heather; she was round and juicy, with a pretty face.

She asked about his roommate at the hospital. Stephen whispered, "Puerto Rican, doesn't speak a word of English. He's all right. I wave to him sometimes so he won't be my enemy."

She wondered what he'd missed most since he'd been hospitalized. "Peace of mind," said Stephen. "Everything is up and down, one day they're your best friend, the next day they're your enemy. Up and down, up and down, it never goes away." He said he'd felt no peace since Vatican II, and Heather, being a good Catholic herself, calculated that was nearly thirty years of torment. "I have been taking communion every day," he said.

"That must help," said Heather.

"It must," said Stephen. "What was I saying? I'm really sick. Oh, right. Some people don't believe it's the host, but with faith you can believe it's Christ's body going to heaven."

After dinner Heather offered to drive Stephen to a park to cheer him up. He chose Tappan Beach in Sea Cliff, the next town over. No one would recognize him there. The park has a playground and Heather coaxed him to ride the swings with her. She made a contest of seeing who could go higher and Stephen was actually laughing as he pumped.

The pass expired at eight. Counselor Charles Winslow drove Stephen back and Heather went along for the ride. She urged Stephen to get well fast because she missed him, and gave him a kiss goodbye on the lips.

"I could just eat you up," said Stephen.

Back at the house in the TV room during a commercial break, Heather said, "I want Stephen to feel welcome here. Very few people reach out to him. I just hope I didn't give him the wrong impression by kissing him. He knows I have a boyfriend . . . It's just that there's something very lonely and isolated about Stephen . . . If it makes him feel special, it's worth it. He kept saying these little comments like he wanted to eat me up. He said he'd like to have a family someday and asked if I'd like a family someday and I said yes."

HEATHER WAS having problems with her oldest brother. She was owed money from their father's estate. Despite several phone calls to her brother, she never received the money. He was worried she'd squander it. It depressed her. For the first time since the hospital she had the urge to cut herself. At the pharmacy she bought a pack of Gilette double-edged razor blades. On a Friday evening she handed a blade to the overnight counselor. "I wasn't planning on using this," she said. "But I've really felt low lately. I'm afraid I might."

The following Monday at the staff meeting, Maureen discussed it with Linda Slezak and the other Melillo group home managers. "She's been good about talking to the staff," said Maureen. "She told me she was depressed but not suicidal, so that's positive."

"This is an improvement," said Heidi Kominsky. "She's coming to us."

"That really is positive," said Linda.

Heather had lied to them. She'd sat in her room that Friday night, the radio on, the door closed, holding the double-edged razor in her right hand and thinking about how she was going to make the cut, which direction she'd go. She'd teased herself with it: would she dodge and just play with it for a while, or be serious and finally do it? Toying like that, taking the razor and drawing it lightly across the top of her left thigh, about three inches, she caught sight of the first drips of blood from the vein, getting that feeling of pleasure, that soothing sweet feeling, just watching the blood drip out, touching the droplets with her fingers, cleaning it off with a tissue and doing it again. It was such a relief to feel something besides emptiness; even pain was better than emptiness. Going back and forth, deeper, seeing more blood, more. Then the thrill receded and the sting set in, that sharp raw bite of finely split skin, and always the final jolt back to reality: What outfits did she have that would cover it?

chapter 8

No One Laughed
in This House for Years

EVERYONE HAD the highest hopes for Anthony Constantine that spring of 1991. Linda Slezak expected he'd be leaving the group home for an apartment in a few months. Jeanne McMorrow, who ran Sara Center, an arts-and-crafts day program for the lower-functioning mentally ill, said, "We don't think Anthony will be with us long. He's clearly getting better." Even Anthony's dad, Dom, who'd watched his son go from being a gifted high school student to long-term institutionalization, who'd been disappointed by setback after setback, said, "It's the best Anthony's been since ninth grade." The father attributed a good deal of the improvement in his twenty-seven-year-old schizophrenic son to the group home.

The credit had to go to senior counselor JoAnn Mendrina. Anthony was her pet. She cajoled and pushed him forward. She taught Anthony to budget his ninety-dollar monthly disability allowance by giving him an envelope with three dollars inside for every day of the week. She showed him how to use a stove, washing machine, and dryer and how to get around on his own. He was now riding two public buses each way to Nassau Community College, where he was getting B's and C's and planning to major in psychology next semester.

There was a boyishness, an innocence, a silliness to Anthony that was endearing. At various points he had crushes on several of the younger female counselors at the house, and they were secretly flattered. It was like being a seventh-grade teacher and having one of your twelve-year-olds fall madly in love with you. He even ate like a junior high kid; he'd have a hot fudge sundae and wash it down with a large Coke. He loved joking around. During a hospitalization, he'd played outfield on the patients' softball team. In a close game against staff, he shouted from left field, "If the patients win, we get discharged, right?" No joke was too juvenile. At softball practice he could fall down laughing if players mentioned they had two balls.

He had a gentleness and openness that was disarming. Every year the group home made a summer trip to Great Adventure Amusement Park in New Jersey. Anthony never went. As he told everyone at a Tuesday community meeting, "Those rides scare me."

Like clockwork, Anthony would come bounding in from program at 4 P.M., yelling, "JoAnn, I'm home!" and they'd sit and talk about how his day had gone. More than once Anthony had said to her, "I wish you were my mother, JoAnn." He called her "the epitome of womanship."

Anthony's own mother, a bright former chairwoman of a junior high school English department, had completely cut him off after he became sick at fourteen. She never visited the group home and would not allow Anthony back in her house. Anthony had told Linda Slezak, "As you know, I don't have a mother. My mother won't have anything to do with me."

On the other hand, Anthony's father couldn't have been more attentive. Every evening Anthony called his dad, a retired shop teacher, from the group home pay phone. Every Sunday, every holiday without fail Mr. Constantine would be at 9 Highland to take his son for an outing. When Linda Slezak learned about Anthony's parents, she assumed they were divorced. When told they were still married, Linda assumed they were separated. It never occurred to her that these two people who'd reacted so differently to their son's illness would still be living in the same house.

But they were. If Anthony called at his usual time, Dom would hurry from wherever he was in the house to make sure he was the one to pick up the phone. When he went outside to work in the yard, he took the portable phone so he'd be the one to answer.

And if occasionally Mrs. Constantine happened to pick up at odd hours, Anthony knew what to say, "Could I speak to Dom please?"

"I'll get him," Mrs. Constantine would answer. That was all the two had said to each other in six years.

NO ONE LOVED the group home more than Anthony. He couldn't understand residents who griped about rules. "They don't know what my life was like in those hospitals," Anthony said one afternoon over a hamburger, large Coke, and hot fudge sundae at the Mykonos, a Glen Cove diner. "They sit around the Tuesday meeting complaining that we don't have the name-brand bologna, we have the store-brand bologna. I never have anything to say—I'm just so thankful to be able to walk around free. Life is so precious. I can go out whenever I want. Every night I go for a piece of pizza and a large grape drink. I'll listen to my headphones when I walk. Once in a while I get a song —I'm dancing in the street. I'm not very good with people but I'll be dancing in the street to this Led Zeppelin. I may not be tall or anything but I'm dancing."

He wanted to get an apartment with a couple of guys and "learn how to be a man. I've seen how bad life can be. I'm ready. I've improved a lot, I lived a lot, a lot of character is developed by me. There's only one last thing bothering me. Do you feel I look like a man? My father says you have to be a man. I'm not that tall or anything, but I feel like a person inside. Is that how you're supposed to feel?"

For years in the hospitals, voices taunted: "Be a man!"

"I had to do certain things or they'd kill me," Anthony said. The voices told him to stuff his face into his pillow and hold his breath until he counted to 100. "God and the Devil were fighting over me."

The voices threatened to turn him into a dog. "You wouldn't believe, I had to do it so many times, hundreds of times, stuffing my face in the pillow, counting to 100. I only did it once at 9 Highland. The voices are much lower now. I can barely hear them. They're much softer."

These days, after dinner, you'd find Anthony up in his room at the group home studying. He put in far more hours than most Nassau Community College students, and had hoped for A's, but was trying to be content with his B's and C's. Reading was difficult since the schizophrenia—the medications and voices interfered. "I spent two years figuring out how to read. I finally stopped on February 11, 1991. I know I have to read in my voice, not the author's voice. I ask people how they read, do they read every word, do they understand every word. They say they don't think about it, they just read. I think a lot about it."

In some ways Anthony's personality was stuck in ninth grade. Mr. Constantine found that if his son hadn't picked up a skill before the illness hit, it was hard to teach now. Anthony became sick before he was old enough to learn to drive. In recent years Dom had taken him out in the car, but found Anthony lacked the proper judgment. There were others with schizophrenia who'd lived at the group home and drove, but their schizophrenia had hit in their early twenties, when they already had licenses.

Try as he might, Anthony couldn't get his brain to work the way it had. People wondered if he was slow. He went for a routine medical checkup at an outpatient clinic in Glen Cove. When Dom got the insurance papers back, he noticed that under medical problems a nurse had written "mild retardation." It angered Dom and he called the clinic. "He's not retarded, he's in college." He made them change it. The illness worked mysteriously, leaving some skills intact and sapping others. As a boy Anthony's memory had been first-rate, but that had deteriorated. He'd just got back a paper in his college communications class. The assignment was an autobiographical profile. Anthony wrote that his life was so awful since the illness, he had considered suicide. When Dom typed up the paper he removed the suicide reference without telling Anthony. Before handing it in, Anthony reread Dom's typed version. "The suicide's not in there," Anthony said. "I guess I forgot to put it in." Schizophrenia had damaged his mind, cut holes in his memory, interfered with his reading, and yet through a heroic effort he could still do college work. He got an A on the paper.

Thanks to the group home, for the first time in years, he said, he had friends. "I don't try to think of bad things in people . . . like Jasper being unbelievably fat. I like to be kind. I like Jasper. He fools around all the time. And Fred Grasso. He's quiet, but he's always making jokes. He lends me his Walkman for twenty-five cents each time. I spent seventy-five cents the last two nights."

Anthony's father had replaced two Walkmen, the last one a week ago. "I was listening to the radio in bed at 3 A.M.," Anthony said. "I took it off my head because I heard voices making fun of me. I thought it was the radio. I flipped if off and it broke against the wall."

"But the voices have stopped," said Anthony. "They're gone.

D O M C O N S T A N T I N E checked *Newsday*'s community events listings for things he and Anthony might do. A Sunday afternoon concert by the Senior Citizens Pops Orchestra of Long Island at Plainview High School gave him an idea. Plainview was Anthony's old school. Anthony still had nightmares about what had happened to him there. Dom figured by taking him back to see it, Anthony might realize the past was gone.

Dom came by before noon. The group home was dead on Sundays —people sleeping late, no organized meals, everyone fending for themselves. In Anthony's early days at the house, Dom used to slip upstairs and straighten up his son's room. He was so thankful about Anthony getting in, he wanted to make the best impression. When JoAnn got wind of this she took Dom aside. "Are you going to continue taking care of Anthony after you're dead?" She'd talk with the father about letting Anthony be independent. Since then Dom had sneaked up to straighten up Anthony's bureau only a few times, though he was still typing all Anthony's school papers on the sly. ("Remember, don't tell JoAnn," he'd say.)

Dom kept the Firebird packed with tennis and paddleball rackets, golf clubs, baseball gloves and games, so he and Anthony would not run out of things to do on their Sunday outings. "Anthony's a good golfer," said Dom, heading for their first stop, a Glen Cove beach, where they'd feed the ducks. "Some Sundays, we go to the driving range. He can hit three hundred yards."

"More like a hundred and fifty," said Anthony.

"With medication, I don't know what it is," said Dom, "but it does something to them. Sometimes now he can't even hit it."

"Yeah," said Anthony. Dom parked in a public lot at the edge of Long Island Sound. He'd brought old bread and hamburger rolls. "There are days we park and just look at the water," Dom said. "One of the things we keep in the car is kites to fly." It was misty. The Sound was still and flat, blurring at the horizon with the gray sky. Seagulls, Canadian geese, mallards crowded around the two of them. "A cardinal," said Dom. Two swans waddled up.

"We like to come to the water and look," said Dom. "It's very restful."

"Yeah," said Anthony.

"See many birds, Anthony?" asked Dom.

"I don't," said Anthony.

"In summer we go to Jones Beach," said Dom. "Walk the boardwalk there. It's one of my favorite things. A good way to use up a few hours." Dom noticed a mallard with a broken leg and he and Anthony tried to feed it extra, but the other birds were quicker and kept stealing the crippled duck's crumbs.

DOM STOPPED at a Burger King in Plainview before the concert. They were a minute's drive from the Constantines' house, a lovely white brick split level, on a quiet tree-lined street.

"Anthony hasn't been home in five and a half years," said Dom.

"I haven't talked to my mother since 1985. It's ridiculous by now."

"You have ketchup on your face," said Dom. "Get a napkin and wipe. Better . . . Anthony's mother is very smart. She was the valedictorian of her high school class. But she's a very fearful person. I've told Anthony he has to understand his mother . . . You want a second cheeseburger? It has lettuce on it."

"I hate lettuce," said Anthony. "It's too good for you."

"I know you're always hungry so I got it."

"One of the hardest things for me is making up my mind," said Anthony. "I can never decide."

"You'll be hungry," said Dom. "Good. I've told Anthony his mother loves him, but she has her own problems."

"She doesn't like me anymore," said Anthony. "It started when I was in high school. She said, 'Anthony, why aren't you getting good grades?' I tried to explain the kids are laughing at me, they're making fun of me. One day I had a fork in my hand, so I threatened her with it. I said, 'I can't talk about it.' I said, 'I can't do it all. I have to live my life.' Ever since, she hasn't talked to me."

What was so strange to Dom, and so hard on Anthony, is that before Anthony became sick, the mother and son had been inseparable. "Anthony would come home from school," said Dom, "and she'd spend hours with him, going over work, talking about things, it was almost too much, their relationship, too suffocating." Dom had always felt like an outsider.

WHILE CURRENT popular theory on the origins of schizophrenia holds that there is a genetic predisposition for the illness which is activated by a stressful crisis, most thoughtful professionals know that is a guess. It could be something else altogether. Dr. E. Fuller Torrey, a leading American researcher and expert on schizophrenia who has served with the National Institute of Mental Health, believes stress has no major role in inducing schizophrenia, any more than it would be considered a factor in Alzheimer's or polio, or other diseases of the central nervous system.

Scientists have headed off in a number of different directions, chasing clues. There is considerable research linking complications during pregnancy and at birth with the eventual development of schizophrenia.

There are respected scientists who believe schizophrenia may be caused by a virus the mother contracts during pregnancy that lies dormant fifteen to twenty years—the way the herpes virus lies dormant.

There are puzzling bits of research that don't fit easily anywhere. Why do schizophrenics tend to have something wrong with their immune systems?

Why are more schizophrenics born in late winter and early spring?

Schizophrenia runs in families, but what does that mean? Does a person inherit a low tolerance for stress and then develop schizophrenia when facing a crisis that a healthy person could routinely handle? Or do genetics operate on a totally different level? Could the fetus inherit a genetic vulnerability to a particular virus infection during pregnancy?

Nor is a great deal understood about the antipsychotic medications that ease some people's symptoms. Thorazine, the first of these medications, was prescribed in the 1950s. Its usefulness as an antipsychotic was a fluke discovery. Previously, Thorazine had been relied on to sedate raving, wounded soldiers awaiting surgery. On a hunch, a Parisian doctor tried it on schizophrenics. In many it controlled the outward signs of madness, the voices and delusions. By the mid-1960s researchers understood that schizophrenic brains have an excess of the chemical dopamine, and somehow Thorazine reduced dopamine levels. But why a single chemical like dopamine is so important, and whether it is the cause or the result of other forces at work, is not understood. And why do the antipsychotics help some schizophrenics a great deal and others not at all?

Perhaps the strongest indicator of how little is known is that the most popular theory of schizophrenia's cause a generation ago—bad parenting—is given little credence today. The popularity of bad parenting theories peaked in the late 1940s. The psychoanalysts of the period postulated that there was a classic type of parent who caused schizo-phrenic children. These parent breeders were labeled "schizophreno-genic." A particular type of bad parent behaved in a particular abnormal way to induce schizophrenia in a child. But strangely, these same parents who were producing schizophrenics were turning out healthy, well-adjusted brothers and sisters, too. Control studies done over the next two decades demonstrated no major differences between parents of schizophrenics and other parents.

Schizophrenia is the most monstrous of the mental illnesses. And yet, as professionals in the mental health system know many decent parents produce schizophrenic children, and many monstrous parents produce children with far less severe problems than schizophrenia.

T H E R E   W A S enough in Anthony's background to give credence to most any theory on the origin of schizophrenia. He was born in the late winter of 1964, February 19. "He's had so much trouble in life, you wouldn't believe it," said Dom. "Even his birth was breech. My wife was in labor two days before they did a C-section." Anthony's legs were bent in, and at six months an orthopedist set them in casts to straighten them. As a small boy he developed thrombocytopenic purpura, a blood disease characterized by a lack of platelets. These children bruise easily. The strong medication prescribed had extreme side effects. "He was so swollen, he looked like a mongoloid," Dom said. "People would turn around and stare at him in stores." Mr. Con-stantine would later wonder if the medication might have affected the chemistry of Anthony's brain.

At nine years old he nearly choked to death when he vomited while being fitted for braces in a dentist's office. Later, as an adolescent he developed extremely severe acne. The Constantines tried several new medications but nothing made much difference. To this day, An-thony's body is badly pockmarked from the acne, with keloid scars. He avoids the beach and pools because it would mean removing his shirt in public.

And yet Anthony and his father both remember the boy's childhood as happy. "Up until ninth grade, we had a good, close family," Anthony says today. He can recall no instance of his parents abusing or mistreating him physically or sexually during those years. His mother had stopped working for several years when the children were young to devote herself to raising them. Through elementary and middle school Anthony did well. His grades were above average. The teachers talked about what a wonderful boy he was, how hard he worked and how well he got along with everybody, says Mr. Constantine. At parent conferences they'd always hear the same comment: "I wish every child was like Anthony." He played Little League baseball and drums in the school band. Dom was proud that Anthony could relate to all kinds of kids—the smart, the not-so-smart, the hostile, the meek. His friends tended to be sports crazy and high achievers. In eighth grade Anthony got honors in math, science, and social studies. The year he was to enter Plainview High, the school launched math and science programs for gifted freshmen. Anthony was placed in advanced biology and algebra.

Dom says, "You could not have asked for a better son. We felt we were so lucky to have him and his younger sister, a girl and a boy. He never gave us a bit of trouble. Never." The family went on camping trips and owned a twenty-six-foot Owens cabin cruiser that slept four. Young Anthony talked of becoming a doctor. He wanted to help people. The summer before ninth grade his parents bought him a used Bausch & Lomb microscope. This two-teacher household placed education on a pedestal. On vacation trips they visited several top colleges, including Brown University and Williams. During their long talks, his mother, who'd earned a master's from Columbia, would tell Anthony how wonderful it would be if he made it to the Ivy League. She hoped he'd do better than his father had.

Dom thought of Anthony as a Johnny Adverse. "He overcame all his problems so well," says Dom. "The only thing is that the mind can take so much and it snaps."

DURING NINTH grade Anthony began spending more time in his room. His parents assumed he was studying. Then they started getting notes from teachers saying he wasn't interested in class, wasn't doing his work. When neighborhood kids hollered, Anthony answered he was busy and didn't want to go out. Dom tried gently prodding at first, arranging a casual get-together with Anthony and a friend. The three would be in the yard playing when Anthony would mention he had to do something for a minute and leave. He wouldn't return, and Dom was left alone with the friend. In time, friends stopped coming. His grades went down. He was cutting class. His parents didn't know it, but while they were at work Anthony was leaving school, walking home, letting himself in with the key, and hiding in his room.

They talked to him. He never said anything major was wrong. The most he would say was that he hated school and that kids were baiting him. Even years later, it was hard for Dom Constantine to separate out how much kids were picking on Anthony as he deteriorated, and how much was the paranoia of the illness settling over his senses.

Anthony made it through the year. There were still bright points. He took the algebra section of the standardized New York State Regents test you must pass to get an honors diploma and scored 100. Dom didn't want to be too harsh. He figured Anthony was going through normal adjustment problems. The boy was in a new school environment with high-powered kids, and these were the beginning of his teen years.

In reality, as Mr. Constantine says now, "it was coming in slow."

This is how Anthony recalls that time: His mind just wasn't operating the same way it used to and he had no idea why. Suddenly, he couldn't do the work in Spanish class, couldn't understand what they were talking about in social studies. It was petrifying. Trying harder didn't help. "I couldn't believe how dumb I was. Before this, I used to just take my smartness for granted. I didn't think it was a big deal." Now he couldn't concentrate for as long. He stopped trying to do the harder work. Soon he wasn't getting 90s anymore, but 80s, then 70s. His mother would ask why. He did not know how to answer.

He'd walk into English class with his head down and his homework unfinished. "I felt very insecure just sitting in my chair. Every day I was so close to tears. Everyone was so different and I wasn't keeping up. I was like a deer in the jungle with tigers all around me. My friends wouldn't talk to me. They thought I was stupid. Everyone else was so smart plus happy. I wasn't smart or happy. I couldn't believe I was this dumb."

He felt no joy from school and spent more time in his bedroom watching his thirteen-inch Panasonic color TV and listening to the radio. Even on school nights he was up until 2 A.M. listening. His parents had no idea. The song he remembered most from that time was "I Will Survive." His room was the only place he was happy. TV made him happy, the radio made him happy.

Anthony says the voices hadn't started yet. He says they didn't start until two years later, in the hospital, when God began talking to him. He also says he wasn't paranoid. But Anthony is probably wrong. Most likely, in ninth grade he began picking up bits of innocent conversation by classmates and turning them against himself. This is the early stage of schizophrenia, when the mind is beginning to lose the ability to distinguish between what's going on around you and what you're thinking to yourself. Anthony may have literally been putting his thoughts into other people's mouths, transferring his own distress about not being able to keep up, his own bad feelings about himself, into his classmates' words. He recalls: "The whole school mood was meanness. I didn't know how to defend myself. I would have liked school if they didn't make fun of me. I liked the school. I didn't like the people.

"People made fun of me every day, every class, practically every minute. I was tortured like crazy. I can remember walking into English class and all the sexy men stayed with all the sexy girls. I wasn't as advanced as they were. They made fun of my appearance. My hair, my nose was crooked, I smelled. I wasn't tall or manly like them."

At the time, Anthony verbalized none of this. To an outsider he appeared sullen, unmotivated, lazy, stubborn. The problem was feeding on itself. Kids have no tolerance for anyone different, and Anthony was becoming very different.

The summer before tenth grade, he stayed in his room as much as possible. Occasionally a friend called or stopped over to ask why he wouldn't join them. Anthony did not respond and soon was totally isolated. He told his parents he needed to be tougher, stronger, taller. He announced a program to eat the right foods. He was so determined, he'd come down to the kitchen and eat a dozen scrambled eggs and drink a half gallon of milk. It made his parents miserable. Then Mr. Constantine would hear him upstairs in his room throwing up, and the two would race to get the bedroom's red shag rug clean so it wouldn't upset Mrs. Constantine even worse.

By tenth grade the parents could not explain it away. They took him to a private psychologist. Once a week, at eighty dollars per visit, the man talked with Anthony about coping with daily pressures. The psychologist gave no name for what was wrong. Mrs. Constantine stopped dealing with Anthony. She had the type of personality that zeroed in on one person at a time. For fourteen years it had been Anthony and his mom. His mother had made him the most important person in the family, centering their world around Anthony. Now his mom spent all her time with Anthony's younger sister Jane. "I can't handle him," she'd said. "You take him, Dom."

Before Dom went off to work, he'd get Anthony up, dragging him out of bed. Anthony did not want to go. He'd be screaming, "I hate school, don't make me, Daddy." Dom recalls: "I'm not proud of this, but sometimes I'd have to throw him out of bed to get him moving." There was awful pressure. Dom was watching the clock the whole time. He had to have Anthony to the high school by 7:00 so he could get to work by 7:15. Anthony felt humiliated, exhausted. He'd been listening to the radio until 2 A.M.—how could they expect him to get up at 6:30? There wasn't one human being who understood.

The boy's shirt would be hanging out, his shoes weren't laced, he'd be screaming, Dom would be screaming. But he'd push Anthony into the car, take him to school, and leave him at the front door. Dom could only imagine what they were saying at school—probably they thought he was on drugs.

The gifted ninth-grader was now in a work-study program aimed mainly at slower students. They went to classes, then to a job the rest of the day.

The paranoid vision turned real. Now kids were picking on him, brutally. Anthony had become weird—a serious offense in high school. In gym, he asked for a paddle to play paddleball and a kid spit on him. Anthony came back from work-study one afternoon and threw down his coat.

"What's wrong?" asked Dom. He showed his father the jacket. Oil was smeared all over. Anthony said a kid from work-study had done it. Dom went to see the teenager's father. A few days later, when Anthony went to get his bike from the rack at school to ride to his work-study job at a warehouse, the rear tire was missing. Dom approached the teenager with a hockey stick. "If you bother Anthony again, I'll use this on you," said Dom, who at five feet, seven inches was several inches shorter than the kid. Dom spoke to the father a second time. "All I ask of you is that he leave Anthony alone."

The father said, "Fine. He'll treat Anthony as if he's dead."

"I don't care how you think of it, just leave my son alone," said Dom.

THE PRESSURE was building inside. Anthony came home one day while Dom was still at work and slammed his books against the wall. He told his mother kids were baiting him and went into the kitchen for something to eat. Every minute they were insulting him at school. He was amazed he'd put up with it so long. Over and over, his stupidity, his acne face, his weak body, their voices harping at him. "I feel like killing everybody!" he yelled, grabbing a fork and pointing it menacingly at his mother. Mrs. Constantine was petrified. She ran from the kitchen into her bedroom, closed the door, and phoned the police. Dom got a message at work telling him to come home immediately. He knew only that it was about Anthony. He drove up the street and saw the police car. When he walked in, Anthony was upstairs crying. The cop told Dom that Anthony needed help. "The boy needs some friends, he's very lonely," said the cop.

Dom had always been troubled by his wife's fearfulness. He felt it was abnormal. Years before, the family was out on the boat in the Great South Bay when the engine began smoking. It was a minor thing, a little seaweed stuck in the intake pipe preventing water from cooling the engine. They were close to shore and right beside another boat that stayed with them until the Coast Guard towed them in. The kids were calm, but Mrs. Constantine was hysterical. She would not ride on the boat again. Dom had to sell it. He could be working in their garage and if Mrs. Constantine noticed he'd left the garage door open, she'd shut it with him inside. "What are you doing? I'm here!" Dom would say.

"It's dangerous having it opened—anyone can get in," Mrs. Constantine replied. "The door should be locked. I guess you don't read the newspapers."

From the time Anthony threatened her with the fork, it was like two different families in one house—Anthony and Dom, Mrs. Constantine and Jane. Mrs. Constantine refused to be home alone with Anthony. If Dom went out to mow the lawn, Anthony had to sit out front in a lawn chair while Dom mowed. If Anthony was at home and Dom hadn't come back from work yet, Mrs. Constantine would drive around or do some shopping or just park someplace and sit until Dom returned.

Through Catholic Charities they found Dr. Henry Brill, a psychiatrist experienced in serious mental illnesses. He was a retired director at Pilgrim State Hospital, donating his time. The man examined Anthony just once for a half hour. Afterward he told the parents: "No question, your son's schizophrenic." Dom recalled that the man was very nice and obviously, from his years at Pilgrim, had much experience delivering bad news. He did not try to sugarcoat it. He said, "Schizophrenics have a certain look about them."

Dom understood the verdict. "There's no cure and your life is ruined." Dom has a cousin with schizophrenia. The man lives with his sister, "rotting his life away," says Dom. He lights candles indoors to ward off evil spirits; he circles their car, blessing it. Dom and the cousin grew up a few blocks from each other in the Bronx. The cousin had worked for the railroad. "He got it after he fell in a pit and hit his head," Dom says. "He was never the same after that."

Dom went back to the psychologist Anthony had been seeing once a week at eighty dollars a pop for two years now, the one who'd been coaching Anthony on how to cope. Dom confronted him with what Dr. Brill had said. "Well, yes, I've felt that Anthony's a little bit schizophrenic," the psychologist replied. A little schizophrenic! Dom was enraged. A little pregnant, a little dead, a little destroyed.

Anthony's care now fell totally to Dom. It was Dom who told the boy he'd have to be hospitalized. He explained it was an illness and the doctors were going to find the right medication so he'd feel better. Dom never said "schizophrenia" to Anthony.

Occasionally, after much effort, Dom would persuade his wife to come along when there was a consultation on Anthony. At one meeting, Mrs. Constantine asked the social worker, "Can you give me any kind of guarantee that nothing will happen to me from Anthony?"

Anthony spent three months of eleventh grade and eleven months of twelfth hospitalized at Long Island Jewish Medical Center. Dom visited every day. Mrs. Constantine visited twice in two years.

During this time, Anthony found himself wishing he had some kind of magic TV machine, to see what his friends were doing, to look into their lives. One of the boys he used to hang out with was going to Brandeis, another to the University of Pennsylvania. It would be fun to turn on the machine and see his friends when he wasn't there.

Anthony finished his studies through a special school at the hospital. There were twenty-five mentally ill kids in the hospital class. He was their valedictorian. At their little graduation, he made the commencement speech to his fellow patients. The theme was "possibilities." He started college at Old Westbury, a state campus on Long Island, and got A's in a few courses before suffering another breakdown. From 1985 to 1989 Anthony was at High Point, a long-term private psychiatric hospital in a suburb north of New York City, in Westchester County. Every Sunday, Dom drove up from the Island to visit his son, always alone. Anthony would write letters home from the hospital asking "When can the whole family visit me, Dad, Mom and Jane?" but the others never did.

O N T H E D R I V E over to the concert at Plainview High, Dom said, "You know what we haven't done today? Listen to your Barbra Streisand tapes." Dom and Anthony shared a fondness for her music. The father bought several of her tapes for Anthony, and when they went on these Sunday outings, Anthony would bring them along and play Streisand in the car.

"Yeah, she's great," said Anthony. "Look! We're going right by our house! I can't believe it! That's where my friend lives. I'd love to have my own room again. I used to stay in my room all the time at home, it was great. I miss my stuff."

"Anthony has a set of drums at home he hasn't played in years," said Dom. "It has a twenty-four-inch bass drum instead of the usual twenty-two."

"I can't believe you're doing this, Dom," said Anthony. "We're going by my house."

They pulled into the high school's parking lot and Dom began the talk he had planned. "All right, how many years ago did you graduate?" said Dom. "1982. A long time ago. Did the building do anything to you?"

"No."

"Has the high school itself ever been bad?" said Dom. "These bad experiences are over. The kids who were there are gone. They're grown up. You go in there, watch the concert, you'll realize there's nothing to harm you there."

"I don't like that building," said Anthony.

"I call it a ghost," said Dom. "When something bothers you, if you confront it, it's not that bad. For instance I used to be real shy. It's hard to believe. I went to teacher's college for education. But I never thought I could be a teacher. And then I taught thirty-two years in the same district. Believe it or not, I made teacher of the year."

"I didn't remember that," said Anthony.

"You focus on it," said Dom, "you stay in school two hours after everyone else goes home."

"Dom, you're the best," said Anthony.

"I don't know about that," said Dom. "But somehow you'll go to the concert, you'll realize what happened wasn't important."

"I tried so hard at school," said Anthony. "I wanted A's."

"The important thing is you tried. It's not important if it's not all A's. You do your best. Pressure is hard on you." Dom mentioned how nervous Anthony had been on the day he moved into the group home two years before. They had to go to county social services to fill out paperwork first. In the midst of it, Anthony went blind. Dom led him into the men's room, where Anthony fainted. After ten minutes his sight came back.

"I remember. That was so scary," said Anthony. "How did that happen?"

"It was like a panic attack," said Dom. "Sometimes he has too high goals."

"Yeah," said Anthony. "Like what?"

"You start hearing voices when you're stressed from school."

"It won't be so bad," said Anthony. "Semester's almost over."

"It's just you put pressure on yourself."

"I'm doing fine at school," said Anthony. "I did a paper, I think I might've got an A. I'll probably get a B or C, but it's really good. Before when I got a C, I wanted to quit college."

"Anthony, you have a lot going for you."

"I know it, Dom."

"Anthony volunteers at the nursing home," Dom said. "He used to volunteer at one of the church soup kitchens. It's part of the group home program, to motivate them. I think 99 percent of them wouldn't get out of bed if they didn't have to."

"I like sleeping," said Anthony. "What's wrong with sleeping?"

"It's not good for your motivation," said Dom. "I try to explain to the kids—kids—men at the group home. When you help other people it makes you a better person. Anthony's a people person. He has a lot going for him."

"You think so Dom?"

IT WAS A glorious spring afternoon. They went inside. A hundred people, mostly elderly or family of the Senior Pops musicians, milled about in the hallway behind the auditorium. "How's it feel being here?" asked Dom. "You're an adult now. It's all different now."

"They painted the doors," said Anthony. "It's homier looking."

They took a seat in the sparsely filled auditorium. Anthony's glasses dropped on the floor and a lens popped out. He looked at his dad. Dom picked them up and pushed the lens into place. During a piece entitled "Pops Hoedown," Dom leaned over and whispered, "Are you all right, are you having any bad thoughts?"

"No, I'm fine," said Anthony. As "Selection from *Les Miserables*" played, Anthony dozed. During intermission he walked through the corridors saying, "I can't believe I'm here." He was smiling. He said he felt a lot better about the high school.

"I feel great," he said, heading toward the car when the concert was over. "There's a nice field over there. If I felt like I do right now, I think I would have played a sport in high school."

As they drove off Anthony and his dad lifted their hands and made a devil's sign toward the school. "Can't hurt me," said Anthony.

Dom dropped Anthony off at the Plainview library for a few hours. Anthony had to study for a quiz. Then they'd go to Christiano's, a local restaurant where the two usually ate their Sunday dinner together. Dom gave Anthony quarters in case of any emergency.

"Thanks Dom," said Anthony. "We're having a good visit, huh?"

A FEW DAYS later Dom sat in the kitchen of the home that Anthony was dying to see again. His wife and daughter were at work. The house was immaculate and amazingly orderly. It didn't seem to be lived in. Though it was midday, the drapes were drawn in the living room, making it dark. There were few personal family photos in view. The off-white wall over the fireplace mantel was bare. The house was dead quiet. Not a sound from the street reached inside.

Dom rarely had an opportunity to talk with anyone about Anthony. When he did, it poured out. "It doesn't bother me shouldering the burden," Dom said. "I tell Anthony we're the A-Team. It's much easier now than when he was back in high school. But what I don't like, Anthony is not accepted by his mother and sister, that bothers me. The sad part is that it doesn't look like it will change. She can't do it. She has a lot of quirks. When Anthony's sick, he says a lot of bizarre things. I know he doesn't mean it, but it scares her. After a while Anthony saw her as the devil and I was Jesus Christ.

"I explain to my son, you don't see your mother but don't get the idea you did something wrong, because you didn't. It has nothing to do with you. She has a problem. She loves you but she can't handle it. Fear's a terrible thing. But unfortunately that works psychologically on Anthony.

"We're the only family he has and I'm his only link to the family. See, the way I feel about it with Anthony, I'm sixty-three, I've had my shot at life. I'm one of his few hopes to bring him around. He's my number-one priority. Nothing is more important than to help him get better. Family is basic. There's nothing more important than family. But I'll tell you, with this kind of thing, it's surprising more marriages haven't broken up. My marriage was hanging by a shoestring.

"No one laughed in this house for years. This whole thing put me in a depression. I went, did my job, came home, and that was it. In summer the only thing I did was mow the lawn. We stopped boating and camping. We haven't had a vacation in twelve years. See, when you have a child like that, no matter what you're experiencing, if you're at the movies, a ball game, it's always in the background, it's there. There's no way for it to go away. Dying would be easier: you grieve, it's over."

When he saw the way his wife was reacting, Dom thought about splitting up. They'd screamed the word at each other in arguments. "Yes, I've considered divorce," Dom said, "and I'm sure she has too. But we bring a background of many years of happiness, raising two children and having joys and sorrow together." Somewhere along the line Dom had decided to keep his marriage together *and* help Anthony as best he could, and this is what his life had turned into, a series of tortured compromises. God knows, he wanted to bring Anthony into the house, even for just a visit. "It would be so nice to bring him home and make dinner here, cook spaghetti, a steak. But there's a feeling we have to draw the line." Dom said his wife believed if she saw Anthony at the group home or talked to him on the phone it would be difficult to say no when he asked to come live at home. "It's easier on Anthony," Dom said. "It would open an old wound. He'd want to know how come Jane's living here and he can't.

"I will tell you this. If I have to choose between staying together and taking care of Anthony, Anthony will take preference. He's the one who needs the help, and I'm his father."

Dom saw little prospect of Anthony making a visit even if Jane and his wife weren't home. "They wouldn't like it," Dom said, "Plus they're here all the time. They never go anywhere."

THAT SPRING afternoon in 1991, in that silent, empty house, it was eerie seeing Anthony's room, so neat and clean and frozen in the late 1970s. In many ways it was homier and more personal than the rest of the house. Everywhere was evidence of a junior high boy who'd been filled with promise and was curious about all the world. A four-piece bedroom set with a dark wood finish took up most of the space, the kind a million suburban parents on Long Island bought at Seaman's or Levitz. The single bed in the center of the room was covered with a blue quilt and had no pillow. It looked like it would barely fit an adult man. A rotary phone sat on the nighttable. Books filled the shelves. There was a big turntable and several dozen record albums, a large number of them by the Beatles. A few tapes were stacked in a corner, but there were no CD's. John Lennon's portrait hung on the wall, along with a photo of Julius Erving flying through the air, when he still had his huge Afro and played in the American Basketball Association. In the closet was the Bausch & Lomb microscope packed in its case and a wooden tennis racket secured with a wooden press. The closet was stuffed with Jane's clothes. She sometimes piled them all over the bed, too.

The clock had stopped at ten to ten. On a bulletin board was a flying horse Anthony had made from sheet metal in shop class. He had last stepped in this room in November of 1985. The calendar was turned to July 1986. For a while Dom had come in to rip off each new month, but then he stopped.

Dom was Anthony's only link to any of this. It scared them both. Occasionally Anthony would ask, "What's my room look like now, Dom?"

"Every once and a while I explain to Anthony that everything that lives dies, that it's not that big a deal," said Dom. On March 23, 1988, Dom had quintuple heart bypass surgery. "I had 90 percent blockage. It didn't frighten me. I figured, whatever happens." Anthony was in the psychiatric hospital upstate in Westchester county at the time. "I took him out one Sunday and explained. I said, 'Don't worry even though there's an element of danger. The odds are in my favor.' I didn't try to hide it. Sometimes when you almost know something, but no one tells you, you have more fear. I wanted it to come from me in case I died. Then my wife would have had to call him and Anthony might not have believed her."

THE THOUGHT of losing Dom had terrified him. That day in 1988, he'd put every ounce of effort possible into saving his father. He knew Dom was scheduled for surgery at 10 A.M. and turned the hospital radio to a classical station to find out how the operation was going. Anthony was sure either God or his dad would update him through music. He worked on blocking any negative thoughts. He was trying to be pure and holy to God. The radio knew what was going on, of course; it could read Anthony's mind and kept shooting out pins at Anthony's heart, trying to keep it from being pure. Fortunately Anthony was able to block them. Then he saw the knives, these pretty little things coming from his dad's heart, and the music kept on saying, "Don't do it, don't do that," and Anthony would adjust the way he was standing and change his thoughts so his dad would be all right. Finally, the music said, "It came close but didn't do it," and Anthony knew the knives had missed his dad's heart and the evil had gone in but missed, and he was greatly relieved and knew his father would be all right.

Four days later, when Dom was strong enough to use the phone, he called and told Anthony the surgery was a success. Dom only missed two Sunday visits upstate to Anthony because of the operation. "I drove myself," Dom said. "I was in pain after the surgery but the main thing was I had to be careful not to sneeze because my chest was stapled together."

SINCE THE GROUP home, Dom said, there'd actually been some joy. "I guess the laughter started again when Anthony got in. The first time I saw the house, I told Anthony, 'We really lucked out, it's nice, it's not like some little dump.' It's the only luck this family has had in recent years. What if there had been no group home available? Or one not as good as this one? The thing I was worried about with Anthony, he was in hospital so long, I was hoping he wouldn't develop an institutional personality. They get used to people doing things for them.

"At the group home, they tended to treat him like a person. That's the advantage of this place and especially that they don't stay in the house all day. It's one of the good things that's happened to Anthony. It's always toward progress. One of the things about the group home, they feel like they're regular people. When you're in a hospital setting, you're a patient. That puts you on a lower strata. Here it's different, like family. I remember his first day at the group home. I called to ask how he was doing. He said the mayor had visited them. They had cake with the mayor! See, I don't think that any person can understand the feeling of coming from a hospital locked room, where every move you make someone has to watch, to a group home, where you go to the store if you want to go to the store.

"He never used to smile. He didn't have too much to smile about. It's nice now, it's like you're going out with your son on Sunday. Before he'd do things mechanically. If I could get one little smile out of him it was a success.

"Want to know something? I think it could be in someone's basement if you have a staff that's as caring."

For the first time in years, Dom was treating himself to a little hope. "I think he could be happy if he finds a nice girl . . . someone soft and intelligent who doesn't aggravate him. The next thing is he has to find some kind of future. If he could find the right niche, he's the kind of kid, he'd work hard for you. Business and government have to form a partnership to put these people to work. There are programs to get criminals jobs, why not people like Anthony? I've tried him on machines, I work on cars, but he's afraid of machines. He's more the white-collar type of person. If I can just help him get that niche. So much in life is finding that niche. If I can give thirty-five years of my life teaching kids who are strangers, I certainly can give time to my own son. Finding the niche is the trick."

A FEW DAYS later, Anthony's voices returned with a new twist: the primary tormenting voice in Anthony's head was Dom Constantine.

On a Wednesday in mid-April, Anthony came home from Nassau Community looking glum. His communications professor had returned quizzes. Anthony told JoAnn he was expecting a 100; he got a 65. At midnight he called Dom from the house pay phone. He said he'd gone to sleep early listening to music—Dom had bought him a third Walkman—but was awakened by the voice of Dom, mocking him. Now Anthony was standing in the hallway, shouting into the phone at Dom: "I don't want you coming to visit me this Sunday. I don't know why you're saying these things about me. Just leave me alone!" He slammed the receiver down. The line went dead and Dom felt sick. He'd feared the voices might be back—the last couple of days Anthony was very quiet and preoccupied when they talked, a strong sign. But this was a first, being inside his son's head.

Staff talked with Anthony, trying to get him to see that the voice was his psychosis, not actually his father. Counselors didn't say it directly. They wanted him to reach that conclusion himself. How could Dom—fifteen miles away in Plainview—be talking to Anthony, when Anthony was in his room alone?

"I know!" said Anthony. "How does he do that? That's the thing." In time he calmed down. "I guess some people hear voices outside their heads," said Anthony. "I'm not like that. That's pretty bad. The voice comes in from in the center of my brain. It's a very low voice, like my dad, maybe because he's the main one I talk to." Anthony called Dom back, apologized, said he was feeling better and wanted to be together on Sunday as usual.

The following Tuesday JoAnn heard Anthony up in his room pounding his mattress and thrashing about. She went up. God and the Devil were at war inside him. He'd had one bad thought and now was sure the Devil would get into his heart. God hated him.

It was exam period, but he said he couldn't go to school Wednesday. "I know something will happen." JoAnn praised him for making a mature decision. She suggested he go down to the basement and work out with his weights to burn off some of the anger. He did and felt better.

Much of Wednesday he spent in his room, tossing and turning. JoAnn and other staff checked in periodically. "The voices were making fun of me," he reported. "I couldn't take it, I just wanted to cry. But I couldn't even cry. I said, "Well, right! You're right, just let me cry.' And they said, 'Oh, crybaby! Go ahead, crybaby! Go ahead, big crybaby.' And I couldn't. I couldn't even cry in peace."

He broke his third Walkman, slamming it against the wall when the voices got inside it. Religion was a big issue. The way he figured, there had to be a Devil, otherwise God would make everything beautiful and everyone happy—and he sure knew everyone wasn't happy. When a counselor tried reasoning with him, Anthony interrupted, "A voice just told me to tell you to stop talking, you'll get in trouble. I can't say too much."

A few minutes later he seemed fine, joking and laughing and deciding to go down for a snack. That night he had cooking duty with one of the newer women at the house. She was quite nervous and carried a notebook and pen with her to write down everything she was told. She wrote in JoAnn's explanation of how to dust the living-room coffee table, complete with da Vinci–style diagrams. She was quite a good artist. "JoAnn's so hard on me," she told Anthony.

"I know," said Anthony. "She's so strict. She has no heart. She goes for the brain."

The new woman felt like crying. She didn't know what to do. "We're supposed to make meat loaf," she said.

"Don't worry," said Anthony. "I'll help you. I know how."

He showed her the way to turn on the stove and she made a note of each step. "It's the medication," she said. "I can't remember anything. I have to write everything down."

"Don't worry," said Anthony. "This is the first day I've been depressed since I've been here."

"Really?" she said.

IT WAS AN exhausting, thankless existence, fighting off hostile voices all day. He had little time left to do anything else. He wasn't man enough for the voices, wasn't strong enough, tall enough, cool enough, or pure enough, and there was no ducking their harangues. The group home staff informed his psychiatrist, and Anthony's medication was upped. He'd moved into the house on sixty milligrams of Prolixin daily, a high dosage that often left him drowsy and drugged looking. During the past two years, Maureen Coley had worked with his psychiatrist on slowly reducing the dosage, eventually reaching forty milligrams a day. Now it was raised to forty-five milligrams. He was kept at Step Five of the house's medication supervision program. This meant he was given two weeks of medication at a time and took it on his own, but at the end of each day he had to check in with counselors who made sure the correct number of pills had been taken.

The extra five milligrams did not stop the voices. Anthony grew more irritable. Stan Gunter, an alum of the house, was dropping by frequently to play the piano and guitar and chat with friends at 9 Highland. Anthony and Stan volunteered at the same nursing home. Stan played the guitar for the old people and they made a fuss. Stan was always acting so cheerful and chatty—his latest thing was learning Spanish. The two returned from volunteering and were in the kitchen at 4:30 when Anthony started yelling at Stan, "I'm going to hit you if you don't shut up." Two of the counselors at the house, Paula Marsters and Jodie Schwartz—neither much over five feet tall— came hurrying in. Anthony was now backing Stan toward the couch, threatening him. He raised his arm as if to throw a punch and Jodie grabbed it. Anthony looked startled, almost scared, and ran to his room yelling the whole way.

Stan said there'd been no words between them, and none of the counselors had heard any. Voices, most likely. Maureen spoke to Anthony. He was so angry, he said, it scared him, but when Maureen tried to find out why he was angry, the only thing he mentioned was his mother. Later Anthony apologized to Stan. "You're my best friend in the whole world," Anthony told him.

Another time, Anthony was baiting Joe, his roommate, who had dinner cleanup duty that night. Joe asked Anthony to help out. "Yeah, right," said Anthony. "You missed this part of the counter, you missed this. This looks like crap."

"Come on, man, give me a break," said Joe.

"You're so lazy," said Anthony.

Fred Grasso was trying to get the Handi-wrap roll started. "You're doing great there, Fred. How pathetic can you get?"

"Hey Joe, don't forget to clean the tray," he said. Joe is a muscular man, a former marathoner and long-distance biker, but he let the comments slide. Anthony went in to watch TV. Nearby, Jasper was having a smoke. Jasper's socks were so vile that a counselor—after several hints—told him to go change them.

Anthony could sit just a few minutes. "The voices are really loud," he said. "Do you hear them?" He went out for a walk. He talked a lot about fighting and acting cool. "I hate being cool. I used to act cool. I used to think it was important. Do girls like cool guys? You know what I hate? These girls, they always talk about their looks. They think they're so great." Anthony wanted to find the right girl. "Catholics don't believe in sex before marriage, right?" he said. "I want to be a virgin when I get married." He said he always tried to do the right thing so his heart would stay pure.

And yet he had been so mean to Joe in the kitchen.

"Joe called me bad things last night," Anthony said. With all the torment, the tossing and turning in bed, Anthony's side of the room was a mess. Clothing and bed coverings were scattered everywhere. "Joe called me another Jasper," said Anthony softly. These were the cruelest words you could say at the group home.

Counselors had suggested he talk about things when they happened, so the anger didn't build. He should have discussed it with Joe then.

"I can't," Anthony said softly. "I can't think that fast. My brain's broken."

He came back to the house and went up to take a shower. Several residents were watching the TV show *Prime Time*, which was running a segment about the antidepressant Prozac, and whether it made mental patients go on rampages. They were all unusually quiet; everyone at the group home was very interested in violent mental patients. The announcer was saying that a few murderers claimed Prozac made them kill ("the Prozac defense") and while no jury had found that believable, you had to wonder. Heather, who was on Prozac, found the show too upsetting to watch very long. Anthony came down from his shower and sat in the back of the room. When Joe walked in, Anthony stood.

"Joe, I'm sorry," Anthony said. "I've been under a lot of strain from college."

"It's OK, man, I understand, it's your illness," said Joe. "We all have problems here."

"You're my best friend in the whole world," said Anthony. Joe went into the kitchen, while Anthony sat in front of the TV a few more minutes, staring downward. He stood to go back to his room. "You don't hear them?" he said.

THE STAFF discussed Anthony constantly. They felt that if they could get him to the end of the semester, the pressure would be off and the voices might subside. They went from crisis to crisis. They might convince him for a day that his father could not be in his head, but the next day they'd have to start all over. They worked at small things that made a little difference: getting him to punch a pillow instead of the walls. He said showers relaxed him, so they urged him to take more showers, two or three a day if it helped.

They tried to catch trouble before he blew. At dinner on May 21, Anthony had said casually, "I've been hearing voices lately."

"Are you hearing them now?" asked JoAnn.

"Yes, they're telling me I said something wrong."

"Anthony," said JoAnn, "the dinner you made tonight was wonderful. Do you see everyone eating the meatballs? Were there any problems?"

"No," said Anthony, "but I'm worried I said something wrong."

"Everyone had a good time," said JoAnn. "It was great. You have to ask yourself, 'Is anyone upset?' "

"I believe you, JoAnn, I do," said Anthony.

That evening at the staff meeting JoAnn told the counselors, "There's definitely something big going on. I used a lot of logic and rekindled his memory and it helped this time."

Though they conferred with Anthony's therapist, they had only hunches about what was at the root of the current crisis. "He says, 'I

can't stop thinking about all the bad things my mother did to me,'"
counselor Sarah Casuto said.

"One possibility," said Maureen, "he's recognizing what he's angry
about and he's angry about his mother." It was possible that Anthony
was frustrated about not doing as well as he hoped in school; that he'd
long wanted to prove to his mother that he could make it and that
she'd been wrong to abandon him; that the current academic disap-
pointment churned up his anger at his mother; and that all this stress
triggered the psychosis.

Or perhaps that was completely wrong. It was also possible that the
illness, the psychosis, the voices, cycled independently of what was
going on around him; that his brain was heading into a down period
on schizophrenia's biological roller-coaster; and that it was causing
him more than the usual amount of trouble now—and staff was noticing it more now—because he needed his mind to be sharp for school.

"Anthony is working with Carol Goldman now in therapy. She's
opening up doors that have been closed too long. And she may be
touching very strongly on the mother issues," said JoAnn. "She goes
deeply."

"Not too deeply," said Maureen. "She's only going to have him ten
weeks." State and county funding cuts had lopped off half the staff
therapists at the Melillo mental health clinic. Maureen was trying
without much luck to find him another therapist. "We talked about
getting him to someone quickly."

"Oh yes, please," said JoAnn. "All the money that was spent for
Desert Storm." JoAnn mentioned that Anthony had already signed up
for the fall at Nassau Community. He was planning on taking two
psych courses—childhood development and abnormal behavior. No
one thought this was a great idea, but Anthony wouldn't be talked out
of it.

Maureen warned them, "Anthony is a volatile guy. While it's very
good for him to express himself, watch out for the physical stuff when
he does. He gets so pent up." She was particularly concerned about
JoAnn and Sarah—they were Anthony's mother's age.

Sarah said to JoAnn: "Anthony tells me you're really nice. He wishes you were his mother."

"You have to be careful," said Maureen. "He may wish you were his mother, but when he's mad and confused and he thinks you really are his mother, he may go for you."

Anthony didn't know this, but JoAnn had tried recently to get his mother involved again. The mother came across as sweet, emotional, tearful, acknowledging that she knew what schizophrenia did to him. On the other hand, she said, "I don't think it would serve any purpose for me to talk to Anthony until he gets well."

JoAnn reported afterward: "It means nothing. He'll never be well."

Maureen arranged a special meeting for May 23 at his day program Sara Center, including the psychiatrist who prescribed Anthony's medication, his therapist, group home staff, day program staff, Anthony, and his father. She wanted to see if they could stop Anthony's deterioration. The meeting did not come a day too soon.

MAY 22, he came home from program and went right upstairs. He was in his room a short while, then rushed into the bathroom and closed the door. You could hear a lot of commotion and the sound of the toilet flushing several times. He hurried downstairs, out the kitchen door, then inside again, pacing back and forth. "Stay away," he warned, "I'm having problems." He watched a music show on TV for a minute—there was a rap group pounding—then went to make a phone call.

His sister answered. "I want to speak to Mom," Anthony said. There was quiet on the line, until his father picked up and asked what was going on. Anthony was adamant. "I want to speak to my mother!" Dom wouldn't do it. "I want to kill her!" Anthony shouted. "I hate my mother and I'm going to do something to her." Dom tried to calm him. "I hate you," Anthony yelled. "I just flushed three of your Barbra Streisand tapes down the toilet and ripped up five others and threw them in the backyard trash."

"Oh no," said Dom.

"Go to hell," yelled Anthony and hung up.

Staff took Anthony into the office. They called his psychiatrist, who spoke with Anthony and added another five milligrams of Prolixin daily. Maureen told him she was putting him back to Stage One —all meds supervised full-time. She had him bring down his pillbox and keep it in the office. He seemed calmer.

While dinner was being prepared he called his parents four more times and hung up each time he heard Dom's voice.

Maureen called the plumber.

A female resident made roast chicken, baked potatoes, and corn for dinner. Anthony picked out two drumsticks and left the table without eating, resumed pacing, returned to his room, came back down. He sat in the living room. Ten feet away, Heather and her boyfriend Larry were kissing and nuzzling. Heather was wearing tight white short shorts and you could see a long scar on her thigh. When someone asked about it, she said, "I was holding the rabbit in my lap and she clawed me."

Anthony stuck his head in the office. "My meds aren't in my room." He'd forgotten. He opened the sliding door and stepped into the backyard, sitting at the picnic table. JoAnn followed him out. He had tears in his eyes and was sniffling, put his head down on the table, and began to cry. "JoAnn, what am I going to do? It was the worst thing I could do. My father loves Barbra Streisand more than anything in the whole world. More than me."

JoAnn smiled. "If you messed up the plumbing, you're dead."

"I know," said Anthony. He said one of the female counselors at Sara Center had made fun of him all Wednesday. "For six straight hours," he said. "All sexual innuendo. I could take it for fifteen minutes, but six straight hours."

"What did she say?" JoAnn asked.

Anthony looked at his watch. "That was six hours ago. I can't remember the exact words . . . It was just there, the sexual innuendo behind every word. They were talking about their vaginas, about putting things in their vaginas. I don't think that's right for a counselor."

"Give me an example of something," said JoAnn.

"They were talking about wearing their shorts up above the knees. But the sexual innuendo was there. I'm not going to be able to defend myself because I can't remember any exact examples. See, I'm just a boy, I don't look like a man for some reason. I don't look like my father. Here's something. She made fun of the size of my penis. All sexual innuendo. She said about the fish under the sea and looked at my eyes watering. She was making fun of my eyes watering—you see it?—fish under the sea. As if I'm not a man. I'm going to get even."

For JoAnn, listening to Anthony's explanations when he was psychotic was like trying to understand one of your dreams the next morning. You know the transitions and logic make sense when you're dreaming them, but afterward, when you lay them out step by step, the rational thread connecting each scene is missing. It was as if in Anthony's damaged, schizophrenic brain, this subconscious dream world leaked into his waking, conscious mind, making his thoughts and speech dreamlike.

JoAnn spoke to him in a soft, soothing tone. She was sensible and concrete. Somehow with schizophrenia, the voices from the subconscious dream world invaded his wakeful daily life. She asked if he was hearing the voices now.

"The voice I'm hearing sounds like my father's voice and the only way I can get it to stop—I don't want to tell everything, I don't want to give away too much—is to kill him. The voice is very sarcastic, 'That's it, crybaby, keep crying.' They make fun of me for crying. I hate my father, I hate my mother. I want to kill them. I feel like taking a knife. My father's going to hate me, I'm embarrassing him, I'm dragging him down with me."

JoAnn urged that he just try and make it through that night, and they'd deal with the rest tomorrow at the Sara Center meeting. "Do you think you could do that for me?"

"All these women at Sara Center," said Anthony. "They'll believe them, they won't believe me. I know they will. They're grown women. I'm a boy. I don't look like a man. My father's a man. I love him. I love my mother. But she didn't treat me right. I hate what she did. I'll get even. I hate my mother. I can't stand my father, but I love him.

"My room at home, it's the greatest place. All my hopes and dreams are there. I have a bunny in there with ears. It looks like a dog. I called him Doggy. When I was home my father tucked me in and put the bunny on the pillow. When I wouldn't get up for school my father would pick me up and kick me out of bed. That was the worst he did. You know, I thought my father was God and my mother was the Devil."

"I know, Anthony," said JoAnn. "How long have I known Anthony Constantine? Do we still believe that now?'

"No," he said softly, head down.

JoAnn assured him that tomorrow at Sara Center she'd be there and Dom would and they'd both be on his side.

"You think my father is just Nice Guy Dom, an industrial arts teacher. There's a lot more to him. There's a lot there. I want my father to get angry. I want to go into the hospital or jail and do something awful so he'll be embarrassed. I want to get even with him."

JoAnn talked about Dom being caught in the middle between Anthony and Anthony's mother, trying to hold marriage and home together and be a good father to Anthony, too.

"You don't care," said Anthony. "This is just a job to you."

JoAnn showed him her watch. "What time is it?" she asked. "What time do I get off?" It was 7:45. JoAnn was supposed to have gone home at 6. Twice more during their talk she did it to remind him. He'd be calm for a while, then grow agitated and start all over. "See, the women at Sara Center are here," he said pointing to a spot on the picnic table. "They'll all band together, so none of the sexual innuendo will come out and I'll be way over here, I'll fall off the end of the table."

JoAnn gently pointed out that the counselor he was upset about was an older woman, and might be a mother figure to Anthony.

"JoAnn, you're like my mother, you run this house, you know how everything works. That's how my mother was. You're the mother of this house." The sun was going down behind the backyard hedge. The warm spring evening was turning pleasantly cool. "No one loves me except Dom, and I threw his Barbra Streisand tapes down the toilet—seventy dollars worth. I'm afraid of my father. He yells at me. He can really yell. There's no peace. How can we have peace in the world? I got in trouble for saying there's no love at Sara Center. I believe what Freud says, the theory of, it's all id."

"Anthony, who are you responsible for?"

"I'm responsible for everything, for my father . . ."

"Stop, stop stop," said JoAnn. "You're responsible for one person, you, Anthony Constantine.

"Just me?"

"And I'm responsible for one person, JoAnn. Promise me this Anthony, promise you'll just relax and calm down and not worry too far ahead."

"A man doesn't cry, right, JoAnn?"

JoAnn knew some who did.

"You'll stand up for me?"

"Yes, Anthony."

"JoAnn, I know you look out for me," said Anthony. "You were supposed to go home at six."

She asked that he not leave the house for his usual walk that night and told the overnight counselor. It was dark when JoAnn went home. She liked Anthony so much. She did not look forward to telling him that her husband was retiring and she'd be quitting next month.

Someone went down the hill and picked up Anthony a chocolate sundae with whipped cream and sprinkles. He ate it in a chair on the front patio of the house, scraping the last drips off the bottom of the Styrofoam cup with a plastic spoon. Then he went in, called his father, and apologized. After hanging up, he said, "My dad thinks I sound better."

ANTHONY FELT the consultation the next day at Sara Center was "the greatest meeting ever," and the psychiatrist and other staff members agreed it was excellent. For the first time, Anthony was able to openly express anger he felt toward his father. "I'm exhilarated," said the psychiatrist. Only Dom left drained and exhausted looking.

Beforehand, Anthony and his dad had talked in the backyard of Sara Center, a large, old, attractive white frame house. There was a bucket with garden plants in it and Anthony kicked it, scattering the plants around the yard. Later he would say, "If you're going to get mad at my dad you have to get really mad; otherwise it doesn't work." Anthony sat at the meeting saying little at first, his hands folded, his head down. He felt nobody loved him, especially his dad because of the Barbra Streisand tapes.

They talked about the Devil and God, and then Anthony mentioned how his father was causing him to hear voices.

"What are these voices like?" asked Dom.

"What do you mean?" said Anthony. "You're doing it to me."

Dom said, "Anthony, it's not me, it's the voices in your head." Anthony didn't buy it, or as he put it, "I believe me."

Anthony in the past had talked about his rage toward his mother, but this was new. He seemed to understand that he'd flushed away the tapes to hurt Dom. He mentioned how angry he was that Dom wouldn't let him go home for even a visit. He recalled being thirteen and fourteen, when he was getting sick and hadn't been diagnosed yet, how he was confined to his room. He'd hold his breath, put his fingers in his ears, his head under the pillow, and hope that if he held his breath long enough he'd be pure and things would go back the way they were, one big happy family. Dom acknowledged it was terrible. "He couldn't come out for days at a time. My wife was screaming to keep him away from her, to put him in a hospital. It was a nightmare."

They discussed trying Anthony on clozapine, the new antipsychotic that was supposed to be so hopeful. Dom said he would check his insurance to see if it was covered.

The staff urged Anthony not to treat his father like a deity. They told him not to worry about being a man, that it happens naturally. They were extremely supportive, praising him for making it through the semester—he finished with a B and C—despite his troubles. Anthony said that this summer while he was off he wanted to learn the guitar. He was going to ask Stan Gunter to teach him.

JoAnn took Dom aside and urged him to keep reassuring Anthony that he wasn't angry, even if he had to do it a thousand times. "We're not dealing with your perception or mind," said JoAnn, "We're dealing with Anthony's. And he's convinced you're in his head and you're angry at him." Before leaving, Dom spoke to his son kindly. "Don't worry about the Barbra Streisand tapes, OK? It's really not that big a deal."

"OK, Dom," said Anthony.

On the way back to the group home, JoAnn told the other counselors that she couldn't understand why Dom had stayed with his wife. "I would have done differently," she said. "But who knows what his views on divorce are." She felt he'd never meant to abuse Anthony, but his decision to hold the marriage together no matter what had cost Anthony terribly.

By the time they arrived at 9 Highland, the plumber was up in the blue bathroom. "You know what clogged that toilet?" he said to Maureen. *The Best of Barbra Streisand.*"

"Yeah, I know," said Maureen.

FOR HIS PART, Anthony felt exhilarated, like he had outshined his father for once. Afterward he said, "I feel better because I can express my personality better. I always had a good personality but couldn't show it to people. I didn't have my whole life together. I feel good."

He'd practically forgotten the Sara Center counselor who'd agitated him so the day before. She'd barely come up at the meeting. "We're friends in a way. We didn't talk directly. She's one of these ladies who can get by because she has nice hair.

"I guess part of the reason I feel better is my dad forgave me. I felt terrible about the tapes. She's so dear to him.

"I used to think I was all heart and no brain. Now I'm thinking I'm smart. I'm not worried. I'm not thinking about my mother. I know I have to be independent. I feel better, I don't even know why, it just happened, I guess because I'm twenty-seven. I'm getting nearer to being a man. But I'm not worried about being a man."

He was hopeful about this new drug. "My father talked to me about clozapine. I hope JoAnn puts me on it. I don't like the Prolixin. I'd rather try something that will work. My dad said clozapine is a miracle drug."

JoAnn had never rated higher in his book. "She and I used to be enemies in a way. She'd make me work and didn't respect me as a person. Just wanted to use me to do all the work and get it over. See, JoAnn is like a mother figure. She's very smart and listened. I trusted her because she's a counselor. She's very close with my dad because I caused trouble on a couple of occasions, so my father talked to JoAnn a lot. They became close friends. I almost wish they were married. JoAnn's all ready to take care of me if I have a problem."

As for his real mother, "I guess she's too busy. I think she's busy bothering my father. I don't want to think about it, I'll get mixed up. I knew I would make it back. I knew in my heart. I know they couldn't squish me down. Wait until you hear me play the guitar. I can play a D chord—that's all I know so far."

THE STAFF HAD explained to Dom that if he invited one of Anthony's friends into the Constantine home, Anthony resented it, since he couldn't go home himself. That day, after the meeting, Dom sat on a folding chair in his driveway with a visitor and tried to sort out what had been discussed at Sara Center.

"He wasn't talking much at first, but by the middle he was sure hot and heavy. I'm not quite sure what his hearing my voice is about. I've been taking care of him a long time and this is the first time he'd said anything like that. The fact that he's venting and getting it all out, how sometimes I bug him—he thinks I want him to be perfect. It's good he's able to say it while I was there. I did my best to explain I'm not mad at him. If that's what's bugging him, fine, he should say so.

"There's been a definite change in Anthony the last three to four weeks. He's been very argumentative. Now I'll say something and he'll snipe. He's got into arguments with people. It's been very disturbing."

At the meeting everyone had talked so optimistically about the new drug clozapine. Dom didn't comment, but he wasn't going to let himself get too excited. Fred Grasso had been on it for several years in that experimental program. "You look at Fred, he's emotionally flat. I don't know if that's him or clozapine. It makes me wonder, will Anthony be that way?"

In the two-plus years at the group home, Dom saw the toilet tapes as a new low. "Naturally I was disturbed. I'm trying to make his life easy. He's already ruined the typewriter I got him. That was two hundred dollars. And the Walkmen. It's a constant thing, bringing them home and fixing them. These tapes run nine and ten dollars each. I know he loves Barbra Streisand. Actually, I like Barbra Streisand. I don't love Barbra Streisand. I put it on in the car because he likes it. To be honest, I'm getting a little sick of Barbra Streisand.

"This is like old times. You hope it won't happen again, but you realize it will sooner or later. It's not too easy to function under these circumstances. There were times in the beginning, when Anthony first got sick, I couldn't function at all. All I could do was mow the lawn. Anything I didn't have to do, I didn't do. Did you ever take a good look at the parents who have mentally ill children? Maybe only another person who's been through it can see it. It's like a beat-up type of look. It doesn't have to be a physical thing. It's an emotional thing you can see in someone's eyes. It's like GI's coming back from war. They don't have to say anything to another GI, they know, they're going through the same agonies.

"The things I've seen in the different hospitals. So many people abandoned. You don't see a mother, father, family."

AS BAD AS this was, Dom felt the group home had handled Anthony's crisis so much better than even the best private hospital where Anthony had been, High Point in Port Chester, New York. Because Dom and his wife had both been teachers in good suburban districts, they had first-rate medical insurance that had paid for top private in-hospital care. In the mid-1980s a psychologist had told Dom, "To give Anthony the best shot at life, I'd recommend High Point," and Anthony had been hospitalized there from November 11, 1985, until February 8, 1989, when he moved to the group home.

The forty-five bed psychiatric hospital is housed in a handsome Tudor style mansion set on a 142-acre estate, and boasts one fulltime psychiatrist for every six patients.

For that three-year-and-two-months' stay, Dom's insurance company had paid High Point $585,099—about six times what it would have cost Anthony to live in a group home. When Anthony started at High Point it was $400 a night for a semiprivate room; in the next three years the fee was raised four times, to the point where it was $650 a night when Anthony left.

And many extra charges were tacked on. The hospital laundry fee went as high as $72 for a two-week period (October 16–31, 1988); at the group home Anthony did his own laundry in the house washing machine and dryer. There was a $21 monthly charge for newspapers at the hospital; the group home subscribed to *Newsday* daily and the twelve residents shared it.

When Anthony needed to go out to an internist it was an extra $75 for the session, plus $31 more to be escorted there by a hospital worker.

At the group home Anthony was never mistreated, never even slightly hurt physically; twice at the expensive hospital, according to Dom and Anthony, he was beaten up. One time, Anthony says, he was very sick, was naked, thought he was a dog, and had decided that he had to lie on the floor, hold his breath, and count to 100 so he'd be a human again. An aide told him to get up and when he wouldn't began kicking him in the ribs, Anthony recalls.

After the second incident Dom got a call from Anthony's psychiatrist, Dr. John Biardi. The doctor said Anthony had injured himself, Dom recalled. Dom made a rare midweek visit. Anthony came into the visiting room and was so happy to see his father he nearly knocked him down, giving him a huge hug. Dom was stunned by how bad Anthony looked. The area around the eye was black and nearly swollen shut, and the eyeball was red. His lip was slit and swollen. Anthony said he'd been put in the isolation room at the hospital for reasons he couldn't remember, and the nurse in charge had let two other patients in who beat him up, punching him over and over in the face. At one point, Anthony told Dom, he had yelled, "Please stop, my father will give you five hundred dollars if you stop." Dom asked Anthony why they'd been beating him. "I don't know," said Anthony. "They're sick idiots."

Dom went home and gave it some thought. "When you're dealing with a person who hears voices and is mentally ill, sometimes it can be hard to decide what's true and not true. But I realized there's no way he could have done that to himself," Dom recalled. "He couldn't hit himself that hard with his fist, and even if he hit his head against a wall, his eyeball wouldn't be all red."

Dom suspected Anthony made some remark to anger the nurse and the nurse then looked the other way while the patients did the dirty work. "I phoned Dr. Biardi. I said, 'It seems so obvious to me that Anthony was beat up.' He said we're going to make an investigation."

The hospital's investigation concluded these injuries "were possibly inflicted by other patients," but found staff had no role in either this incident or the time Anthony claimed he had been kicked in the ribs. High Point officials also reported that Anthony had twice hit staff, including once breaking a male nurse's glasses.

"I suppose I should have made a report or sued," says Dom. "But if I complain, you don't know how Anthony's going to be treated. . . . I needed the place."

What Dom came to see, as time passed, was that the fancy hospital had no cure for schizophrenia. "They'd say he's getting better but he needs more time," says Dom. "After a while I felt they were just keeping him because I had insurance." And Mrs. Constantine wouldn't let him home.

It was Dom who found the group home. "The hospital's social worker said she didn't know much about Long Island. You'd think these people would have a list of group homes. I found it from a story about the Glen Cove house in the paper."

Dom was amazed at the way he could call the group home staff whenever he needed to. A letter mailed to parents from High Point Hospital had informed Dom he was permitted to call Anthony's psychiatrist, Dr. Biardi, only on Monday between 12:30 and 1 P.M.

"At the group home, I couldn't even say which staff members are good . . . They're all so concerned. At the hospital he went through episodes of bad things, he was put in the isolation room. Here five or six people talk to him. I feel the hospital, they react after the fact, once there's a crisis. The group home, they see it coming."

THE THING Dom was thinking now was that maybe the group home had let him get too hopeful. The Streisand tapes were a reminder not to underestimate schizophrenia. "Now we have to go through the whole process of building Anthony up again. It's like you're building a house and a storm comes and rips it down and you have to build it again. It's hard."

A car pulled up and Mrs. Constantine got out. It was late afternoon by now. She was done with work. She's a short, plump, plain woman with straight gray hair, who looks sweet and grandmotherly. Dom got up out of his folding chair in the driveway and explained that he'd been discussing Anthony.

"Anthony was the most kind, wonderful boy," said Mrs. Constantine. "There's not a thing you could say against him, but his illness changed him." She excused herself and went in the house through the garage entrance, which Dom then closed immediately.

Dom returned to his folding chair. "What gets me the most—this time, my wife heard what Anthony was saying about killing her. For years I've been doing my best to pave the way for a short visit. I know in five or six minutes that was all gone. There are a lot of firsts here. I saw it all going down the drain. There's no future now as far as him coming home. Not only my wife's scared, but Jane, his sister, too.

"I see these people different. I'm with them. What they say and what they do are two different things. She's fearful of him. She's full of fears.

"You don't know how hard it is not being able to bring him home, driving around every Sunday with that trunk full of games, thinking up things to do with your grown son. The worst thing is holidays. You know what it's like trying to find something to do Christmas Day? . . . It's hard to find any restaurant open. Thank God the Chinese restaurants are open. But I'll tell you, it's a terrible feeling.

"This is a tragedy. Things happened yesterday that never happened before. This is new, killing his mom. My wife talks about moving someplace where Anthony couldn't find us. Maybe one of these places that you have to go through a guardhouse to get in."

Then Dom folded up the lawn chairs, put them away, and went back inside. It was about time for the afternoon call. Dom wanted to be sure he was there to answer the phone.

chapter 9

IF MAUREEN WANTS ME TO GO, I'LL GO

WITH THE pleasant warmth of May and June, the house seemed to expand. You could sit outside on the front patio, or in the backyard, at the picnic table or along the concrete retaining wall. These evenings they often cooked out on the gas grill donated by one of the original resident's parents. With the windows open you could hear the fire station horn down the hill on Brewster sounding at noontime, and the distant whistle of the Long Island Rail Road trains pulling out of the Glen Cove station every hour, the rustle of the tall maples that towered above the house, and the drone of crickets at nighttime, hiding in the backyard grass. Residents enjoyed relaxing out front, smoking after dinner, watching people pass by on the way home from downtown. On these balmy evenings, counselor Donna Rubin would sometimes drive several of them to the high school field, and other times they gathered on Douglas Drive, the side street in front of the house, to lob around a softball. Occasionally a neighbor a few houses away would come out and pretend to be gardening in her front yard while she peered at them playing catch, but nothing ever came of it. The most serious complaint in a couple of years by a neigh-

bor—phoned in anonymously to Linda Slezak's answering machine—
was that two staff members had been seen kissing and hugging in front
of the house. In reality this was Heather and her boyfriend Larry from
3-West. They apparently looked too good to the neighbor to be mentally ill. Maureen felt the complaint was insulting and did not mention
it to Heather.

Melillo arranged for reduced-priced memberships at the local
YMCA, and several residents took advantage. JoAnn in her typical
motherly fashion made sure everyone interested had bathing suits. She
took Jasper to a Big Man's shop in Carle Place that was having a sale
and bought him a swimsuit, several summer shirts, and shorts. Each
year most of the miscellaneous cash fund at the house went to buy
Jasper new clothes. He'd put on so much weight he was constantly in
need, and his mother never came around anymore. At the shop he tried
on size 56-inch-waist shorts. "They're fine," he said. The crack in his
butt was showing. "Too tight," said JoAnn, pulling out a tape measure.
The biggest size in stock, 62, barely fit.

"These are good," he said trying another pair. "They stretch. I
won't split them." He seemed in a great rush to be done. Jasper would
never say, but JoAnn assumed he was embarrassed and she moved
along as fast as possible. She wrapped everything up in fifteen minutes,
and that included a cigarette break outside for Jasper. When she made
the purchase she pulled out a tax exemption form for nonprofit organizations, to save paying the 8 percent sales tax. At Modell's JoAnn
bought him a pair of Reebok sneakers on sale for forty-five dollars.
Jasper had trouble reaching down to try them on. Walking to the regis-
ter, he got stuck between two T-shirt racks.

Fred also claimed he didn't know how to buy himself a bathing
suit, but in this case JoAnn pushed him. "We'll give you your money,
Freddy, and you can go into town," she said. He went off himself and
came back twenty minutes later.

"How'd it go Fred, everything all right?" asked Jasper.

Fred nodded nonchalantly. He was wearing sunglasses and a
windbreaker. A tall, dark, handsome, silent man, Fred appeared to be a
very hip individual. Some new women at the house always had a crush

on him. He showed JoAnn his bag. "These will be fine," JoAnn said. He'd bought shorts instead of a swimsuit. "You can wear underwear with them," she said. JoAnn never knew with Fred. She'd watch him fix a complicated gearshift system on the house's ten-speed bike and then she'd see him dusting the living room with Windex.

"Use Pledge, Fred."

"This Windex works good," said Fred.

"Dear, use the Pledge, trust me."

Several went to the Y pool regularly, including Eve, who'd competed on the Howard University swim team before her illness forced her to drop out. At dinner, Jasper would make a big deal about swimming. "I'm not eating more than three pork chops tonight," he'd announce. "I'm going swimming and I don't want to feel slouchy." He caught sight of Fred (six-one and 160 pounds) helping himself to a second chop: "Watch it, Fred you'll get slouchy."

Inevitably, after dinner, Jasper would seek out JoAnn. "Excuse me, Jo Ann, but have you seen my bathing suit?" He liked to talk about the pool with her. "There's only one lifeguard," he said. "What do you think would happen if three people are drowning at the same time?" He'd sit and wait patiently for a counselor to drive him over to the evening session. "I'm going to shower and soap myself all up," he said in the car. "It's nice there."

EVERYONE WAS in good spirits on the day of the weekly grocery shopping trip. There was plenty of snack food, cookies, soda, juices, green grapes, and fresh cold cuts in the house. A counselor and a resident would go to Finast supermarket together and then the whole house helped put away the two dozen bags, forming the grocery sack equivalent of a bucket brigade from the counselor's car into the house and down to the basement, where the frozen meats and bulk nonperishables were stored.

State guidelines permitted Melillo to spend about $325 a week on food for the house, which was deducted from the residents' monthly disability checks. To stretch the budget, four or five times a year JoAnn and another counselor, usually Jodie Schwartz, would make a half-hour drive to BJ's Wholesale Club in East Farmingdale, where they stocked up on giant economy sizes. There they could get a forty-five roll carton of toilet paper for $10.68, eighty ounces of iced tea mix for $3.99, and a one-and-a-quarter-pound bulk pack of Vienna fingers. JoAnn was very much the general on these expeditions, stopping to figure everything to the last penny. They went down one row, and Jodie put an $8.98 carton of sixty Glad trash bags into the carriage. They rolled on a little way and JoAnn lifted it out, replacing it with a carton of one hundred Iron Clads for $7.85. "Sorry," said Jodie. "I missed that." JoAnn was very coupon oriented, and with her $.50 off on Fig Newtons, $.40 on Gatorade, $.30 on Hunt's ketchup, she was usually able to keep the total under $300.

On shopping nights people felt a pressure to eat a lot of the new food, fearing they would not get their share and knowing popular items would disappear in a few days. While four of them sat around the dining room dealing a hand of spades one May night, they each had several cookies stacked on the table beside them, like poker chips.

Stan Gunter was visiting again. Since leaving the group home last year, he'd stopped back to say hello periodically, occasionally staying for dinner. His apartment was an easy walk away, just down the hill and across Brewster. Lately he seemed to be at 9 Highland more—this was his fourth night in a row. Everyone liked Stan; he was the easiest-going guy in the world and sensitive to the group home rules, formal and informal. When the regular Tuesday community meeting started Stan would leave—no outsiders were permitted, not even former residents. He understood, too, as a visitor to the house that on a shopping night, you do not take a cookie unless offered. When he came he played the piano or the guitar or both. Maureen particularly welcomed that—he was professionally trained, played beautifully, and it was good to have the TV off.

Still, she was starting to get a funny feeling—nothing she could put her finger on, but when a former resident like Stan stopped by so frequently it was sometimes a way of asking for help. At a staff meeting she suggested that the others keep an eye on him. If he continued to visit, they should probably make sure everything was all right. Of course, it might also just be that Stan had a crush on the lovely Paula Marsters, a bilingual counselor he often practiced his Spanish on during these visits.

Stan played some classical piano, then "Whiter Shade of Pale," "Ob-La-Di, Ob-La-Da" by the Beatles, "Nobody Knows the Trouble I've Seen," "Amazing Grace."

"I could listen all night," said Joe. "It's so restful." Joe was watching the spades game and trying to get them interested in a day trip he wanted to put together to Atlantic City, about a two-and-a-half hour drive away. "If we can get enough to fill a bus, it doesn't cost much, twenty to twenty-five dollars," he said. "I'm going to be announcing it at my pre-voc program. I know a lot of people will be signing up." No one seemed interested at the house, money was so tight.

Jasper overheard. "What's there to do in Atlantic City?" he asked Joe.

"Jasper!" said Joe. "Gambling. You can walk on the boardwalk, you can go to the beach, all for twenty-five dollars."

"How many days?" said Jasper.

"Seven days at Trump Taj Mahal for twenty-five dollars."

Jasper nodded. He'd think about it.

THE SPADES game went on quietly. Heather and her partner were winning by so much they could not contain their glee, and it was getting to Eve, so as so often happened at the house, she kicked the dog. "You can smell it out here," Eve said. "Someone should do something about it. They should make him clean it in there." Jasper's room was on the other side of the house from the dining room, but on these hot nights odor traveled.

"I can't take it, I can't take it," said Joe. "No wonder Stephen went to the hospital. Can you imagine being Jasper's roommate? He was asphyxiated. Poor guy got blown out of there. We need fumigation."

· · ·

THERE WASN'T much letup in Maureen's job. She was constantly juggling staff turnover, scheduling problems, a tight budget, and of course, crises among residents. The beauty of the house was its small scale, just nine full- and part-time staffers, so everyone knew each other well. For Maureen, staff supervision was never a serious problem. The drawback to the house also was its small scale; one counselor leaving or out sick could gum up everything. If you wanted to take your vacation you had to find another staffer to cover for you those weeks. It was bad enough that the state only allocated $16,640 a year for a counselor's job; but on top of that, to go hunting for a vacation replacement for your Saturday overnight shift was depressing.

Maureen lived with all the daily budget irritants of anyone running a government-funded program in this era. As summer approached she gave her annual electric-bill speech. The house did not have central air conditioning, but there were two box units downstairs, and a few residents—Heather, Fred, Joe—had their own units in their bedrooms. "Last year we used 18,397 kilowatt-hours of electricity," Maureen said, reading from an old bill. "That's 67 percent more than the average customer. We can't be blasting the air conditioning." She did not permit air conditioning during the day, and at night required that units be kept on the "energy saving" setting.

Her most immediate staff concern right now was replacing senior counselor JoAnn Mendrina, who would be leaving in a few weeks to move to Vermont with her husband. Maureen relied heavily on JoAnn. They meshed nicely. Maureen was relaxed and laid-back about domestic matters like chores and the house's appearance; JoAnn was fanatic about making sure chores were checked off and the house was clean. On the other hand, JoAnn had an authoritarian streak that was softened by Maureen. Most important, JoAnn was experienced—she was that rare older counselor in a field dominated by young people working for entry-level pay. She brought heart to the house, particularly to the sickest residents. Before 9 Highland, she'd worked with retarded adults. To her, people with severe schizophrenia like Jasper, Anthony, and Fred were high functioning. She watched out for them. It was JoAnn who made sure that each year on his birthday Jasper got his favorite food, a lobster. (She'd cook it for him.) When Heather went out to the doctor for her asthma, it was JoAnn who'd say, "Bundle up, sweetie, don't get in a draft." Maureen did not know where she'd find another JoAnn at a senior counselor's salary of twenty thousand dollars.

As for residents, Maureen rarely had a smooth stretch. As one improved, another veered downward. Heather appeared to be sinking. Twice in two weeks she'd handed in razor blades to the staff, the last time a whole pack's worth.

Anthony, on the other hand, seemed to Maureen to have bottomed out with the end of the school year, and survived his crisis without a hospitalization, a victory of sorts. He'd signed up for a library card in Glen Cove so he could check out psychology texts over the summer and get a jump on fall classes. Upping his meds had helped, although there were consequences. "Anthony's a little slower," Maureen told Linda Slezak. "But decrease the dosage, the voices get louder." She wanted to find him a male therapist to discuss the rage he felt for his mother, but state budget cuts kept Anthony on a waiting list for any therapist at all. The Melillo clinic staff told Maureen that the best they'd be able to do would be a female student-intern therapist. It made her angry. These were typically twenty-two-year-old kids in the first year of a master's program and were very green. Anthony would probably be the first schizophrenic the student intern met. "The stuff is coming out, it's coming up," said Maureen. "Anthony doesn't have the greatest impulse control. He's gone after a few people in the house and I'm afraid what might happen if no one's around." She lived in fear that the state's fiscal crisis would detonate at 9 Highland one day.

Maureen was also pressing to have Stephen DeRosa put on clozapine at Glen Cove Hospital. He would be the first clozapine patient there. "Medicaid is supposedly picking up clozapine this week," Maureen announced at each staff meeting for a month. In 1990, clozapine had gone from the trial stage to approval by the U.S. Food and Drug

Administration. It was now considered the best hope for people with severe schizophrenia who'd not found relief from other medications. Twenty-three states had cleared it for Medicaid reimbursement by 1991, but not New York, despite editorial support from papers like *The New York Times*. There'd been no great philosophical reason behind New York's opposition; it was simply a budget saver. Clozapine cost about five thousand dollars a year and without Medicaid reimbursement most people were shut out.

New York once had a reputation for being enlightened about such matters; now the bottom line ruled. It wasn't until the New York chapter of the National Alliance for the Mentally Ill, an advocacy group, sued, that New York finally agreed in principle to compensate Medicaid patients. The state would be one of the last to cover its use.

LINDA SLEZAK was pushing hard now to move Jasper out of the group home, and Maureen was ready to stand up to her boss *if* Jasper wanted to stay. Yet try as she might, Maureen could not read Jasper. Would he mind moving to a lower-functioning program? What if it was a big adult home where there was nothing to do? How would he feel about leaving his hometown of Glen Cove? Maureen asked him several times, and Jasper's answer was, "Maureen, if you think I should go, I should go." Maureen had other staff talk to Jasper, including Michael Perry, one of the black counselors at the house, whom Jasper felt quite close to. ("We're both men of color," Jasper would say.) Jasper told Mike, "Looks like I may be leaving," but when Mike Perry pressed Jasper about how he felt, the answer was the same: "If Maureen wants me to go, I'll go." Jasper trusted Maureen totally. It was a curse.

Maureen was quite clear on how Linda Slezak felt. At a recent meeting with the house managers, Linda discussed a state proposal to permit group homes to be permanent residences in some cases. The idea was to change the current model, which anticipated people leaving for a more independent setting after two years. Since a group home was as independent as some people could be, why shouldn't they be able to stay long-term? Why move them out just for the sake of moving? They all agreed the idea made sense. Maureen mentioned that Stephen DeRosa and Fred Grasso would probably fall into that permanent category. "Fred's good," said Maureen. "He gets something from the house."

"Maintaining is progress for these people," agreed Heidi Kominsky.

"They've just hit their plateau," said Maureen. "Even Jasper, if . . ."

"I don't know about Jasper," said Linda.

"I said, maybe, maybe . . ."

"I don't know about Jasper," Linda repeated. The longer this thing dragged on, the more Linda was convinced the group home was not for Jasper. When he first moved in, he did well, Linda felt, because he looked at it as a place to get better so he could go home. Now that he saw he wasn't going home—his mother wouldn't even visit anymore —he'd lost motivation. Plus, the illness had clearly worsened. Some very good people had tried and given up on Jasper, like Mike Long, director of North Shore Day Treatment, one of the best programs in the New York area. "He snored in group therapy," Long said. "He could barely make it to lunch each day. Some afternoons, I'd find him sleeping under a table in the back. Jasper has done a lot of drugs and who-knows-what. He's very sick." Long's verdict: "He's not going to make it."

Several residents hoped he'd leave. His cigarette bumming was worse. Even Fred, who would give anything to anyone, was tapped out from all the times Jasper had asked, "Can you advance me a pack until Friday?" His odor and hygiene were now an issue almost every week at community meetings. It was getting harder to placate the others.

"We need to do something," Joe said at that week's meeting.

"I used some Lysol in the hallway," said JoAnn, "and I'll hang an air freshener strip out . . ."

"That's not solving the problem," said Eve.

"It's not something that can be taken care of with spray," said another. "Something has to be done about Jasper's room."

In one of his many nervous gestures, Jasper rubbed his hands over his face; with his hygiene problems he was constantly giving himself eye infections. On nights when he cooked, Heather would not eat the food.

Jasper was a drain on the house. Just by sitting down clumsily, he'd bent a couple of kitchen chairs to the point where they were no longer usable. Two of his beds had collapsed. Linda Slezak had tried to get his county caseworker to get them funds for a special heavy-duty bed, but it had been over a year and they were still talking. So Jasper was sleeping on a mattress on the floor.

The house had spent more of its small miscellaneous cash fund on Jasper than on the other eleven residents combined.

Jasper embodied every resident's worst nightmare of mental illness. Many felt he was pulling them down by association, resented him and bullied him for it. Jasper and another resident, Richard, had both gone to Glen Cove High in the early 1980s. One afternoon, Jasper picked up Richard's high school yearbook, which had been left on the coffee table in the living room, and started leafing through the photo pages.

Richard walked back into the room, saw Jasper with it, and glared.

"I think my picture is in here," said Jasper.

"I looked," said Richard. "It's not."

"Really? For me?" said Jasper, continuing to browse.

"I told you, I checked," said Richard.

Jasper looked surprised, then got the hint. He delicately handed the yearbook over. Richard realized he'd been mean, and offered the book back. "You can look at it more," said Richard.

"It's OK," said Jasper. "You said I'm not in there."

JASPER BROUGHT out the protector in Maureen, but there was also a principle at stake. She felt the group home should be a diverse place, with people of all capabilities. The healthier residents would give Jasper something to strive for, and Jasper in turn would make them realize there were others worse off who needed their help. It was a way of teaching people to be more accepting. Maureen was angry about the attitude of some of the so-called high-functioning residents like Heather, who were so intolerant of Jasper. "Here are people," said Maureen, "who look at Jasper and say 'low-functioning' and yet they're cutting themselves and can't get out of bed in the morning for program—problems Jasper doesn't have."

Maureen felt staying in his hometown was important. Jasper had toured counselor Mike Perry around Glen Cove when Mike was new. He had taken him over to the projects and introduced his street friends who still hung out there. They'd treated Jasper respectfully. Maureen worried that if Jasper went to another program he might never get back, would quickly become a target for long-term hospitalization. One criterion for justifying long-term institutionalization was several short-term hospital stays in a year; Jasper had had two already in 1991 and the year wasn't half over yet.

There was one other factor driving Maureen that she did not speak about much: guilt. At the start of the year she had agreed to move one of the men, a severely ill schizophrenic, out of the house to a lower-functioning group home, where everyone was very sick. You didn't have to go to the program there if you didn't want, didn't have to do chores if you weren't up to it—didn't have to do anything. Now he often called, asking Maureen when he could come back to 9 Highland. She felt like she'd deserted him. She wasn't going to make the same mistake of shuffling Jasper off just so the agency's turnover record satisfied state auditors.

THE ONLY program Maureen and JoAnn could find that would take Jasper was a transitional skills residence thirty miles away, in the next county, on the grounds of Pilgrim State Hospital. One day in late spring, JoAnn drove him out for a look. Together they toured Building 70, where the program was located. JoAnn made polite conversation. She was surprised that they made residents sign in and sign out. The agency tour guide emphasized that even though this program was on the grounds of Pilgrim and in an old hospital building, clients were not hospitalized; this was community-oriented care aimed at strengthening independent living skills and returning people to society.

Afterward JoAnn drove Jasper around the hospital grounds. The two silently took in Pilgrim, an isolated, sprawling, brick complex that had once been the biggest mental institution in the world—ninety-two brick buildings holding sixteen thousand patients in the 1950s. Nine miles of underground tunnels connected the buildings so patients of that era could be moved about with minimal risk of escape. In its heyday, four hundred straitjackets were used a day.

Now most of the buildings were boarded up and in disrepair. Three decades of deinstitutionalization had reduced the patient population to sixteen hundred. The grounds were littered, the grass overgrown, an occasional poor soul walked head down along the buckling sidewalks. In spring, with all the windows open, you could hear the screams coming from the locked back wards.

JoAnn asked Jasper if he wanted to go for a cup of coffee.

"I don't have any money, Jo," said Jasper.

"I didn't ask you about money, I asked you if you wanted coffee." JoAnn was normally very strict about lending residents money. She believed that they had to learn how to make their ninety-dollar Social Security allowance last all month, even if it meant sacrificing. "My treat," she said.

JoAnn did not believe in letting her guard down with residents. She believed a staff member should keep a professional wall, let residents make their own judgments. "It reminded me of an Army barracks," JoAnn told Jasper. "I'm not impressed. It's very depressing."

They finished their coffees and Jasper said, "When you budget my money for me next month, Jo, make sure you take off this coffee."

JoAnn's mind was made up. As she told one of the other counselors, "I'm going to call Mrs. Slezak and make an appointment." She would not waste her time speaking with Linda's assistant. JoAnn's brother ran a Naval base in California, her husband was an ex-Marine, and JoAnn had the military wife's respect for the chain of command, but this was too big. "Mrs. Slezak knows me well enough, that if I bypass authority to go to the top, there's a reason."

Linda said, "Of course JoAnn, come on over." She had a good idea what was up from the nervousness in JoAnn's voice. JoAnn sat in Linda's small, stuffy office. "I realize this is what I'm being told to do," said JoAnn. "I realize that I'll be leaving in a few weeks, I'm just an observer, I'm not a decision maker and I have no right to override the director." And then JoAnn proceeded to make all the arguments for keeping Jasper. The one that struck Linda most was, "That other place is not good enough for our Jasper."

Linda still thought they were wrong, but by the time JoAnn had finished the speech, about all she could say was, "Thank you, JoAnn. You go back and tell Maureen you're off the hook." Linda loved the women that ran that house. If they were so determined for another shot at this 350-pound man who smelled like hell and did not himself appear to care, she could not tell them no.

JoAnn and Maureen started over with Jasper. They assigned him a primary counselor they felt he could relate to better, Robert Kouril, a very masculine type in his early twenties who liked weight lifting and cars and was new to the house. JoAnn explained to Robert about being very concrete with Jasper. "If he's doing his chores and he says, 'Give me a break, Jo,' I want to know how long. Then I go back to him and say the time's up and he'll say, 'OK Jo, I'm ready.' "

Maureen planned an all-out assault at cleaning up Jasper. "Jasper has to take a shower before he leaves the house and he has to take one when he gets back," she told staff at a Tuesday night meeting.

"When I was in the kitchen with Jasper, preparing the chicken," said Jodie Schwartz, "I thought I'd pass out."

"Last night I made sure he had the soap and baby powder," said Charles Winslow. Charles had opened the shower door and watched, to make sure Jasper cleaned himself everywhere.

"You have to," said Jodie. "He even smells when he comes out of the shower. I feel funny telling him to take a shower."

"It's worse to let him stink in front of his peers," said Maureen.

"Sometimes I feel like taking rubber gloves and washing him myself or disinfecting him," said Jodie.

"I think that's exactly what we have to do on the nights there's a male on duty," said Maureen. "You really have to get in and do it with him," she told Charles. "I used to do it with old ladies in the homeless shelter. You do it and you do it right and do it with dignity, they appreciate it. We'll broach it with him tomorrow."

"I don't think Jasper gets upset about it," said Charles, "and if he does, he doesn't show it."

"He doesn't show much," said Maureen. "But this has to be done with sensitivity."

JASPER GREETED all this news with a calm demeanor and his usual comment: "Whatever you say, Maureen." She never knew how much of an impression she was making, although that night after dinner he went into the living room, turned on the stereo, put on his headphones, and began sashaying around the room. As he danced his eyes were closed and he sang a little ditty they'd never heard before, "Doo, doo, doo, doo, take my meds . . . Doo doo, doo doo, soap it up . . . Doo, doo, doo, doo, socialize . . . Doo doo doo doo, watch TV."

chapter 10

SOMETIMES IN LIFE,
YOU HAVE TO MAKE SACRIFICES

STAN GUNTER WAS visiting the house five or six days a week now, and Maureen suggested it was time for Jodie Schwartz to take him aside to make sure nothing was wrong. Jodie had been his primary counselor when he lived at 9 Highland and knew him well. After he finished off a set of a dozen songs at the piano with "Georgia on My Mind," Jodie called him into the office. She didn't want to say, "Why are you coming so much?"—too insulting. "How you doing, Stan?" Jodie asked.

Stan said he hadn't been feeling well, his medication was causing him anxiety, but the doctor had changed it and he was fine now.

Jodie asked if it made him feel better to come to the house.

He said his apartment was lonely since one of his two roommates was hospitalized. He enjoyed having an audience to play for at the house, he said, plus he was trying to learn Spanish—Stan already spoke French, Italian, and Danish—and it was fun to practice with Jasper and Paula Marsters.

The group home staff was concerned that Stan had a crush on Paula. Most males at the house did at one time or other. He was seeking her out, suggesting they go for coffee, and acting slighted when she wasn't more responsive. At times in his past, Stan had been obsessive. Jodie asked if everything was all right with his fianceé Jenny. "You know how it is when you've been seeing someone for four years," Stan said. "You can get in a rut." Stan and Jenny had met at day treatment program. She was quite shy and he'd won her over by making her a cup of herbal tea with the bags he carried in his shirt pocket. They'd lived in nearby group homes at first and now both had supervised apartments in Glen Cove. Lately Jenny had been mentioning marriage a lot. They were in their late thirties and she wanted kids. Stan didn't feel he could be much of a guide for children since he was still looking for the answers himself.

"Do you have your eye on someone else?" Jodie asked.

"No," said Stan, "but I'm trying to do different things."

"Are you still engaged?" Jodie asked.

"Oh, yeah," said Stan.

"Well, that's great," said Jodie.

"Yeah," said Stan.

She took one last shot. "I'm glad everything's OK with your meds now. And you're feeling well . . ."

"Yeah," said Stan.

JODIE TOLD Maureen, but had no confidence that Stan was being honest. In the two years they'd known each other, Jodie had learned how private he was. He would tell you his history, discuss past breakdowns, talk until two in the morning about Beethoven and Mozart, but he would not say how he was really feeling *now*. You found out the truth after the fact. Though he appeared quiet and gentle, he had a fierce will. He would yes her to death and then do what he pleased. Stan had a way of answering questions that stopped you from asking more.

Jodie was quite sure she wasn't getting the whole story, but she got that feeling a dozen times a week at the group home. You could only do so much. Stan wasn't in the group home anymore and had a good deal of support—a therapist and counselors who visited him seven days a week at his supervised apartment. Jodie had no standing to pry further.

As it turned out, her instinct was right. Stan had been lying to her. It wasn't the first time. But the consequences would be disastrous this time.

STAN WAS viewed as one of the group home success stories. In 1990, when Linda Slezak was battling the East Hills community to open the Melillo agency's third house, *Newsday* did a human interest article on group homes, accompanied by a photo of Stan at the piano. When the Glen Cove *Record-Pilot* finally wrote a positive piece about 9 Highland, it featured Stan and Jenny prominently.

He'd always liked the group home, found it "comfortable," "cozy," "homey." "In a way it was like a miracle for me," he'd said. "I was stuck in my parents' house and applied and they said you can live here." Stan was of the house's most creative cooks, sometimes spending two hours preparing an original vegetarian dish complete with "secret spices" from the local health food store. He landed an impressive job with an optical company. Using his French, he handled consumer complaints from clients in Canada. He was also a ham radio operator, and kept his equipment at the group home and later at the apartment. He gave guitar lessons to people at his day treatment program.

Stan took advantage of living in Glen Cove, first at the group home and now in the nearby apartment. Opponents of 9 Highland had once argued that a new business development planned for downtown would overwhelm the mentally ill and that was another reason not to open the house. Stan was a regular customer at the nicest restaurant in that new downtown development, Avanti Pizza. He became a friend of the owner. They'd chat together in Italian. The owner was so fond of Stan, a few times the man refused to let him pay for dinner.

Stan was a bit the artistic bohemian. He'd lived in Greenwich Village a few years, and had a knack for finding the bits of that life scattered through suburbia. Recently he'd made friends with people who ran a little Spanish café in Glen Cove. Several nights in May Stan played guitar there, trying out his Spanish, drinking coffee with the owners until 2 A.M. "That's the way to learn a language," he told Jenny. "It's like jumping in a pool when the water's cold, when you break through that ice."

That was Stan at his best. But there was another, less promising side. He was fired from his job at the optical company after six months. The pressure was too much. At first he'd leave after lunch without telling anyone, and later called in sick several days in a row. Since then he had resisted efforts, first by Jodie at the group home and then by the counselor at the apartment, to help find him another job or a day program. He always had an excuse. Lately he'd been volunteering a few hours each afternoon at a nursing home in town. Counselors felt it would be healthier for Stan to be more occupied, but he resisted.

His diagnosis was "schizo-affective," a fuzzy label applied to people who at times have schizophrenia's symptoms, at times the symptoms of manic-depression, but who can also go for long stretches without problems. The illness had surfaced late, when Stan was in his mid-twenties. Until then, he'd been the most artistic, outgoing child in a very dynamic family of six. Growing up, Stan had lived all over Europe. His father had an impressive career as an engineer, holding top positions with companies in New York, London, Paris, and Denmark.

There was often friction between Stan and his father. Mr. Gunter is a big, domineering man with a first-rate mind who had the engineer's confidence that any problem could be solved. Stan viewed life as less rational and controllable and at times felt overpowered by his dad. They had clashed repeatedly over Stan's choice of a career in music. Mr. Gunter felt it was impractical.

But Stan also described his childhood as happy and exciting. His mother, an intelligent woman with a gentle manner, knew how to soften her husband's rougher edges. The children were exposed to classical music and art and all sorts of sports. The family sailed together, around the Mediterranean and the Caribbean. There was no reason to believe Stan wouldn't be as successful as his two younger brothers, who became computer specialists, and his sister, a Wall Street executive. Of the four, Stan was the most aggressive about mixing in where he lived. When he was fifteen, he had an eighteen-year-old girlfriend in Paris and played in a rock band there. He taught himself Danish by sitting in bed at night with a dictionary, translating Hans Christian Andersen's works. ("Andersen was a perfect teacher," Stan would say. "He wrote in simple language, but expressed great things.") Stan was the son who'd learned to swim by jumping in over his head in the pool. As a boy he would enter a room and announce, "Here I am." At thirteen he begged his parents for a motorbike. When they told him he was too young, he found a junked one and fixed it up himself.

Music was his passion. A framed picture of Beethoven hung in the kitchen of his Glen Cove apartment and a Beethoven symphony, concerto, or string quartet was likely to be playing on the stereo. Stan composed both classical and folk-style music. His folk songs were full of humor, with titles like "Speed Queen Henry," inspired by an old man he'd met at a laundromat. After graduating from a state college he was accepted by an impressive music academy in England, the Royal College of Music. Stan had talent, but in England it soon became clear he wasn't talented enough for his dream—to be a concert pianist and classical composer. Others would have settled for being a high school music teacher. Not Stan. A professor at the academy said that to succeed you must work night and day, even if it meant going without sleep or food, and Stan took him literally. He grew obsessed, turning himself into a zombie. When he suffered his first breakdown at twenty-four, he was thin to the point of being emaciated, and exhausted. He'd stopped eating and sleeping. In the fifteen years since, he'd been up and down, bouncing from jobs to hospitals to a brief failed marriage to his parents' beautiful antique-filled home on the Gold Coast of Long Island.

The Gunters had read extensively about schizophrenia and attributed the illness to genetics plus stress. Stan's aunt—his father's sister —had schizophrenia. The genetic odds in such a situation are one in ten. As Stan's father said, "The numbers are right; there are about ten nieces and nephews. The statistics are very clear." The father was particularly hard on himself for not recognizing it earlier and for failing to help his son reduce the pressure in his life. He was convinced that if Stan had set more modest goals, the schizophrenia never would have surfaced.

Stan's stay at the group home and apartment was the most stable he'd been in a long while.

OTHERS WERE noticing that he didn't seem himself lately. Dom Constantine, Anthony's father, spotted it during a Sunday visit to the house in late May. Stan had "that faraway look" and was talking a lot about religion. "After a while you get to recognize the signs," Dom would say later.

Stan was slow to respond to questions. Anthony asked Stan to teach him guitar. "I could pay you maybe fifteen dollars, and you could give me lessons," Anthony said. "I could come over to your apartment."

Stan looked right at Anthony but did not answer.

"Like maybe now you could give me the number?" said Anthony.

"Yeah, I could do that." Anthony stared at him. Slowly, Stan recited his phone number, pausing at each digit.

"You live in the Glen Cove Arms Apartments?" said Anthony.

". . . Yeah . . . yeah . . ."

"So we could do it next week? A couple weeks?"

". . . Yeah."

"I'll call you? Or you call me?"

". . . Yeah."

Joe from the group home was seeing Stan a good deal. They went to the Spanish restaurant and over to Stan's to watch cable TV. For the first month, as an introductory special, Stan and his roommates were getting all fifty stations for the basic fee. The Playboy channel was Joe's particular favorite. Joe watched Playboy and Stan discussed his religious ideas. He respected Joe—Joe kept his own Kosher food at the group home. Stan casually mentioned one evening that he'd seen Jesus Christ sitting in the apartment, talking to him.

"Are you sure?" Joe asked.

Stan said, "Yeah, he's talking to me." Stan was surprised that everyone couldn't hear him.

Joe did not believe in intruding, but one of the apartment roommates was alarmed. The roommate had been released from the hospital after several weeks, and was struck by how much Stan had deteriorated in that time. Stan admitted to his roommate that he was hearing voices. On four different occasions, the roommate told the counselor who visited their apartment daily that Stan wasn't doing well, wasn't talking to them and admitted to hearing voices.

An apartment counselor does not know her clients the way the group home staff does. The program is designed for more independent living. The assumption is that the person is healthier and needs less professional support. Every evening the counselor comes to the apartment for a half hour or hour to talk, make sure everyone is coping, and arbitrate any disputes between roommates. At a group home, staff observes twenty-four hours a day and troublesome behavior is usually picked up quickly. In an apartment program, a person's problems would be harder to detect, especially if he did not wish to reveal himself.

Stan's apartment counselor worked for Long Island Jewish Hospital's independent living program and visited three or four other apartments each evening. She reported Stan's condition to her director, Steve Ronik, who oversaw the 64-client program. Ronik would later say that hearing voices isn't in itself that alarming, that Stan had given no indication recently of being violent to others or himself. Ronik happened to see Stan at an agency get-together that last week of May. Though Stan seemed quieter and more reserved, Ronik noted that he was still functioning and fulfilling his responsibilities.

Ronik and the other Long Island Jewish officials weren't alarmed enough to press for a hospitalization on their own. But they were concerned about Stan's deterioration, and during the last two weeks of May made four extra calls to Stan's therapist. They felt if Stan needed a hospitalization, the therapist would pick it up.

Until very recently Stan had been seeing a highly experienced therapist, Dr. Jo Rieben, a psychiatrist. For five years they'd met weekly.

Dr. Rieben was that rare psychiatrist in the mental health system who would do more than just prescribe medication for a chronically ill person with schizophrenia. Most psychiatrists prefer treating the worried well; it's considered more satisfying and hopeful and is far more lucrative. Dr. Rieben had a commitment to serving the chronically ill. She'd chosen to do her residency at Bellevue Hospital, spending four years there working with the sickest mental patients from New York City's streets. A decade later she was still caring for the chronically ill at a day treatment program at Queens Hospital. Dr. Rieben talked to Stan about his relationship with his father and his music, about coping and feelings of depression. Stan told Maureen and Linda Slezak how much Dr. Rieben meant to him: "Dr. Rieben doesn't talk about meds too much, she's not a complete medication freak," he said. "When you're there, she's on a personal level trying to help you with everyday practical things." She made Stan feel human. Sometimes they'd just go out for a cup of coffee to chat, like friends. She had copies of his music tapes at home and enjoyed playing them. Dr. Rieben saw him for the Medicaid rate, twenty dollars a session. Privately insured patients paid seven times that rate. During Stan's whole time at the group home, Dr. Rieben was his therapist. Stan was generally open with her and when he did conceal, she was good about picking it up, she'd known him so long. She'd learned the hard way. In 1987, before they knew each other well, Stan had taken an overdose of pills mixed with wine. She'd recorded this suicide attempt on Stan's original referral records that were sent in 1990 to the Long Island Jewish apartment program.

As she got to know him better, Dr. Rieben learned from Stan that voices had commanded him to kill himself that time and the only way he could quiet them down was by getting himself drunk. Since then, the psychiatrist had kept a careful tab on the voices, questioning Stan regularly.

But when he entered the Long Island Jewish apartment program, Stan was told he would have to find a new therapist. Steven Ronik said that Long Island Jewish Hospital officials wanted all their apartment residents to have a therapist associated with their hospital's clinic or a clinic that had a reciprocal agreement with Long Island Jewish. This angered Linda Slezak, who argued the point with Ronik and lost. The Nassau Support and Advocacy Center, activists on mental health issues, had also written letters of complaint in previous years to Long Island Jewish and the state protesting the policy. As long as the therapist was licensed and certified, why couldn't a person like Stan see whomever he preferred? Dr. Rieben wrote a letter to Long Island Jewish, saying she wanted to keep Stan as a patient and would be responsive to the apartment program's needs. "Switching therapists at this time would adversely affect his continuity of care," she had written. "I am hereby requesting that an exception be made in this case so that Stan and I can continue our work with one another." She pointed out that she was affiliated with Long Island Jewish Hospital and had admission privileges there.

Still Ronik was adamant. To Linda and Maureen it was a crazy, inflexible policy. Until the very day Stan moved from the group home to the apartment, they were stalemated. At the last minute a compromise was worked out that pleased no one and seemed absurd. Stan could not see Dr. Rieben. But since he was living in Glen Cove in the apartment, and since Long Island Jewish's clinic was on the other side of the county, he would be allowed by Ronik to see a therapist at the Melillo clinic in Glen Cove. Long Island Jewish officials said they knew and trusted the Melillo clinic. Mr. and Mrs. Gunter were skeptical about the arrangement, but Stan so wanted to advance to an apartment program, they agreed. Their grown son resented if they interfered too much in his matters. Stan dropped the psychiatrist he knew so well and started over at the clinic with two people he would never get close to. One was a psychopharmacologist, a doctor who specialized in medication. The man saw Stan once a month for a few minutes to check on whether there was any need to alter medication. Stan's main therapy was provided on a weekly basis by Joanna Mandel, an unpaid student intern getting her master's degree. She was one of the half-dozen inexperienced student interns the clinic relied on as a means of coping with budget cuts.

To satisfy the apartment program's policy, Stan was forced to trade a forty-one-year-old medical doctor who got her psychiatry training at New York University, one of the finer programs in America, for a master's degree candidate at a local school.

Stan had finally reached the point in therapy where he talked to Dr. Rieben about the voices. He did not tell his student-intern therapist. "We never got around to it," Stan said.

A T T H E S A M E time Stan was preoccupied and faraway, when he did speak he was more opinionated and angrier. He was frustrated when he tried talking to Jasper in Spanish at the group home, and Jasper was so busy hallucinating he didn't respond. Stan blamed the group home for not doing enough for Jasper. "They should try harder with Jasper."

He was critical of Paula Marsters for being too distant with residents. "There are some counselors, they stereotype residents. The counselors feel they know what's right and that's not always the case. They're too aloof. They should tell you a little bit about their own lives. I've tried to talk more with Paula recently, but she said there are certain rules and they're not allowed to break rules, they have to keep a distance. If you took her out of the setting, she has a nice smile, she'd be nice. Certain counselors, they keep the office door closed too much. I had a book of flamenco guitar music in Spanish. Paula was there on duty and not doing anything. I said, 'Can you help me with the Spanish?' She acted as if it was a big pain in the butt. I got discouraged, you know?"

T H E L A S T W E E K of May was the beginning of a record hot summer on Long Island. Every day that week was sunny, humid, and in the mid-nineties, twenty degrees above normal—sticky, miserable weather. Even the occasional thunderstorms did not break the heat. On May 28, when a visitor arrived at the apartment around noon, Stan was home alone, sitting on the couch, soaked in sweat. His face was flushed pink, his forehead glistened, his hair was so wet you could see through to his scalp. Large circles of perspiration showed through the front and back of his shirt and stained his pants at the thighs and knees. The apartment was baking. When asked, Stan said the air conditioners weren't working right. It did not occur to him to open the windows. After it was suggested, he said, "Maybe I ought to open a window." He spoke like a 45-speed record on 33, then stood slowly and opened the sliding glass door leading from the living room out to the balcony. If he wanted to escape the heat, Morgan Park, a gorgeous town beach, was just a five-minute drive away, on Long Island Sound. "It would be too hot," Stan said. To get a little relief, Stan and his guest sat on the balcony overlooking the parking lot, surrounded by Stan's ham radio antenna and wires.

Stan offered little, although twice in twenty minutes he mentioned he was going to give Anthony guitar lessons. He said that he'd been having trouble sleeping and would get up in the middle of the night to work on his music. Stan kept his Casio PMP-600 electronic keyboard in the apartment and could plug in earphones so there was no noise to disturb his roommates.

He briefly grew animated when he played a couple of sweet pieces he'd written, one called "Jenny's Song," for his girlfriend; another "Thank God We're Alive." "Listen," he said, "you'll feel like you're in heaven."

These visits usually lasted a couple of hours, but keeping anything going was so difficult, this one ended after an hour. At 1:30 he volunteered at the nursing home. On the car radio the newscaster was saying they were forecasting at least three more days of record heat, with scattered thunderstorms.

THERE WERE many hints of what was to come, if you were looking for them. He talked about how, in the past, he had stopped taking his medication because it interfered with his creativity. "I didn't like the idea of medication. I kept thinking about God. The thing that bothered me, it appeared your mind was not just a bodily organ—your soul was in there and taking medication would affect your soul, too. It would upset God. It didn't seem the right thing to do. I've been disturbed about that." But was he disturbed enough to stop taking his meds now? "No, no," he answered.

Another time he mentioned how the meds flattened him out so he didn't feel his sharpest. But when asked if the side effects were bothering him now, he answered. "Oh no, no."

He was feeling creative again, he explained another day. "I used to sit at the keyboard and feel tense. Now I say, 'Don't worry about it.' My brain—I could feel the rust in the wells of my brain starting to move. It starts coming together. I'm writing this piece now, I was worried it sounded a little bit like Mozart, but then I thought, What the hell, man, so what if it sounds like Mozart a little bit, so what if it's archaic? This is something my parents never understood. So what if I don't sound like Billy Joel? It's me. I've come to accept it. I think one of the most important things in life is happiness. Life is simple, really, all you have to do is figure out how to be happy."

Stan told no one, but during the second week of May he had stopped taking his medication, Narvane, an antipsychotic. The meds left him drowsy in the morning and he also felt they undermined his creativity.

H E D I D N ' T like to discuss the voices. He'd been let in on something special and was supposed to keep it secret. The difficult part was trying to concentrate on the important messages from the voices and at the same time listen to what the people around him were saying. It exhausted Stan. The solution was just spending more time alone so he could devote all his energy to the voices. They were more exciting anyway.

On May 30 he was startled awake at around 3 A.M. by a deep voice commanding, "Get up! Get up!" He went into the living room, put on his earphones, and began composing. He worked for a couple of hours, then went back to bed. He was pleased. He was doing some great music. Being off the meds really helped. When he woke, it was like he'd written the song in a dream. A lot of the time lately he'd felt like he was in a dream.

He'd been hearing a high-pitched voice, a woman's voice, and wasn't sure who it was. One afternoon while volunteering at the nursing home, he accompanied the elderly residents to a mass there. He happened to look up at Jesus on the cross, and suddenly the high-pitched woman's voice said, "It's me, it's me!" That's how he knew it was Jesus. Stan was beginning to put things together. This high voice he'd been hearing for so long was Jesus. It was making sense now.

The deep voice that woke him—that had to be God the Father. Stan had been listening to "Nights in the Garden of Spain" that hot sticky morning at the end of May. He got it in his head that he and Jesus were supposed to protect the garden. Stan was on a horse with a sword—it was like a dream, but it was much more real, he could see it far more clearly than you see a dream, he really was on the horse. He was riding alongside Jesus and together they were protecting the garden. They weren't supposed to let anyone into the garden.

Jesus confided in him that the Father was a bad God. Stan believed him. It was amazing how things were coming together. God said he wanted to come into the garden. Jesus said, "No, we don't want to let him in." Stan was on the horse guarding the garden. His orders were clear: he was not to let God in.

Stan realized he had been let in on something of considerable magnitude: Jesus and God were at odds with each other.

Stan took a break and began practicing the guitar. He wasn't depressed. He felt good and loved having the apartment to himself at times like this. God and Jesus were encouraging him to practice. Then they said he'd been so good, they would show him Heaven! All Stan's hard work was paying off. So they lifted the apartment building into heaven—not just Stan's apartment, number 21—the whole building.

There was light all around. The sky was an extraordinary blue, dazzling over the clouds. Plainly this was Heaven. Stan asked God about meeting Beethoven. In an instant Beethoven was walking toward him saying, "Play something, son." Stan started playing a piece he'd composed himself, "Return to the Garden," but stopped in the middle. He couldn't remember all the chords. Then God said in a deep voice, "He's weak! He has this mental disease. Your brain is defective." God was very angry and told Stan he shouldn't smoke anymore. Some time passed; Stan became preoccupied and lit up a cigarette. God was enraged.

And this is where it started getting tricky. Jesus said, "Let's call up the Exchange." Stan didn't know what that was, but he could tell from the tone of the voice, it meant trouble. Then he realized God and Jesus were talking about releasing energy at each other and causing the universe to explode. Stan was right in the middle of the conflict. It was a hell of a mess. Why did Stan have to be singled out? It made so much sense, though—the Exchange—it was like nuclear war. One side fires and the other fires back. The Exchange was big. Stan was afraid of this thing the Exchange. At one point when Stan really thought they'd do it—call the Exchange—he heard a thunderclap in the distance. Stan thought, Oh shit, it's starting. It was so clear, the Exchange was nuclear war. There'd be nothing left.

Then God told Stan he had to jump to save the world. If he didn't everyone would perish. Be blown up. Stan thought about Jenny and his family, and himself. And he weighed that against the whole world's destruction. Sometimes in life you have to make sacrifices for a greater cause. He wanted so badly to make everything all right. Stan opened the sliding door and stepped out onto the balcony, past all his ham radio equipment. He normally didn't like heights, but the Exchange erased his fear. He climbed up onto one of the vinyl chairs.

AT 1:01 P.M. on Thursday, May 30, City of Glen Cove patrolman Steve Vetrone got a call on his car radio: Man lying on the ground in parking lot of Glen Arms Apartments. The patrol car pulled up about thirty seconds later. Vetrone didn't know if it was some homeless character or what, but when he got close, he saw how serious the situation was. The guy was bleeding all over. Fluid from his brain was coming out the ears. Officer Vetrone thought the subject was dead, but was startled to see him stir. He immediately radioed for the rescue squad, a code 3 emergency—lights, sirens, the works. "This one's real bad," Vetrone, a six-year veteran, said over the radio. The body was in a heap, the clothes skewed all around. Nose was split down the middle, eyeglasses had cut his brow. Blood covered his forehead. The legs were twisted in all the wrong places; the left one seemed pretty much destroyed. He had black-and-blue marks everywhere and Vetrone could tell from the crazy way the hip was turned, it had snapped. The left ankle bone was sticking through the skin a couple of inches.

The man was moaning. He tried to lift himself up and when Vetrone told him to relax, help was coming, he weakly attempted to fight off the patrolman. Clearly the subject was in shock. As Vetrone worked to keep him calm and still, a woman came over and said she had seen him. Maria Olabado, a downstairs neighbor, happened to be looking out her living room window when she saw something hurtle past. She'd called the building superintendent, who called the police.

The emergency medical squad is located just a few blocks away at the firehouse on Brewster, and arrived at 1:08 P.M. They wrapped him in one of those high-pressured "M.A.S.H. suits," developed during the Vietnam war to keep wounded soldiers from bleeding to death. At 1:20, siren wailing, the ambulance raced toward North Shore University Hospital.

Detectives from the Glen Cove Police and then Nassau County arrived to work the scene. They entered the empty apartment four floors up and were struck immediately by the stifling heat. There was no air conditioning, no windows open except the sliding door. They found footprints on one of the vinyl chairs on the balcony. Glen Cove Police Sergeant Robert Kormoski's initial impression was that the man had been working on his ham radio antenna, lost his balance, and fell.

Detective Frank Mauro of the Nassau County Police looked for a suicide note, but found none. On a table near the keyboard he did recover a recent letter informing Stan that one of his close friends from college days had died. Detective Mauro saw this as evidence that Stan may have been depressed.

They took measurements. The body had fallen thirty-five feet and hit the parking lot thirteen feet out from the edge of the balcony. "The distance from the building leads you to go for a jump," said Detective Mauro. At the point of first impact, a long, heavy railroad tie supported a grass berm at the edge of the parking lot. Stan had hit with such force, he'd chipped the railroad tie on his way down.

Police used yellow chalk to outline the spot where the body had landed. "Not your typical body outline," Detective Mauro remarked. It looked more like a circle than anything with arms and legs.

H O S P I T A L E M E R G E N C Y room surgeons pumped him full of intravenous fluids and blood immediately and the anesthesiologist put a tube through his mouth and into his windpipe to control his breathing. His blood pressure was very low—it had almost fallen off the charts: 50/30. He was in shock. They took X rays of his neck, chest, and pelvis, and a CAT scan of his brain. Doctors checked the fluid from his abdomen for signs of internal bleeding and that test came back negative. They put in a brain monitor—basically a bolt screwed into his skull to keep track of blood flow and swelling.

Then they did an arteriogram, a dye study to see if there were any ruptures of major arteries. In about 95 percent of jumps and crashes of this magnitude—or "deceleration injuries," as they're called in the medical textbooks—the heart's aorta is damaged. There is a ligament that holds the aorta in place that is positioned in such a way that it is vulnerable to being ripped from the body wall. It is a structural weakness in the human heart that emergency room doctors know too well.

A plastic surgeon worked on the nose, which had split down the middle and "butterflied." Through the wound they could see the back of his throat. They were concerned about infection spreading from the nasal area to the base of the brain. It required stitching on several different levels.

When the arteriogram came back it showed a laceration of the aorta, the major artery leaving the heart. The aorta carries the blood to the body's limbs and most of the organs. A hole there means that instead of blood reaching the arms, legs, kidneys, liver, it spills uselessly through the torn aorta into the body cavity. Before long, a person bleeds to death. In emergency rooms, where time is so precious, everything gets reckoned in percentages. With a ruptured aorta, 50 percent die at the scene; 90 percent die soon after; 95 percent die if it is not surgically repaired within twenty-four hours.

The surgical team was split on what to do about Stan Gunter. A couple wanted to operate on the aorta immediately. A couple felt he wouldn't survive such an operation and the general anesthetic that went with it. The senior surgeons decided to let him rest until morning. They were quite sure he would not make it through the night. Stan's parents were informed it was extremely bleak. In medical lingo, he was not viable.

THE NEWS traveled quickly. Within an hour Maureen heard and told the group home staff. JoAnn called a special house meeting that evening without giving a reason. Everyone was griping—people wanted to know why they had to have a meeting when it wasn't Tuesday.

Maureen said she knew many residents were close to Stan and explained that he'd had a bad accident. "He either fell out of a window or jumped out of a window," she said. "It was either suicide or he fell." The room grew eerily quiet. JoAnn and Maureen had positioned themselves so that between the two of them they could see everyone's face. "We know it's a serious injury, we don't know how serious."

Maureen glanced around for anyone who wanted to talk.

"I don't think Stan would jump, you know?" said Jasper. "He's been in too good a mood. We been talking a lot of Spanish. I think he was pushed."

Anthony kept clenching and opening his fist. "Stan was going to give me guitar lessons," said Anthony. "We're good friends now. We're really good friends." Later, JoAnn told Anthony he shouldn't feel guilty about the time he'd shoved Stan around. "You think he forgave me, Jo?" Anthony asked.

"I know he did," said JoAnn.

"I suppose when he's well enough," said another, "he'll go into the psych unit."

"This is not the time . . . ," Maureen said.

JoAnn tried to get Fred Grasso to say something, but twice he didn't respond. Finally he said, "I feel very sorry. I hope he never does it again." Fred was hugging a pillow.

That night both Maureen and JoAnn stayed late. Heather barely knew Stan, but said she was very upset and depressed by the news, plus the windshield wipers on her car weren't working and her closest friend was being held in constraints on 3-West at Glen Cove Hospital. Heather kept asking Donna Rubin and Paula Marsters if she cut herself would she automatically be rehospitalized. She said a rosary for Stan.

Anthony wrote a letter and brought it into the office to show JoAnn. He wished Stan the best luck in the whole world and said he knew God would take care of him. Every other sentence was underlined for emphasis. He told JoAnn that on Sunday, when his father Dom came, he'd like to visit Stan at the hospital.

Staff talked about it among themselves. "It's hard to know," said Maureen. "If Stan seemed out of it, it might not have been suicide. He might have been working on the antenna. He was always fiddling with gadgets; he might have got dizzy in the heat and fallen."

"They're leaning toward him jumping," said Debbie Dombrowski, manager of the Glen Head house. "If he'd fallen he would have hit the balcony below. But he landed fifteen feet from the building . . ."

"I wonder if they can tell," said Linda Slezak.

"They can tell," said Debbie. "I have a friend in forensics. It's like a science. They measure everything, all the angles. If you fall you don't go out fifteen feet."

ON A DAY when *Newsday*'s two lead stories were about county workers being put on furlough because of budget cuts, and William Kennedy Smith looking the judge in the eye in Palm Beach and pleading not guilty, an inside story on Stan appeared under the headline MAN FALLS 4 STORIES. It said police had ruled out foul play "but were still trying to determine how Gunter fell," and gave a number to call for anyone with information.

. . .

JENNY, Stan's girlfriend, was devastated. When they broke the news to her, both Stan's family and counselors were vague about Stan's condition. As a precaution, she left her supervised apartment and spent a few nights at the Melillo group home in Glen Head, where she used to live. Staff could watch her closely there. People kept telling her they knew Stan would be fine. Jenny was sure God would take care of him.

Several years back she'd had a boyfriend who'd killed himself.

IT HIT TWO others hard. Joe, the current group home resident closest to Stan, had tears in his eyes when told. He figured Stan was depressed about his apartment. "He told me he didn't like it, he wanted to get an apartment with me," Joe confided. "He said he wanted to move out in the worst way, he felt confined, cramped. He was a warm person. He had a good heart. I figured he'd get married to Jenny. He said, 'Joe, I can't work. I don't know what I'll do. How could we support ourselves?'

"My opinion—I think he attempted suicide. He lost all hope, I guess. He didn't sound depressed, but I guess he was. There was no way out of there. He didn't like the living conditions. The main thing I remember, he wanted to get out. He said, 'Joe, I'll get an apartment with you.' I said, 'right, who'll pay for it?' He said, 'My parents will pay.' I couldn't do that, man.

"I hope he comes out of it. It happened to someone in my family. He was in a coma six months. I said, 'Let my brother die in peace with God's help.' I used to go and cry for my brother and that's why I can't visit Stan now. My brother has schizophrenia, he jumped from the fourth floor at Pilgrim. With Stan it's like living it all over again. These people, they don't understand. They say he'll be fine. He fell on his head on concrete. This girl at day program said, 'Joe, you're a friend, but you're chicken, you won't visit him.' I can't take it. I could have a nervous breakdown. It'd break my heart. Most people don't realize he could be lying in a respirator with casts all over his body."

· · ·

JULIE CALLAHAN was shocked, too. She and Stan had moved into 9 Highland at the same time. They were the two night owls, sitting up watching some awful movie together until 1 A.M. He'd be in the big soft chair, Julie would be on the couch, and if she got tired she'd just curl up and go to sleep. She felt comfortable with him. The thing she liked about Stan was he respected your privacy. He never asked leading questions about what was wrong with her. He was so musical and yet he was patient when they played together and kind about her ability. She was planning to phone him to arrange some lessons when she heard the news. She hadn't understood how serious it was. Then she called again to get the visiting hours and they said he was in intensive care and she was heartsick.

Julie was competitive with Stan. He was always being held up as the group home success. Stan had the good job, Stan had the fiancée, Stan had the car, Stan had the talent. They'd both graduated from the group home about the same time, in the fall of 1990, anxious to be out before the two-year mark.

Now Julie was the supposed success story. Julie had the good job, Julie had the car, Julie had her own apartment. And Julie had a great fear. The more she moved away from the mental health system and on her own, the more she dreaded discovery and public humiliation. Stan's terrible fall reminded her how quickly it could happen. She hated when people called her a success because she realized it was so fragile. She was managing the multiple personalities, but she could not control them. The ordinary suburban life she was trying to build might be stripped naked at any moment. Literally. How many times had she woken to find herself walking some strange suburban street in the rain, late at night, with no shoes? Or worse, wearing nothing but a raincoat? Or worst of all, in bed with a man she did not know? Understanding it did not protect her. She had learned how vulnerable she was at the end of the summer of 1989, at the group home, just as she began to accept that she had this strange multiple personality disorder.

Her others appeared one night for everyone to see.

chapter 11

JULIE,
SUMMER/FALL/WINTER 1989

TWO SUMMERS before, in 1989, during her first year at the group home, Julie Callahan had seemed a highly unlikely candidate for a success story. On August 17, 1989, she was discharged from Glen Cove Hospital's 3-West. It was her second hospitalization that summer, her fifth in three years. She'd just turned twenty-one and had spent thirty of the last thirty-nine months on psychiatric wards. At discharge, the hospital psychiatrist noted that Julie needed long-term treatment for her multiple personality disorder, though no specialist had been located yet. On her exit assessment, her prognosis was listed as "extremely guarded."

Julie looked terrific. A lot of that was getting off the meds. She was no longer being doped into a stupor. The stay on 3-West was a turning point in one respect: they'd stopped labeling her schizophrenic. It meant the hospital psychiatrists had no easy justification to medicate her, and though they still tried, this time she was able to resist them. Dr. Melamed, the chief of staff on 3-West, could see that the antipsychotic that had been prescribed, Trilafon, wasn't working, and decided to switch her to another antipsychotic, Stelazine. He spent two weeks weaning her off the Trilafon, reducing the dosage gradually. The less medication Julie had in her system, the better she was. She felt like she'd come awake again. When Dr. Melamed tried to start her on Stelazine, she'd refused. "You can't see how much better I am?" she said. At a group therapy session on 3-West, the patients were asked to grade themselves on their progress. Julie gave herself an F for medication. The therapist wanted her to discuss it with the group, but Julie cut it short—"I don't think that's such a good idea." She wasn't looking to set off an anti-med revolution on 3-West. Alone with the therapist later, Julie was firm: "I feel human again, you have to see it. I can get up in the morning. I am not taking this fucking medication."

She never had to again.

BACK AT THE group home that summer, Julie had hoped to pick up where she'd left off. She hated the idea of anybody knowing her diagnosis—she felt like such a freak—and several times asked house manager Tim Cook if any of the other residents suspected. Tim hadn't even told most of his staff. He understood how important Julie's privacy was. He and Linda Slezak were searching for a specialist. In the meantime, he asked Julie to stay close to the home and promise not to go off by herself on walks. He hoped this would curb the incidents. When she was feeling "disorganized"—like she was about to switch into another personality—Tim wanted her to immediately come to the staff. Julie agreed, but even Tim had only a dim understanding of how little that meant. The other personalities hadn't agreed to a thing.

On one level Julie accepted the multiple personality diagnosis. On another, she resisted. It just seemed too weird. There are some people with multiple personalities who achieve co-consciousness—they become aware of what the other personalities are doing and thinking and can communicate with them and control when they will appear. So, for example, a childlike personality is not permitted to come out during the day at work, but may appear at night, in the safety of the home. Reaching co-consciousness is often a key goal in therapy for people with the disorder. It allows them to plan and bring order to their lives. Julie did not have co-consciousness. The periods when other personalities emerged was simply blacked-out time for Julie. She was only able to piece together what the other personalities were doing by what Tim told her and by the circumstantial evidence. She was like a detective, deciphering what the other parts of her had been up to.

Outwardly she seemed fine. She was going to program, speaking about college again, hanging out with the other residents. After she'd been back a couple of weeks, she asked permission to go for a walk on her own. She assured Maureen Coley that she didn't feel crazy and would return in fifteen minutes, and she did. On Labor Day the house sponsored a picnic. Julie invited over a male friend and seemed in great spirits, singing and humming along with Tim's guitar music.

The next day Julie slipped out after supper. She came racing back into the house forty-five minutes later, crying. Her clothes were ripped; her hair was all wet and matted on one side. She ran up to her room and would not say much to Tim, Maureen, or JoAnn. She told them she'd "wound up" at the train station and was "sitting there" and then she tried to get away. But she would not be clearer about what happened. She'd had no warning signs that she was going to leave the house, she said.

She explained more to Tim later. She'd come to in the backseat of some car at the train station with two men, was terrified, bolted out of the car, and raced home. Tim asked if it was sexual, and Julie was sure it had been. Tim believed that Marlena, the wild, teenage personality, had some sort of sexual encounter with the men, and when things got ugly, retreated inside, leaving Julie to deal with the consequences.

This was a nightmare, although she had been through worse. At least she wasn't beaten up this time. Long before she knew anything about her disorder, when she was a sixteen-year-old teenager in foster care, she'd come out of a blackout in a strange basement apartment. She was naked except for a pair of men's underwear; her wrists and upper arms were black-and-blue, and she was bleeding between the legs. The young Julie surmised she'd been raped. She dressed quickly and was about to slip out when she heard footsteps on the basement stairs. An old man came down into the room, looked around at the mess, and screamed, "Who the fuck are you? Where's my son?"

"I don't know," Julie had sobbed. "I don't know." The man grabbed her by the arm, yanked her up the stairs, and shoved her out the front door, throwing her onto the sidewalk. She'd had no idea what town she was in. When she'd finally figured it out, she was fifteen miles from her last memory and a day had passed.

THE NIGHT OF the train station incident, around midnight, Julie came downstairs and was wandering the house aimlessly, her head down, hair in her face, arms folded tightly against her body. JoAnn, the overnight counselor, asked if she was feeling all right.

"I'm fine, how are you?" Julie answered sharply. She went upstairs to bed and in fifteen minutes JoAnn checked on her. She was lying awake in the dark. "Are you all right, honey?" asked JoAnn.

"I'm fine," said a voice.

TIM AND Linda Slezak were in a bind. What to do with Julie while they tried to find her the right treatment? Julie dreaded another hospitalization, and none of them wanted that for her unless they could find a facility that specialized in multiple personalities. But they feared she was heading for some terrible trouble. She was continuing to see her therapist—Dr. Blank, the one who'd been so sure she was schizophrenic—though he wasn't much help.

In order to treat multiple personalities, a therapist must identify and get to know all the personalities, winning their trust one by one. A person with the disorder can have more than a dozen personalities, each formed in childhood to cope with a different crisis too awful for the abused youngster to confront head-on. The book *Sybil* described a woman with sixteen personalities. There may be a personality created to deal with repeated rape by the father; another created to deal with a mother locking the child in a closet; another to cope with a resulting disaster at school. Some personalities are childlike, some adolescent, some adult. The therapist must eventually find the trauma at the root of each. The usual goal is first to help the patient to attain co-consciousness, and in time integrate and fuse the disparate personalities into one. It is a long, slow process that may take years. Sybil spent over a decade in psychoanalysis before the fusing process began. With a multiple personality patient, one therapy session often goes on for hours and deals with several personalities.

Dr. Blank was seeing Julie for two traditional forty-five-minute sessions a week. Tim had a feeling that she was actually coming back worse off from this traditional therapy. It was as if Dr. Blank knew enough to release some of the demons, but then couldn't close her up by the end of the session.

On September 8, the Melillo group homes were scheduled to go on a two-night camping trip on the eastern end of Long Island. Tim had arranged it personally, at his old Boy Scout camp, Camp Baiting Hollow in Wading River. Julie wanted badly to go, and everyone felt it would be good for her. It was one of those events that made the group home special.

TIM LED THE caravan of cars in his 1981 Toyota. The camp is on the North Shore, about an hour and a half's drive from Glen Cove. It was a balmy Friday afternoon, one of the last warm days of the year, and it felt great to be heading off for a weekend adventure. Tim's car windows were all open. As he drove he held a comb in his hand, trying to keep his sandy blond hair under control. Julie and her best friend at the house, Peggy, were in the car behind him, joking about the vanity of their fearless leader. "I bet he's combed his hair fifty times," Julie laughed. They were excited about the weekend. Tim had told them about the lake nearby and how it was an easy walk to Long Island Sound, where they'd go swimming.

Few of the group home residents had ever been camping before. They were surprised by the rustic accommodations. A good-sized cabin, equipped with just a refrigerator and coal stove, sat in the center of a clearing. That was for counselors. Six plywood lean-tos were scat-

tered around the clearing's edge. They weren't much bigger than closets, had no doors, were unlighted, and each held two double bunks
inside. Up a hill a considerable way from the clearing were flush toilets. In the opposite direction, about seventy-five feet from the cabin,
was an outdoor cold-water sink. Jasper spoke for many when he said,
"We're supposed to sleep here, Timmy? Outside?" Julie's friend Peggy
was more direct: "You have to be fucking kidding me."

They unpacked the coolers and shopping bags full of food, chose
lean-tos, and put their bedding in the bunks. Tim sent them out to
gather firewood. Jasper chopped logs down to size. He was good with
an ax. Others strolled along the sandy paths. Julie wandered across the
bluffs to the Sound and tossed rocks in the water. It was pleasant. A
few took late-afternoon naps.

As night came, Tim the Eagle Scout built a roaring fire. They sat
around it on four log benches and toasted marshmallows. Trees towered above them, making a leafy roof that blocked out most of the sky.
Two small gas lanterns hanging from the cabin, along with the fire,
provided the only light. The darkness made Julie uneasy.

"You're really very safe here," Tim said.

"I'm really scared, I'm really uncomfortable," she answered. "I
don't like that there's animals, wild animals."

"There's nothing to worry about," said Tim.

"I hate the woods, I hate it."

Tim left to talk to some of the others, telling counselors to keep an
eye open. He noticed Julie take Anthony Constantine's hand and walk
off to Anthony's lean-to.

Oh no, this is great, thought Tim. He let a few moments pass,
hoping he was wrong, then wandered over to the lean-to. They were
making out on a bottom bunk. Tim wondered if Julie had switched to
Marlena. "OK guys, come on," said Tim. She shot up. "I'm fine," she
blurted, then hurried over to the picnic table at the other end of the
clearing by the three oaks and put her head down on her arms.

Her friend Peggy joined her, but Julie didn't seem herself. She was
withdrawn, restless, pacing, head down. Suddenly Julie bolted up the
dirt road into the night. Several searched, called her name, but couldn't

find her, and then a few minutes later she just showed up. Tim took her aside. "Julie, where'd you go?"

"I don't know," she said. "I just found myself out there." She'd blacked out, and when she came to she was standing in total darkness, surrounded by trees. She didn't know how much time had passed. Minutes? Hours? She didn't know how far she'd run. She heard noises in the woods that terrified her. Even in broad daylight, Julie is scared of animals—dogs and cats included. She was afraid if she moved in the dark, she'd step on something wild. She started yelling for help, then heard Peggy's voice far off, shouting "Julie!" Thank God.

TIM FED THE fire and pulled out his guitar, singing for over an hour: some Cat Stevens; Crosby, Stills, Nash & Young; Dylan; "Bye, Bye, Miss American Pie"; "If I Had a Hammer." He had the right kind of voice for a campfire. Jasper wanted a Spanish song and Tim belted out the only one he knew, "Feliz Navidad."

It was a great kick watching Jasper singing along, snapping his fingers and clapping. Julie loved it, but suddenly felt strange, spacey, light-headed.

She was switching, and she would have no further memory of that long night.

SHE PUT HER head down on the picnic table and stayed like that for twenty minutes, at times quietly weeping. It was past midnight.

"She's really out of it," Maureen whispered to Tim, "she won't talk to me." When Tim went over to check, she leaped up, racing around the cabin and down the dirt road that led to the lake and Sound. Tim weighs well over 250 pounds, the road was sandy and hard to get any footing on, but he peeled off and caught her about a hundred feet past the cabin, near a boulder. Tim tried to carry her back toward the cabin. She fought ferociously, swinging her arms, kicking and punching, and though he is nearly three times Julie's size he could not move her more than a few feet without her squirming free. He'd get her ten feet closer to the cabin, by a large beech tree, and then she'd fight free and he'd have to hold on to her for dear life with a bear hug. Back and forth they went, between the boulder and the beech tree. He tried to lift her and lost his footing in a gully, twisting his ankle and wrenching his back. The pain was piercing. He could barely stand.

At times Julie would curl into a fetal position, resting, and Tim would stroke her hair, trying to soothe her, the way you would a baby. Then all of a sudden she would scramble free, screaming, "Let me go, you bastard."

"Julie, don't fight, relax, calm down, it's all right," Tim said over and over. For a half hour he attempted to handle the situation himself. She'd be calm, then suddenly hysterical, yelling that the man in the black hair had her. During other stretches she seemed to have no idea where she was, asking, "How did I get here? Are these the woods?" Tim tried to hang on as the personalities rapidly switched.

He spotted Maureen in the soft light of the cabin's gas lamp and signaled to her. "I've got Julie," he said, and asked her to bring a sleeping bag and flashlight. If he couldn't calm Julie enough to walk her back to camp, maybe he could zip her into a sleeping bag and they would carry her that way.

The night was warm and humid, with no breeze. Tim was drenched with sweat. During a quiet stretch, while he waited for Maureen, he maneuvered Julie over to the outdoor sink and grabbed it, hoisting himself up with one arm, holding Julie with the other. But she fought back wickedly and he finally just sat down, his arms and legs locked around her, her back against his stomach.

Maureen returned with the sleeping bag. The best they could do was to get Julie to sit on top of it. When they tried to ease her feet inside, she twisted and rolled free. Tim kept waiting for it to pass, for the Julie personality to reappear. He had Maureen hold her upper body and he took her legs—he was trying to minimize any contact that might seem like a sexual assault to a personality. The two counselors talked about getting her out of the woods as quickly as possible; obviously something she'd seen here had connected with her past and set her off.

Julie's friend Peggy heard the commotion and stood nearby, eavesdropping. It worried Tim. The last thing he needed was to lose control of the group. When Julie seemed calm enough so Maureen could handle her alone, Tim spoke with Peggy, suggesting she go back to the campfire with the others. "This is no big deal," he said. She insisted on staying and Tim figured it was worth seeing if a friend might snap Julie out of it. Peggy talked to Julie about the walk they'd taken earlier. It was like Julie didn't know her. Just because you were friendly with Julie didn't mean the other personalities would have anything to do with you or, in some cases, were even aware of you. At one point Julie stopped whimpering, lifted her head, tossed her hair back, stared dead on at Peggy, and in a composed voice announced, "Would you please leave me the fuck alone?"

Peggy shuddered. She looked like she'd seen a ghost. "It seems like she hates you," Peggy whispered to Tim. "This is weird—is she possessed?" Tim tried explaining, but Peggy was crying, "She's possessed! I want to go home! I want to go home!" Maureen helped Peggy back to the campsite.

A COUPLE OF hours had passed. Tim felt like he'd been restraining Julie all night. He tried something different. "Can I speak to Julie?" he said to her.

"No, this is Marlena, who wants to know?"

"I'm her friend Tim. Can I speak to Julie?"

"You want me to disappear, you're like all the rest."

"Can't Julie come out?" Tim said.

"No, I'm in control and she can't come out."

"Is she all right?" asked Tim.

"She's fine, she's inside."

"Can't you get her outside?" asked Tim.

"You just want me to go away. You're hurting me." Tim said he'd ease his hold if she sat still, and she agreed, but as soon as he did she tried escaping. Finally she seemed exhausted, then calm.

"Are you there?" Tim asked.

"Yeah, where am I?"

"You're just on the other side of the cabin going through quite an evening," said Tim.

"What happened?" she asked.

"You don't remember?" Tim said. "What's the last thing you remember? You ran into the woods and got scared. You remember talking by the table?"

"Not really," she said.

"You were afraid of animals and we tried to calm you down," said Tim.

"I don't remember."

"Do you know Marlena came out?"

"Marlena? Marlena came out?"

"And a baby crying," said Tim.

"Yeah, there's a baby, what did she say?"

Tim told her he'd help her figure it all out. He didn't mention that she'd been abusive or hurt him. Together they walked back toward the light of the cabin, Tim limping beside Julie and Maureen. It was nearly 3 A.M. "Everything is fine, fine, it's just hard on you," he said. "We'll be here for you, don't be afraid." He was relieved to have Julie out and back in control of the personalities.

It wasn't Julie, though.

THEY WENT into the cabin and set up an extra cot for her with the counselors. Within minutes her eyes were closed. "She's asleep," Maureen whispered. Tim and Maureen poured themselves mugs of coffee, Tim took his sneakers off and they sat on their cots, on the far side of the cabin, whispering.

"Holy shit, I can't believe it," Maureen said. "Each is like a separate person. How'd you know what to do?"

"I didn't," said Tim. "I just went with it. I don't know if what I did was good, bad, or indifferent." Tim still believed there were three personalities besides Julie—Marlena, the profane teenager; Patricia, a mournful girl of maybe ten, who seemed to be Julie's dead sister; and Didi, the young girl-baby personality.

"I was scared to death," said Maureen. "I didn't know if she'd run in the woods and kill herself." She kept thinking about how different Julie looked with each personality shift—the rage and defiance in the teenage Marlena's eyes; the uncontrolled high, thin weeping of the baby who'd rolled into a ball and sobbed herself to sleep. It was eerie. Tim and Maureen were talking about how Peggy and the others would take it, when suddenly Julie sat up, jumped off the cot, and raced out the door. "Grab her!" yelled Tim, and Maureen hurtled after her while Tim laced up his sneakers.

TIM RAN down the dirt road a quarter of a mile, past the sink, beech tree, and boulder. He found one of Maureen's sandals in the deep sand. There was no sign of her or Julie. He stood in the dark and listened. He could hear Maureen's voice calling, "Julie, Julie, come on Julie . . ." The voice was getting farther away. It sounded like they'd left the road and gone into the woods. Tim knew the terrain backward and forward from his scouting days. When he was older, he'd even taken girlfriends parking at good old Camp Baiting Hollow. Between the lake and the Sound was a swamp. The Scout leaders used to tell them to stay away, the swamp was so dangerous kids had drowned there. Maureen was an expert camper; she'd backpacked all over the country, had even come face-to-face with a bear in the Rockies. But she did not know these woods. Tim had an image of the two of them in the pitch black running pell-mell into the swamp and never being found again.

Maureen could barely see a few feet in front of her. It was lucky that the night was clear, and she was able to get glimpses of Julie's hair as it tossed back and forth, catching the moonlight. Mainly, though, Maureen followed the sounds of Julie careening past bushes and underbrush. Tim limped along the twisting path, far behind, calling their names. He was just at the crossroads between the path to the Sound and the path back to the camp when Maureen yelled, "She's coming back your way." Tim limped behind a tree and waited. As Julie raced by, he pounced and tackled her. It was awful. She looked like a scared little animal, sweating and shaking. He wrapped his legs and arms around her and sat down, leaning against a berm, the only way he could sit because of his back.

"This is it, you have to go back to the ranger's for help," Tim told Maureen.

"What if you can't hold her?"

"This is it, I'll just have to hold her," said Tim. Maureen had lost the one sandal and held the other in her hand. Julie was barefoot. "Do you know where you are?" Tim asked.

"I think so," said Maureen.

"You go straight up the road to the top, then follow it around right to the ranger station."

"OK, OK, OK," said Maureen and she ran off barefoot into the dark. Julie was on Tim's lap, facing away from him. He kept talking to her over her shoulder, trying to be soothing. When she was a young personality, he'd rub her head and shoulders, trying to calm her. She'd never use his name. She fought, fell asleep, woke, cooed, cried, and fought again. They were both soaked with sweat. Tim could see through Julie's white shirt to her bra. At one point Marlena screamed, "You just want to touch me, I hate men, I hate you," and she squirmed around and kneed him in the crotch. Then she fell asleep again.

Around 3:30 he saw two Suffolk County Police cars bumping their way slowly down the uneven sandy road, rocking back and forth like big animals, their blue and red lights flashing wildly through the dark forest.

"All right, miss—shit, what's happening?" said a cop.

"Shut up," Tim said. "Don't talk to her that way. We have to get her personal belongings. You can help get us back to the cabin. I need her chart."

"What's wrong with her?" the cop asked.

"The person is having a psychiatric emergency and needs to get to the hospital and what you can do for her is just have an ambulance at the ranger's station. Can you do that for us?"

Tim and Maureen wedged her into the backseat of a patrol car, sitting her between them. As they got close to the cabin, Tim said, "Do we really need the flashing lights? I got thirty people here I don't want to scare." The police turned them off. Tim grabbed Julie's chart with all the phone numbers and hospital contacts and her shoes. He wanted to get her onto 3-West at Glen Cove. Anywhere else it would be a nightmare trying to explain.

Julie was screaming, "I'm not fucking going! Let the fuck go of me!" The ambulance was waiting when they got back to the ranger's station. Two of the men grabbed Julie's shoulders, the other two her legs. It took all their strength to strap her onto the ambulance stretcher.

She was taken to the nearest hospital, Central Suffolk in Riverhead, which does not have a psych ward. There Tim spent a couple of hours making calls, while Maureen and a very large nurse held Julie down. She'd be calm, then suddenly struggle ferociously. They wanted to avoid putting her in a straitjacket, and at times the only way to control her was for Maureen to lie on top of her. Glen Cove Hospital was full. So were several of the others the group home usually relied on. The only place they could get a bed was Nassau County Medical Center, the county hospital—a step above Pilgrim, but not anywhere Tim wanted to send someone he cared about.

Julie was totally uncooperative. A doctor at the Suffolk hospital scribbled, "Agitated, wants to leave. Claims she does not like anyone." Tim rode a taxi back to the camp while Maureen made the hour-and-a-half ambulance ride with Julie to Nassau County Medical Center. Maureen had lost both shoes and was wearing Julie's size 6½ sneakers, which were quite painful on size 8 feet. Maureen didn't look forward to explaining Julie's situation to the hospital's emergency room psychiatrist, and thought she might seem a little more convincing with shoes on.

"Where's Tim?" Julie kept asking. "Is Tim all right?" Maureen took it as a sign that the Julie personality was back.

She wasn't, though.

THE TAXI left Tim off at the top of the dirt road leading to Camp Baiting Hollow. The sun was just coming up through a clump of tall pines. As he hobbled back toward the cabin, he found Maureen's sweater rolled in a ball and fifty feet later, one of her sandals. He retraced their wild chase and noticed the spots where the dirt and sand were scratched and scattered. The air was cool, the morning still now except for the birds, and Tim remembered how he'd loved this place as a boy, how big and mysterious it had seemed then. No one was awake. Walking back into the silent clearing, it was as if nothing had happened. Tim lay down on his bunk and slept for a couple of hours. He dreamed that he, Maureen, and Julie were racing through the woods.

BY THE TIME they got to the county hospital, Julie seemed fine. She'd slept the whole ride and now was calm and in a chatty mood. They wheeled her in past the main emergency room to the psychiatric section. This is the poor people's public hospital, and emergency was filled with the leftover havoc of a Friday night—bullet wounds, stab wounds, car crashes.

Maureen and Julie were taken onto the locked psychiatric section, where they spent hours fidgeting on the vinyl chairs, waiting for processing. The only other person in the waiting area was a confused homeless man. Maureen was called into the interview room first and gave the psychiatrist a sense of what had happened. The doctor wanted to know whether Julie had really been violent—she seemed so appropriate and calm in the waiting area.

"Look at me," said Maureen. She was caked with dirt and mud, her hair a mess. She showed the psychiatrist bruises on her arms from the night in the woods. "This is all from Julie."

At one point as Maureen and Julie sat together in the waiting area, Julie suddenly broke into a chorus of "Feliz Navidad." Maureen smiled, then joined in. "Maureen, you better watch it," said Julie, "you'll wind up in here, too."

Maureen didn't know it, but the Julie personality was back for the first time since Tim's sing-along at the campfire the night before. She'd picked right up where she left off, so to speak—hadn't missed a beat in Jasper's song.

Maureen stared at her. Julie looked better off than she did. Julie wasn't half as bedraggled from the chases or the wrestling in the dirt. She seemed rested. Had Maureen been right to push so hard for a hospitalization? Julie was clearly in control again.

Who knew how long it would last?

Julie's whole body ached, but she had no recollection of the night. It was not Julie's way to just come out and ask what had happened, and Maureen did not realize the Julie personality had been gone so long. Maureen gave her the basic story, but before there was a chance to fill in the gaps, the psychiatrist took Julie off to be screened. She spent the next three days at the county hospital with little idea of what had happened. She didn't know if she'd hurt anybody or how much the others had seen.

Julie tried to explain to the emergency room psychiatrist that locking her in a hospital did no good, that once she "woke up" from one of these spells she was fine and that a hospitalization actually made her worse, but the psychiatrist kept saying things like "So you really think you're OK?" or "So you don't think anything unusual happened last night?" Julie tried for a three-day voluntary stay, but they insisted on involuntary commitment. It teed off Julie; if they were going to commit her, why didn't they just do it instead of pretending to be taking the screening seriously.

Before she was moved up to the fourteenth floor, Maureen came in to say good-bye, hugging Julie and handing back her sneakers. It was almost ten on Saturday morning. As the barefoot Maureen left through the locked door, she had to step to the side. Three big men in orange jumpsuits were being led handcuffed and chained into psych emergency. The door closed and Maureen looked back through the window at Julie waiting there surrounded by inmates from the county jail.

THE LOCKED ward was circular, with a large, glassed-in nursing station in the middle, connecting 14-East to 14-West. Most of the patients sat by the station all day. They were required to dress in hospital gowns. Attendants wore blue scrubs and hogged the televisions so you had to watch *their* favorite shows. A few patients kept coming up, begging for quarters for the pay phone.

Julie walked round and round the circular ward, past the nurses' station and the Ping-Pong table, trying to get the time to pass. She pressed her face against the sealed windows. This was the tallest building on Long Island for miles. Fourteen floors below, the cars and houses looked like toys. She felt like she was going mad. She knew this was wasted time, that these people could not help her with her problem. There was so much she needed to figure out. For starters, she had to talk to Tim to find out what had happened, but he was still away on the camping trip.

A male patient, an obsessive type, began following her around. If she sat to watch TV, he'd sit beside her; if she took a seat at the nurses' station, he did too. "Can I sit next to you when you eat?" he asked.

"If you stay away for the rest of the afternoon, you can eat with me," Julie said. If nothing else, she'd learned plenty of survival tricks in the system. She kept circling the ward, hoping someone half normal would talk to her or ask her to play Ping-Pong. She wanted to scream or cry or punch the wall over this insane, useless lockup, but couldn't, so she paced faster and faster, trying to get some of the feeling out. The more she circled, the more she felt trapped, like a zoo animal. There was a psychiatrist with a bow tie and freckles and suit pants that didn't match his jacket, and every few hours, so he'd have an entry for his charts, he asked if she was hearing voices.

Just your stupid voice, Julie thought.

She kept reminding herself that she was on a psych ward and shouldn't tell anyone she wanted to kill herself.

This was her third hospitalization in four months. She was afraid they'd kick her out of the group home. She could not stop worrying that they'd send her to Pilgrim this time.

She called her therapist and the house asking when Tim could come visit. She was counting on him Monday, but JoAnn explained he had to go to the doctor. My God, Julie thought, what did I do to him? She stood by the pay phones for long stretches, waiting for a call back.

Dr. Blank came to see her. They had a nice talk. He apologized for thinking she was schizophrenic. "I misjudged things," he said. It meant a lot.

On Tuesday, Tim limped onto the ward and told her everything after "Feliz Navidad."

The next few days Julie called the house regularly to inquire about Tim's health. "Did Tim tell you I need long-term?" she asked counselor JoAnn Mendrina during one call.

"Yes," said JoAnn.

Julie said she supported this, it was time to take care of her problem once and for all. "Do you think I'll be able to come back to the group home afterwards?" she asked.

"What did Tim say?"

"He said yes. But what if it's a year?" Julie asked.

"Think positive," said JoAnn, "Think in terms of months."

"You know how much I like the home," said Julie. "It's the best home I ever had. Would you tell the staff thank you for me?"

"I'll put it in the log book in red," said JoAnn.

September 15, 1989, at 3:30 Julie was transferred by ambulance to Glen Cove Hospital's 3-West. The plan was to keep her there until Tim Cook and Linda Slezak could find a long-term facility that specialized in multiple personality disorder.

LINDA CALLED psychiatric hospitals all over New York State for Julie. They either didn't treat multiple personality patients or wouldn't take Medicaid payment. The costs at the private facilities were astronomical: Four Winds Hospital upstate charged $960 a day—not including doctor's fees, testing, or medication.

She contacted the National Institute for Mental Health in Washington and got names of hospitals that specialize in the disorder. There were five in America, all out of state (in Illinois, Texas, Georgia, and two in Pennsylvania). A New York Medicaid patient would have little chance getting in any time soon.

Fortunately, the National Institute was able to provide the names of two New York City–area therapists in private practice who specialized in multiples—the only two in the region on the Institute's referral list—and this time Linda Slezak got lucky.

Dr. Deborah Deliyannides of Manhattan agreed to assess Julie. Several times in October, Tim picked up Julie at Glen Cove Hospital and drove her the hour into the city for sessions. The psychiatrist confirmed that Julie was indeed a multiple. Julie sat through these sessions with her hair down over her face. During one long silence, the doctor asked if "parts of the mind were arguing about whether or not to talk," and Julie answered yes. The doctor also noted that Julie exhibited amnesia for large parts of her life—times when other personalities undoubtedly were in control; for events in the hospital; and for matters they had discussed together only minutes earlier. On the other hand, the doctor noted, both Julie's short- and long-term memory were good for "neutral details."

Dr. Deliyannides was optimistic. But she also sounded a warning: "There is no doubt in my mind that if left untreated Julie's condition will deteriorate; her level of functioning and her overall sense of well-being will diminish."

Dr. Deliyannides felt Julie needed one double session a week and agreed to see her for $150—$75 per session, half her normal fee. For the first couple of months Julie would stay in the Glen Cove hospital, travel to Manhattan to see Dr. Deliyannides, and then, when she was stable enough, move back to the group home, continuing her therapy from there. Once back at the group home, if Julie had an emergency, Dr. Deliyannides had privileges on the new wing at

North Central Bronx Hospital, meaning that for once a hospitalization would not be wasted time for Julie, it could be used for treatment.

Both Julie and Linda Slezak were delighted with the plan. Julie liked Dr. Deliyannides, found her sensitive and insightful. She'd never had a therapist who'd questioned her about her history of abuse in such a delicate manner. Linda was pleased to have arranged for quality treatment at a fraction of what a specialized in-hospital care would have cost (assuming they could have even found a receptive long-term facility). This was precisely what community mental health was supposed to be: quality care at reasonable cost.

There was one final hurdle: funding for the therapist. Dr. Deliyannides already had several Medicaid patients and could not afford to take Julie for the government fee of twenty dollars per session. Julie would need supplemental funds from Nassau County to pay for the therapy.

Linda did not expect it to be a problem. The New York State mental health commissioner, Richard Surles, had created a "flexible service dollars" program to fill exactly these kinds of gaps in the system. He had also initiated a new type of super social worker, the intensive case manager, who was to make sure that particularly troubled people would not fall through the cracks. These emergency funds had been used by intensive case managers to get clients' cars repaired so they could continue getting to work, pay security deposits on apartments, and buy appropriate clothes for job interviews.

Advocates gave the commissioner's innovations high marks; implementation was less impressive. The local counties controlled the actual purse strings, and in a prosperous suburb like Nassau, where social services were a low priority, anything could be turned into a battle.

Linda Slezak filled out the forms for Julie and attached several pages describing their search for an appropriate therapist.

At the start of November, Beverly Green, the county's assistant commissioner of mental health, called asking for more information and suggested trying several local psychiatrists instead of Dr. Deliyannides. County officials did not like the idea of Julie going to a therapist in New York City—all of thirty miles away. Linda contacted all the locals suggested. Only one worked with the multiple personality disorder; she charged $160 a session and was taking no new patients. The others told Linda they weren't qualified to treat the disorder. She got letters from Dr. Melamed at Glen Cove Hospital and Julie's therapist, Dr. Blank, saying how lucky it was that someone of Dr. Deliyannides's caliber had agreed to treat at a reduced fee. Dr. Dan Vogrin, director of the Melillo clinic, wrote that Julie met all state criteria for a high-priority care, including the fact that she'd been homeless and had been a heavy user of hospital services for years. He pointed out that the state was trumpeting a "consumer-driven system" and this was precisely what the consumer, Julie, wanted.

Linda and Dan Vogrin marshalled their troops. The state had set up regional committees of program heads, and the one for northern Nassau County also wrote endorsing the plan for Julie to be treated by Dr. Deliyannides.

On December 12 they got the answer to all their letters, appendices, and phone calls: a three-paragraph response that boiled down to, no. "Not consistent with the philosophy of the program." Of course, none of the powerful people that Linda or Dan had pleaded with signed the rejection letter—not Isidore Shapiro, county commissioner of mental health; or Beverly Green, assistant commissioner; or Robert M. Blume, county director of mental health, mental retardation and developmental disabilities; or John Iafrate, director of the state's Long Island regional office of mental health. These high-paid county and state bureaucrats knew to remove their fingerprints from such a cold, nasty, mean-spirited business. The rejection was signed by one Harleen Ruthen, county social worker.

JULIE HAD made up her mind to keep a positive attitude about this hospitalization. Her determination was touching and she quickly became the hospital staff's favorite. A group home counselor brought his portable typewriter over and paid her to type his college papers while she was on 3-West. She typed a nursing assistant's job résumé and cover letter. Julie still had her old speedy touch; as a star business student in high school she'd maintained a 97 average her senior year.

Everywhere she went Julie made friends—hospitals, too. She developed a friendship with an attendant, and helped him get a job as a part-time counselor at 9 Highland.

Staff from the house visited her regularly. JoAnn baked brownies. Most residents came at least once, and a few like her good friend Peggy stopped by often. Even Jasper showed up, though he didn't say much except, "Do you think I should go in, too? I was thinking I should. The food's good here."

Being under such close observation in a confined, locked area made it hard to deny her disorder anymore. The other personalities couldn't come out in privacy by sneaking out the side door in the middle of the night, as they'd done so often at 9 Highland. This wasn't for lack of trying. A young personality, screaming that the man in the black hair was after her, had wedged herself halfway out a barred window when staff hauled her back in. It was horrible to watch; you were looking at the face of a child, locked in the past, being raped. This five-year-old personality called herself the Scared One. She seemed to have been created to absorb the father's brutal attacks and was now condemned to relive them nightly. She believed she was back in the family home and had no understanding that the window she was trying to get out was actually three floors up on a hospital ward.

Attendants kept her company through the many nights when the haunted personalities emerged. She'd sit on the bed in room 9, repeatedly banging her head against the wall. From the ward's hallway it sounded like a workman hammering. Often the only way they could calm her was with a shot in the behind. Some mornings she woke in restraints. Julie had no recollection of these nights.

Other patients got glimpses of what was going on. The sickest were often the least guarded in their comments to Julie, and that played a role in getting her to accept it. A very psychotic fat woman said, "I know you're grown up, but I know there's a little girl inside you, too.

You're both." A male patient who'd flirted with Marlena about her shapely bottom told her, "Sometimes you're quiet and sometimes you're wrestling on the floor. Are you Julie or are you Derriere?"

And finally, her sessions with Dr. Deliyannides convinced her. The specialist thought this was it, pushing Julie beyond a reasonable doubt.

SHE WAS FURIOUS when she heard of the county's rejection of the plan to see Dr. Deliyannides. The entire fall, three months, had been spent locked up, waiting, for nothing. "See," she said to Maureen, "I told you I'd be screwed over." At Mellilo they felt the same way, although Maureen assured her they'd come up with another plan and she just had to be patient a little longer.

After ninety days in the hospital, Social Security disability no longer compensated the group home for holding the bed. Linda Slezak decided they'd keep it open anyway and worry later about making up the lost revenue. In an era of tight budgets it was a real kindness. Julie was relieved, and yet, she was beginning to have mixed feelings about the group home. Hospital staff didn't want her going back too often— they were afraid of incidents—and Julie felt she was losing touch with people. When she did visit, residents asked her diagnosis and how soon she'd be back for good. Several times in November and December, after getting passes, she'd tell the house counselor who came to pick her up on 3-West, "I can't do this today."

Julie was accustomed to the constant changes at the group home— residents leaving, staff leaving—but in November, Tim quit as house manager to take a job with another social service agency, and Julie was heartbroken. Maureen Coley would be taking over and Julie liked her fine, but Tim was special to her, he'd put so much of himself into the job. There'd been a bond between them since he'd figured out her problem, and he was the only one she could really talk to openly without feeling like a sideshow act.

She normally didn't go to occupational therapy at the hospital, it gave her a headache, but for several days she labored quietly painting a ceramic bear for Tim, his going-away gift.

. . .

JULIE HAD WORKED so hard to build some direction and dependability into her life, and it was being yanked from her. Tim was gone and they'd come up with no long-term plan for her. The people she had trusted her life to weren't coming through. As Julie grew confused and less confident, the other personalities began asserting themselves.

The hospital saw she wasn't doing well and became increasingly restrictive with passes. In mid-December she was allowed to come back to the group home for a two-hour evening visit, from 6:45 to 8:45. Residents were exchanging Christmas gifts that night. Julie was fine at first; then at 8:15 JoAnn noticed she'd taken her eggnog and slipped up to her room. JoAnn posted another counselor by the front door and went to check. She knocked and called, but there was no reply. So she walked in. At first glance there was no Julie. Then JoAnn spotted her, crouched behind the door, her head down. She had changed from jeans and a sweater to a dress.

"Julie," JoAnn said. "Julie." No response. "This is important. I need to speak to Julie." She looked groggy, like she was just waking up. JoAnn guessed she was in transition to another personality when interrupted.

"Julie?"

"Yeah?" said Julie. JoAnn explained it was time to leave for the hospital and asked her to change back into her jeans and a sweater since it was so cold out. Julie did.

A FEW DAYS later JoAnn drove her from Glen Cove Hospital to her appointment with Dr. Blank, who was seeing Julie while the search for a specialist continued. Julie was in good spirits, chatting about getting her hair cut and asking JoAnn for help budgeting her money.

She had a 1:30 appointment. JoAnn took a seat in the waiting room, starting on some paperwork she'd brought along. Ten minutes passed and then suddenly, Julie raced by, out the waiting room and through the door. Poking his head out of the office, Dr. Blank asked, "Is Julie with you?" The counselor and doctor chased after her, to the parking lot, but couldn't find her. JoAnn was irritated—Dr. Blank seemed so calm about her disappearance.

JoAnn started back to the group home, then spotted Julie walking on the opposite side of a four-lane boulevard. Without missing a beat, the counselor popped a U-turn and parked ten feet behind. "Hello," said JoAnn as she got out of her car.

Off she ran again. JoAnn pursued her four blocks, but couldn't keep up—the counselor was thirty years older—went back to the car, drove around, found her, parked, and approached her again in a bank parking lot.

"Julie?" said JoAnn.

"Stay away."

JoAnn did. "This is JoAnn from the group home. Who are you?"

"None of your business." It was the Marlena personality.

"Remember we talked about your getting a haircut?" said JoAnn.

"I never told you that!"

"Julie told me that," said JoAnn.

"I don't care what Julie does. I'm not going back to that fucking hospital or that fucking doctor." She said she was going into New York City and warned JoAnn not to follow.

JoAnn found a pay phone, called Melillo, explained what was happening, and went hunting for Julie. The counselor practically bumped into her; Julie was walking back into the bank to make a call herself. JoAnn got on the phone to Melillo a second time. "She's right beside me," JoAnn whispered. "I want help right away." Julie was now sitting on the floor of the bank lobby, talking on the pay phone in the voice of four-year-old Didi. Didi called Dr. Blank—"my favorite person in the whole world"—and he phoned the police, too.

Again she fled, hopping a fence and disappearing. JoAnn lost her. Three Nassau County Police cruisers soon arrived. My God, they sent the Army, JoAnn thought. She rode with one of them. In fifteen minutes they found Julie crouched down near a storefront, like a timid animal. The three squad cars pulled around her, so she was trapped, and JoAnn kept thinking, I hope they don't push her over the edge. The police were going to take her to the county hospital, it was standard procedure, but JoAnn pleaded that this would be worse for Julie, that she already had a bed at Glen Cove Hospital—and won out.

The ambulance ride back to 3-West was quiet, and later Julie had no recollection of the afternoon.

It would be months before Julie got another pass.

A COUNSELOR from 9 Highland visited 3-West the next day and Julie explained how worried she was. "You don't want to face it yourselves," Julie said, "but you're not going to find me anything and I'm going to wind up at Pilgrim State. It's better for me to just get out of here and get my own apartment." Julie knew they'd be watching her closely when she returned to the group home, that she wouldn't be able to sneak out so easily any more. She feared that her inability to abide by the house rules would lead to yet another hospitalization, and it wouldn't be Glen Cove next time. "I'm not stupid," she said, "I know what happens if you overuse these private hospitals."

The other personalities had lives they wanted to pursue. Tess, a ten-year-old personality, needed to leave the group home to go to church; Marlena had a busy social life. At times the Scared One was so sure she was about to be raped by the Daddy person, she had to flee the house. None of them felt bound by group home curfews, chores, or other rules. "It's not like I can say, 'Shit, I'm in trouble, I better shape up,' " said Julie. "I can't control this."

THAT CHRISTMAS OF 1989 at Glen Cove Hospital was the fourth in a row she'd spent on a psych ward. It had always been the most important holiday to her. Partly it was the child in her—literally. Didi loved Christmas. Partly it was that she'd never had a true Christmas growing up and longed for one like in the books. The

Callahans had either ignored it or bought a handful of presents that were put away in the basement right after they were opened, because the parents said the kids would just break everything anyway.

Julie and another young woman on 3-West created a fireplace, complete with logs and bricks, from construction paper and taped it to the front of the nursing station. In occupational therapy they cut out felt stockings and stitched them together. Julie sewed extras for the ones who couldn't do it themselves. She went from room to room, hanging them on all the ward doors.

Everyone got a few gifts that Julie assumed had been donated by some charity—stuff like toilet water. A nurse who'd been particularly touched by Julie took her aside discreetly and gave her a new ring. Another nurse surprised her with a dress pin in her stocking.

Julie remembered little of Christmas Day 1989, and assumed it had belonged to the young ones inside her.

chapter 12

TWO GROUP HOME STARS

WHEN THE SURGEONS arrived for work at North Shore University Hospital early on the morning of Friday, May 31, 1991, they were surprised to hear that Stan Gunter was alive. The damage from the previous afternoon's jump had been so extensive they assumed he would not last the night. The hospital called the Gunters and told them to be there by nine to sign papers authorizing an operation.

Repairing a torn aorta is simpler if it is the patient's only injury. In that case he can be connected to a heart-lung machine, which bypasses the damaged aorta and maintains the flow of blood around the body throughout the operation. Unfortunately, deadly blood clots will form if a person is placed on a heart-lung machine; an anticlotting agent must be administered. This was not possible for Stan. He would have bled to death from his wounds if given anticlotting medication.

So the operation on Stan's aorta was high risk. The surgeons would be under intense time pressure. The aorta is the main pipeline carrying freshly oxygenated blood in two key directions: upward, into the brain; and down the left side of the body to the limbs, organs, and spinal cord. The force of Stan's jump had ruptured this pipeline at the spot where the aorta curves downward and is attached to the body wall. Freshly oxygenated blood could still reach his brain, but the descending pipeline was leaking. The surgeons' job was to cut open Stan, clamp the aorta above and below the tear, remove the ripped section, and replace it with a Dacron sleeve—a man-made piece of aorta tubing. It was like fitting a new section of pipe onto a broken water main. However, by clamping off the descending aorta, they were depriving the lower body of freshly oxygenated blood. The spinal cord can survive about thirty minutes without oxygen. If the operation took too long, Stan would be a paraplegic (assuming he survived).

Stan was given general anesthesia and his body temperature was lowered, reducing his need for oxygen during the operation. When they opened him up, they found a three-quarter-inch rip, nearly all the way across the aorta. It looked like a hot dog sliced through except for the rear skin, which was still clinging to the body wall. Dr. Mark Gilder, one of the surgeons, found it remarkable that Stan hadn't bled to death.

Throughout the procedure the anesthesiologist kept calling out the elapsed time: five minutes, ten minutes, fifteen.

The surgeons were shooting for twenty-five minutes and hit it.

That afternoon the doctors told Stan's parents that the aorta would be fine. Just a decade before, Dr. Gilder explained, the technology had not existed to do the procedure.

Over the weekend Stan communicated with them for the first time. He couldn't talk. He had tubes everywhere: in the mouth to breathe; in the nose to drain his stomach; in his wrist to monitor blood pressure; in his penis to monitor renal function. He motioned and his parents handed him a pad and pen.

"Coffee," he wrote.

H I S   P E L V I S , left thigh bone, left elbow, and left heel were all broken. The pelvis was split clear through, but since he'd be bedridden for a long period, they decided to leave it alone and see if the two pieces would mend on their own. The femur, or thigh bone, was broken in several places and couldn't be set with an external splint. The week after the heart operation surgeons administered a general anesthetic again, cut a foot-long incision down the side of his left thigh, pulled the femur out of his hip socket at an angle, drilled a hole in the top of the bone, installed a stainless steel rod to serve as an internal splint, pushed the femur back, and sewed up his thigh.

Instead of trying to rebuild his shattered heel, they repacked it the way you would mold raw hamburger, then placed it in a cast.

The forearm has two bones. One was pulverized. The arm was opened and the destroyed bone was replaced by an internal stainless-steel prosthesis.

Doctors felt Stan would lose flexibility in the left arm, and would walk with a limp, perhaps permanently, but were delighted by his progress. Word of his recovery spread. Surgeons at this first-rate suburban hospital called it a near miracle. He'd been saved by the latest medical technology.

A week after the heart operation the breathing tube was removed. Stan could talk. He didn't appear to have brain damage. It was extraordinary, more than his parents had let themselves hope for. In one week they'd gone from assuming he'd be dead to rooting for a complete recovery. The doctors believed he'd be able to resume most activities, including driving and playing the piano. The mother and father asked Stan what caused the accident.

He told them about God and Christ battling in his apartment, the Exchange and the end of the world.

The parents had guessed it was voices. "It was just a hallucination," said his mother.

"Don't be too sure," said Stan.

"It's all in your mind," said Mrs. Gunter.

"You don't know that," said Stan.

There were limits to modern medicine.

.   .   .

NINE DAYS after the heart operation the Gunters got a call at home. Stan had taken a sudden bad turn. Doctors weren't sure he'd make it.

He'd been eating lunch when he lapsed into unconsciousness. His blood pressure plummeted, his temperature shot up. Monitoring lights flashed, bells rang. Dr. Gilder, the chief resident on the trauma unit, came running.

Had Stan swallowed something that went to his lungs? Did he have a clot? Was it the heart? He was too sick even for a pulmonary angiogram—they feared moving him. After several sophisticated tests and a CAT scan of the abdomen, Dr. Gilder still didn't know the cause, but his lead theory was septic shock, a vicious bacterial infection that rapidly spreads and can kill a patient. In Stan's case the infection could have invaded the body from several locations: the catheters they'd hooked up to him; the Dacron sleeve in the heart; the rods in his limbs; the broken heel; the nose injury near the front of the brain. In desperation, they pumped him full of antibiotics.

He responded within hours but continued to have a low-level fever and high pulse. They did CAT scans of all the organs. Dr. Gilder kept reviewing the sophisticated, three-dimensional X rays. The case preoccupied him. He was only twenty-nine, the hospital's senior surgical resident. In his nine years of medical training he had never been so challenged. He spotted something near the kidneys and consulted an expert in interpreting CAT scans. There seemed to be hemorrhaging by the top of the kidneys, where the two adrenal glands sit. An adrenal gland is the size of a pea but extremely important. It produces cortisone, an anti-inflammatory crucial in helping the body heal itself.

Dr. Gilder reviewed his textbooks. In very rare situations—5 out of 100,000 reported cases—severe trauma like a jump can destroy the adrenal glands. The injured patient's blood pressure is so low, the blood doesn't reach the glands. The glands are so small they don't hold much blood in reserve and die. Only since the era of the three-dimensional CAT scan—about fifteen years—had doctors been able to pick up the damage by observation. In the past, patients usually died.

As the texts pointed out, until recently the connection between adrenal damage and trauma was mainly known from autopsies.

Once pinpointed, the problem was correctable. Stan would have to take cortisone pills for the rest of his life.

MODERN MEDICINE saved Stan's life once more. He still had a low fever, low blood pressure, abdominal pains, didn't want to eat, and was vomiting. Dr. Gilder feared septic shock again, and worried Stan wouldn't be able to withstand a second attack. If a patient's intestine is not stimulated for a long period, a gallbladder infection may develop. Stan fit that bill; since the incident he had relied primarily on intravenous feeding.

Dr. Gilder ordered up a hepatobiliary scan, a nuclear medicine study that measures gallbladder function. The test indicated trouble, but the surgeons worried whether Stan's heart and lungs would withstand more anesthesia. They decided to use an exploratory gallbladder procedure that was new, faster, easier on the patient, and did not require general anesthesia: a laparoscopic cholecystectomy. Four small holes are punctured in the abdomen and a ten-millimeter camera is forced through one of the holes. Stan's insides were flashed on a high-resolution TV screen in the operating room. The surgeons could see Stan Gunter's gallbladder clearer than they'd see Ted Koppel at home on their TV screens talking about the crisis in health care. It was gangrenous. Through two holes they inserted their surgical tools, severed the diseased bladder, and pulled it out. Then they sealed the incision and eased the camera through the hole they'd made in Stan's belly button.

STAN DID NOT have another medical emergency. His parents marveled at how he'd been pulled back from death four times. As a gifted engineer, Stan's father was particularly impressed by the role technology had played and appreciated the surgical ingenuity.

Saving Stan was the high point of Dr. Gilder's young medical career.

The surgeon took a special interest in Stan and tried getting him admitted to the hospital's psychiatric wing. But the psychiatric staff would not take Stan. They pointed out that he wasn't hearing voices and was no longer a danger to himself or others.

The psychiatrists did visit Stan on the medical floor and struggled to come up with a treatment plan. One wanted to try him on the new medication for schizophrenia, clozapine. Another pointed out that clozapine's side effects could damage bone growth, and Stan's bones were in none-too-good shape now. The psychiatrists ultimately decided to continue him on the same antipsychotic he'd been taking before the jump, Navane.

Dr. Gilder was disappointed. The young surgeon had just been at the center of a string of exhilarating successes demonstrating medicine's extraordinary power to mend. It momentarily allowed him to think that this power applied to the brain, too.

"We spent a couple of months putting him back together," Dr. Gilder said later, "and if you think about it, we never fixed the cause of his problem."

IN LATE June of 1991, soon after Stan was out of danger, Julie visited him at the hospital. He was asleep when she walked in. She stared at him for a moment, her fellow success story. Much of Stan's hair was shaved off. His face was so drawn, she thought all his teeth had been knocked out. (In truth, he was just painfully thin, having lost forty pounds at the hospital.) He still had a tube in his throat. They'd told Julie how great he was doing. Terrific. Life was so damn cruel. This poor, gentle guy. She was about to leave when his hospital roommate said, "Wake him. He likes having visitors."

It took a few moments for Stan to zero in on Julie, but then he smiled. "How you doing?" he said in a whisper. She looked like a beautiful ballerina, dressed in a black cotton blouse and fitted yellow toreador pants, her hair pulled back tight in a high ponytail.

She was surprised at how openly Stan discussed the jump and the dispute in his living room between Jesus and God.

He commented on the thin line between reality and fantasy and said he'd have to pay closer attention in the future.

Julie mentioned that her fifteen-year-old car had finally died, and Stan laughed. It was a total piece of rusted junk with a rag stuffed into the gas tank in place of the missing cap. People at the group home used to joke about how long it would be before Julie blew herself up.

"I was going to call you and ask about lessons," she said. Her therapist thought it would be good for Julie to get back to music. "I figured you'd give me a good discount." They agreed to do it when Stan was better.

She stayed twenty minutes and said good-bye without telling him the best news. She knew Stan didn't need to hear it. If the situation had been reversed, she wouldn't want to know. Plus, she wasn't saying much about it to anyone because she didn't want to jinx things.

Just days before, she'd cut her final tie with the mental health system. She was living like a regular person now. She'd come so far in the last year and wondered if she'd be able to keep it up.

IT HAD BEEN such a long haul. The seven months Julie had spent at Glen Cove Hospital after the camping trip, from September of 1989 to March of 1990, were wasted time. The hospital psychiatrists were sympathetic, but acknowledged that they didn't have anyone to treat her on 3-West. The county diddled three months before deciding to reject her request to see the multiple personality specialist in New York City; several more months passed while an alternative treatment plan was debated. The tortured scheme officials finally came up with when they were preparing to discharge her back to the group home in March 1990 was a classic case of bureaucratic bungling. It wasted tax dollars, did not provide the necessary treatment, and showed a fundamental lack of understanding of multiple personality disorder. Linda Slezak and Maureen Coley groaned when they heard the plan, though they tried to put their best face on things so Julie would at least give it a chance. Julie saw right through it and was furious.

The new treatment plan assigned Julie to a psychiatric resident in training at a local hospital. The young doctor had never worked with a multiple before. This was a huge undertaking for someone just starting out. Treating a multiple is like handling a dozen patients at once. Quite often one personality will not like another personality and the therapist walks a tightrope, trying to win each personality's trust without alienating the others. Sometimes the therapist is a mediator between personalities. Marlena's sexual adventures upset Julie; Julie's willingness to submit to psychiatrists and counselors who did not know what they were talking about upset Marlena. If the therapist sympathizes too much with Julie, the Marlena personality may emerge, take control of the body, and run out of the room. End of therapy session.

From the county's point of view, the advantage to this plan was supposedly money. The psychiatric resident was still in training and would see Julie for no charge. To make up for the young doctor's inexperience, the county paid a veteran psychiatrist $100 a week to supervise the trainee. However, this did not mean that Julie got to see the experienced psychiatrist. The experienced psychiatrist was being paid the $100 weekly fee simply to consult with the trainee psychiatrist.

For $150 Julie could have seen a top multiple-personality therapist two sessions a week; for $100 a week she was getting a novice. But not even that small amount of money, the $50 a week difference, was really saved. If she'd been allowed to start with the New York City specialist when she was ready, Julie would have been released from the hospital five months earlier. Those five wasted months (covered by Medicaid) cost the taxpayer an extra $79,500 (150 days at $530 per day).

To save $50 a week—$2,600 a year—the county wasted $79,500. (The county didn't have any incentive to care; Julie's prolonged hospital stay was paid for by the state and federal governments via Medicaid.) Julie could have been treated by the New York City specialist for 30 years, and it still would have been cheaper for taxpayers.

Julie quickly gave up on the psychiatric trainee. Unlike a lot of other therapy, a psychiatrist for a multiple has to be flexible about the time spent. Sessions often spill over as various personalities spill out.

This therapist wanted to see Julie once a week for thirty minutes. Julie went to three sessions and stopped. She had too many problems to be someone's guinea pig.

IN MARCH 1990, right before she was discharged, Julie got a hospital pass from 11 A.M. to 3 P.M. to visit the house and prepare for her return. To accommodate her need for privacy, house manager Maureen Coley switched room assignments around, giving Julie one of the two singles, the second-floor room above the office. After lunch JoAnn suggested she tidy up her new room.

Julie's clothes had been removed from her old closet and scattered on the mattress in the new single. Several pieces dropped onto the floor, which wasn't clean. There were a few things on that floor that she couldn't identify. This had been Jasper's room before and he had never kept it clean. It wasn't horrendous, and someone else might not have minded, but Julie is fastidiously neat and just seeing her belongings this way made her skin crawl. "I felt like my stuff had cooties," she said. "It skeeved me." She was going to have to wash all of her clothes now.

She didn't feel great being back. In many ways she was no better off than when she'd gone into the hospital. She had no therapist to rely on and could not stop thinking about a commitment at Pilgrim State.

"I can't do it," Julie told the senior counselor. JoAnn suggested Julie try to clean up for fifteen minutes and then JoAnn would be done with her office work and could come up and help. Julie went back up but felt overwhelmed. She blacked out. When JoAnn came up at 2:25, Julie was gone. JoAnn searched the house, then called the hospital to report her missing.

JULIE CAME to in a pizza parlor. It was night. She was sitting at a table eating with three guys she did not know in a place she'd never seen before.

Dropped down on another planet again. Immediately she began a discreet search for hints of what the hell was going on. The three were very relaxed, talking about a band they played in, as if she knew all the ins and outs, too. They seemed Spanish. She glanced out the window. Oh shit, she thought, I'm in the City. Julie did not know New York City at all. Marlena must have taken control, left the group home, and ridden the train into New York.

"What's the matter?" one said. "You got so quiet."

"I don't know," Julie said. "I got to go home."

How was she going to get back? She needed to figure out their names, find a transition. They were talking about driving.

"Let me see your license photo," she said in a teasing way to the one who seemed to know her best. His name was Juan. Another was Juan, too.

They'd take her to Penn Station, they said. She had to make a quick decision. Could they be trusted? And what were her alternatives? Julie didn't know the subways—she didn't even know where the hell in New York City she was. She felt she'd be risking her life taking one. They seemed OK and appeared to know her from more than just that night. Apparently they were friends of Marlena's. She said she'd appreciate a lift.

When they reached the car Julie started getting into the backseat. "Get out of here!" one said. "Get in the front seat." At this point she realized that the driver assumed he was going out with her. She sat next to him and he put his arm around her while he drove. The trip to the train station was spent distracting him. "The City's really pretty . . . what's that building? . . . when is the band's next date? . . ."

"Are you sure you don't want to stay over?" he said. He wanted to know when he'd see her again. "It's not going to be another six months, is it? Can't I have your phone number?"

"You haven't had it so far," Julie said, and they laughed. They did seem OK. At the station, he leaned over and gave her a whopper on the lips. She coyly squirmed free and closed the door behind her, waving as she passed the newsstand and disappeared down the escalator to the trains.

There were more homeless people than commuters in the station at that hour, sifting through the garbage, wandering with pull carts full of ragged clothes, bathing in rest room sinks, sleeping in doorways. As a teenager Julie had been homeless after fleeing her brutal parents. She used to hitchhike back and forth on Long Island all night to keep warm. (She'd had this crazy idea that some good person would like her and take her in.) Some nights she'd slept in the parks, waking with her feet so cold she thought she was paralyzed. Her greatest fear in life was being homeless again. Even Marlena, as cocky a personality as she was, admitted a fear of homelessness. It was the main reason Marlena had tolerated Julie's staying at the group home.

Julie went to the bank of pay phones along the wall, pulled out a stack of quarters, and called Glen Cove Hospital. One of her favorite nurses came to the phone. "Where are you?" the nurse asked. "You have money to get home?"

"I don't want to be sent to Pilgrim," Julie said.

"We'll try to keep you here," said the nurse. "You want me to come pick you up?"

"I'll never make it standing here that long," said Julie.

She raced and caught the next train back to Glen Cove. It was nearly deserted. Some guy tried picking her up and she worried Marlena would pop out and take him up on it.

Marlena didn't, though.

JULIE'S RETURN to the group home in March 1990 was as difficult as everyone had expected. At moments Julie was the star she'd been when she first entered the house. They went ice skating and she was the best. A few times on weekend mornings when residents usually fixed meals for themselves Julie made everyone French toast. She was still the one who helped with going-away parties and got worked up about coloring Easter eggs.

But basically Julie felt the program had nothing for her anymore. She had no patience for their goal setting or their rules. She wanted a job, a therapist, and a place of her own so the personalities could come out in privacy. The state mental-health office was planning to start a new subsidized housing program that would give you an apartment, with a caseworker you could call whenever you needed support. It sounded perfect for her, but like all new projects in this period of budget cutting, it was taking longer to get started than expected.

At the group home now she felt on display. She hated that all the counselors—even new ones—knew more about the other parts of her than she did. They'd find her pacing in circles in her room, and when they tried speaking to her, the personality out at the time wouldn't respond.

They'd call to her through her closed bedroom door and a masculine voice sometimes answered, though Julie was alone. Did she have a male personality, too?

They'd ask if her stomach was feeling better and Julie didn't remember having had a stomachache. Had she? Or was it a young personality reliving a sadistic kick in the stomach from fifteen years ago?

The overnight counselor checking the house before going to bed ran into the sweet, bubbly four-year-old Didi in the upstairs hallway one night. "Hi! Who are you?" said Di. "What are you doing?"

He explained he was making rounds.

"Me too!" said Di.

SHE WAS violating curfew about once a week, often staying out all night. Counselors worried she'd be hurt. When Maureen asked where she'd been, Julie had no answer. She wasn't the personality leaving the house. Repeatedly in the group home's daily progress notes during these months there'd be a description of some problem and the entry: "Julie could not remember what happened." Sometimes she missed meetings to discuss these incidents with Maureen because another personality had made the appointment.

When they spoke to her after a late night out, counselors never knew what Julie's attitude would be, and it depended at least in part on what personality they were talking with. "I'm sorry, I'm sorry, I know I should be punished, I should stay in another night, I'm sorry," she said once, sounding like a junior high kid home late from a date.

Other times she was laughing and haughty, like the whole thing was too Mickey Mouse for words. She explained to counselor Jodie Schwartz that she'd purposely been doing her cleaning chores lackadaisically for weeks just to see if staff noticed and no one had picked it up, "so you guys failed the test."

Or she might switch right in the middle of discussing it. She slipped out at 11:45 one night, returning at 2 A.M. She said she didn't remember leaving, had ended up near Morgan Park on the other end of Glen Cove, and called a friend who drove her home. "I'm just so tired of not knowing when I'll switch," she told Paula Marsters, whom she liked a lot. "It's frustrating to seem to be doing well, then suddenly switch." And then she switched, to Marlena, who complained about "what bastards guys are. If they come near me I'll cut off their balls, pour salt on them and let them fucking die."

It was confusing to everyone, especially to Julie. Before program one morning she came into the office. Her hair was wet from the shower and hung in front of her face. She was holding her head, as if in great pain. Jodie Schwartz asked if anything was wrong. "It's the rain . . . I don't know . . . I better go."

"Did something happen last night?" the counselor asked.

"Why?" said Julie. "Did something happen to me?"

"I don't know," said Jodie, "I wasn't there. Do you remember?"

"I don't know," said Julie. "Do you know?"

ON MAY 28, she returned at 5 A.M., knocking on the office door, weeping. She was a little child personality who kept telling Paula Marsters, "I don't want to be out here, I want to go inside." Paula said she'd leave her alone in the office ten minutes and when she came back she wanted the Julie personality out and in control. Julie responded to her name when Paula returned, but soon switched and the little child was out again, moaning, "That man is going to get me, the man with the black hair."

"What's your name?" asked Paula, but she got no answer. By now the counselors understood that Tim Cook's original assumption of three personalities was wrong. Besides Didi, there were plainly several childlike personalities, though staff didn't know them by name yet. This child was afraid to sleep in her bedroom because the "man is going to get me. I'll jump out the window if he comes." She suddenly fled the house, returning in an hour, still crying. She wanted to sleep in the office with Paula. Paula watched her doze off, then went out to lie on the living room couch.

At 6:45 Julie woke and questioned what she was doing in the office. Paula was vague and Julie said she'd like to stay, because "for some reason I feel safe here." Most residents were still asleep. As the counselor went into the kitchen she noticed someone had thrown up on the floor. She went to the laundry room for a mop and saw a jug of Clorox on top of the dryer, its top off, and more vomit on the floor.

A suicide attempt? Paula talked to Julie, who had no recollection of getting sick or drinking bleach. As a precaution they went to the emergency room, where a physician said he didn't think she'd taken much, if any, and suggested Julie drink milk and rest.

Later that morning Julie complained her stomach hurt.

The next day she questioned Paula about how often a woman was supposed to get her period. When the counselor asked Julie if she'd missed, there was no reply. Paula couldn't be sure how old the personality was and later, when another counselor brought it up, Julie had no recollection.

This was their great fear—and Julie's—and like a lot of worst fears in life, it was never spoken aloud.

She told the counselors little things like how she'd find herself at the train station in high heels, a short tight skirt, with no recollection of how she got there. She did not tell them that on some of her overnight disappearances she'd awakened in strange beds with men she did not know. She felt it was more than they could comprehend. It certainly was more than she could comprehend. She never knew how she got there, whether these guys would hurt her when she tried to leave, or the best way of getting out of there fast. She felt like she'd been raped, although another personality, probably Marlena, could have consented or even had a relationship with the guy.

These horrors filled her mind, then she'd come back to the group home and Maureen would ask, "Are you all right? Where have you been? Why didn't you call if you were going to be out past curfew?"

They were the exact questions Julie wanted answered, too.

She found she could say very little, it was just too hurtful to talk about, so she'd give some superficial answer to get by. But her mind was racing: Great, Maureen, you think this is fun for me? Do you know how alone I feel? How can I tell you the truth—every counselor at the group home will be informed, I'll be a spectacle and I can't do anything about it anyway and neither can you.

Maureen was in an impossible bind. She understood Julie couldn't control the disappearances, but how could the house manager hold eleven other residents to curfew and not Julie? Mainly she tried to pressure Julie to follow the rules, hoping a stern message would filter through to the other personalities.

But a multiple doesn't work that way; each personality needs to be consulted individually regarding her behavior. That was one of the purposes of therapy and why it was such a sin that the county had blocked Julie's request for a specialist. It is hard to know exactly what was going on with the personalities at the time, but Marlena's acting out and flaunting house rules may have been a way to force an issue. She was fed up with being confined. In the best of times Marlena tolerated the group home. Now that Julie had misgivings and was less sure of what to do, perhaps Marlena had more sway among the personalities. Marlena was a personality of action. She was the personality who, as a teenager, had made the courageous decision to run away from the brutal parents' home, and though Julie suffered for it in the short run, it was the right thing to do.

A few times Maureen grounded Julie for a night or gave her extra chores, which incensed Julie. How could they punish you for your illness? "They were very punitive at the house," Julie said later. "They didn't know how to handle it." And it was true, they didn't. Who did?

.   .   .

THE LESS Julie could control her other personalities and the more "public" they became at the group home, the harder she worked at controlling the piece of her life that was still hers—Julie. She strived to have the group home staff know as little about her outside pursuits as possible. She prohibited her primary group home counselor from consulting with her day program counselor, and her intensive case manager from consulting with the group home staff. Julie knew she seemed paranoid, but this was a way to preserve a modicum of privacy and dignity in her life.

In mid-June, when Julie announced she wanted to leave the house, she accused Maureen of sabotaging her efforts to get into the new, unsupervised supported apartment program. "Behind my back, you're not going to recommend me," said Julie.

Maureen showed a rare flash of anger. "If you have any doubts," said the group home manager, "you apply for the program yourself and we won't say a thing." Maureen believed Julie should get one of these apartments—if the state could ever get them open—and told her so. She knew the group home was the wrong place for Julie now and hated that community mental health was so limited. At one point, in desperation, they offered Julie another more restrictive program, a supervised apartment with one or two roommates that would be visited by a counselor daily. The only one available in the area at the time was a two-bedroom apartment with a man living in it already. Julie could just imagine what the presence of a strange male roommate would do to her young, fearful, sexually abused personalities. Worse yet, the man had dark hair, like her father, who still appeared to the young personalities nightly, to rape them.

She was holding out for a place of her own.

THE AMAZING thing about Julie was that even in the worst situations, she advanced herself. Who knows where *will* comes from, but Julie's was ferocious, and through all the chaos of these months, she never lost sight of what she needed to do.

Telling no one, she started at the Glen Cove Library with the card catalog, found *Through Divided Minds*, a good book about multiple personalities, and called the author, Dr. Robert Mayer, a New York City therapist. He gave her a name on Long Island, and slowly she built a list of five specialists in nearby suburbs to call. She started attending a multiple-personality support group in New York City.

At the same time, Linda Slezak was searching again. Through the American Psychological Association, she found Dr. Hilda Sandler, who lived in the county and treated multiples. Without telling Julie, Linda Slezak called Dr. Sandler. She wanted to see if Dr. Sandler was accepting new patients and would take Julie for the twenty-dollar Medicaid rate. She did not want to give Julie any false hopes. Linda Slezak spoke with the therapist twice without divulging the patient's name. Dr. Sandler was clearly experienced in the field and did not seem surprised by any of the stories she heard. And she was receptive, which was no small thing. Dr. Sandler understood what she was undertaking.

Linda Slezak was delighted and visited the group home to tell Julie, who acted uninterested. Julie had been disappointed too often; the therapist was something she wanted to arrange herself. But Linda Slezak persisted, returning a week later and again urging Julie to call.

Julie didn't tell anyone at 9 Highland for weeks, but she did go to see Dr. Sandler at her office-home and liked the therapist. One of Julie's finest attributes is her ability to judge people. In the next months Dr. Sandler would let sessions stretch on past midnight as she began developing relationships with the sixteen personalities.

JULIE TOOK driving lessons and got her license. She also enrolled in a vocational training program considered one of the most demanding in the system. She was determined to brush up on her secretarial skills and land a job. For the first five weeks she took a battery of screening tests and generally did quite well. She couldn't type the eighty words per minute of her Future Business Leaders of America days, but still did fifty and knew she'd get faster with practice. Her clerical marks were high, too. The achievement tests showed an ability to do well in college. Aptitude tests indicated an interest in working with children as a social worker.

The tester noted that Julie could be moved along quickly and recommended the fast-track thirteen-week word processing program.

On a few tests, like reading comprehension, there were crazy scoring variations, but this time the tester could make sense of them. Years before, when Julie was first hospitalized, they figured the huge variations reflected psychosis; now they knew there must have been a younger personality popping out during the test.

In retrospect, Julie had figured out that the childish self-portrait drawings she had done during her hospital screenings must have been four-year-old Didi's.

The director of the vocational program, Barbara Green, knew from the records that Julie was a multiple, and was quite taken by her. "Isn't she adorable?" she'd said to her secretary. She wanted to start Julie right away on a two-day volunteer clerical job, but was concerned the young ones might pop out on the job.

Julie assured her they only came out at night.

She was very serious about the volunteer job and even when one of the personalities had stayed out all night, Julie insisted on going to work the next morning. When Maureen said it was OK to stay home, Julie answered, "I have to go." She knew she did best in a regimented work environment. From the beginning she received good reviews, the office supervisor describing her as quite eager to learn. And the young personalities did not interfere, though it was a different story the other three days of the week, at vocational training.

JULIE WASN'T getting along with people at the group home, didn't know her therapist well yet, and needed someone to confide in. In early July, she was sitting in Barbara Green's office at the training program, discussing moving out of the house, when her voice began to fade. She was looking at the floor. "I'm all messed up," Julie said, growing distant and woozy, like someone about to faint. Her speech became confused: "I don't think we should talk about the room spinning around . . . I don't think we should be floating up in the air . . ." Her shoulders slumped, her hair fell over her face. When she looked up, she was Didi.

Didi opened up the big pocketbook Julie always carried, rummaged around, and merrily began pulling out toys: a wooden car, a stuffed yellow bear, a coloring book, and a jumping frog. Barbara Green used to keep the toy frog on her desk. Julie would fiddle with it endlessly while they talked and finally Barbara had said, "Take it if you like it so much." Now Barbara could see why. Didi.

People asked why she carried such a big bag and Julie would answer truthfully, "I have no idea, I just have this attachment to large bags for some reason." Didi's toys.

Di sat on the office floor, chattering happily and making up stories about the toys. Barbara stared at the attractive, well-dressed twenty-two-year-old at play under the desk. The counselor understood, but seeing it the first time scared her. All she could think was, I'll never get Julie back again. I'll be with this four-year-old all night, I'll have to take her home with me. How to explain it to her kids?

"Do you want to play with me?" Di asked.

Barbara sat on the floor and made the wooden car go. What if one of the clerical supervisors walked in? "Di, sweetie, this is an office. It's a grown-up place . . ."

"I know my numbers," said Di. "You want to hear? 1-2-3-4-5-6 . . ." She could count to 15 with one mistake. "And I'm only four. Pretty great, huh?"

"Didi, this isn't a place for children . . ."

"I don't know my letters," said Di. "You know what? You can teach me. I want to learn to read." Di saw a "Speak and Spell" game in the filing cabinet and asked if they could play.

"I don't think that would be a good idea," said Barbara. "I need Julie back. She has to work on her typing."

"I can't get Julie back," said Di. "I don't know how."

Di was out an hour. Barbara Green needed to go to the bathroom but was afraid to leave. God knows what she'd find when she came back—or who. She took a different tack, explaining there were dangerous machines in the office that weren't safe for little girls. And then, while still on the floor, Di switched. She stood, then sat in the chair. "What happened?" asked Julie. They discussed it and decided she could make it through, until the therapy progressed with Dr. Sandler.

IN THE NEXT weeks, Julie worsened. She was switching rapidly, in ways that interfered with her daily life. Barbara Green got a call one afternoon from a childlike personality in some phone booth, but too young to explain where. Barbara could hear trucks and cars in the background, like a highway. She kept her on the line, asking for landmarks, but the best the young personality could do was, "I see a big building." Barbara found her not far from the office. She wanted to take Julie to the emergency room, but Julie resisted. The two had tried the emergency room at a nearby hospital a few weeks before, and even with Barbara explaining about multiple personalities, the psychiatrist on duty didn't get it, asking questions like, "Are you hearing voices?"

Julie reluctantly agreed to try the emergency room again, and Barbara arranged for an office off the main waiting room with a security guard. With no warning, Julie stood and raced out, past the guard. Barbara Green was stunned at her speed. It had to be the Marlena personality. She ran from the hospital, along a major roadway to a golf course, with three guards in pursuit. They found her sitting under a bush. Barbara and the guards were red-faced, huffing and puffing. Julie didn't look the least bit winded despite the run. She was a young personality now.

"You just ran as fast as lightning," said Barbara, breathing heavily. "Aren't you tired?"

"It wasn't me who ran," said the girl under the bush. They walked back to emergency, where they sat a few more hours. Barbara gave her a surgical glove to play with and the young personality blew it up like a balloon.

By the time she was seen, Julie was in control, and went home again. She did not tell them at the group home and made Barbara Green promise not to.

E V E R Y   D A Y brought a surprise. Barbara Green was in her office, meeting with a client who was complaining about not getting enough attention lately, when Julie suddenly poked her head in and said, "Are we going to play with the toys again?" and ran off. Didi! The client looked shocked, but Barbara acted like it was just another four-year-old woman, and finished off with the scheduled interview, promising to be more attentive in the future.

A clerical instructor pulled Barbara aside. "Something very bizarre's going on with Julie," said the instructor. "She's sitting at her word processor babbling." Didi! By the time Barbara got to her she was typing away in adult fashion.

As Barbara headed off to lunch with three other staffers, Julie ran by and ducked into a training room. These rooms were off limits during lunch. Didi! The supervisor made an excuse to get out of the lunch date and tried reasoning with Di about going back inside. "I want someone to play with," said Di. "I never get to come out." Barbara led her into the office and they played on the floor again.

Eventually Di went in, but another young personality popped out. This was the five-year-old that other personalities called the Scared One. She was crying about the darkness and how they kept her locked up. She trembled and curled into a little ball. "They're going to hurt me because I made a messy on the floor," she cried. "I couldn't hold it. I tried, I tried. They're going to lock me in the dark. It's dark!" There was no darkness, no mess, but Barbara promised to clean up everything and said it was safe to go back inside.

Julie emerged and Barbara started dialing Dr. Sandler for her, but before she finished another personality was out. This one had blank eyes, and was about ten—Tess, the churchgoing personality. She'd apparently come into being to absorb the trauma of the death of Julie's younger sister from illness thirteen years earlier. Tess felt complete despair and told Barbara she wanted to return to the group home, pick up the big knife and go to the cemetery, take the knife, and cut out all the people so they could freely and individually fly up to heaven to be with God and their dead sister.

"You can't cut people out with a knife," Barbara explained; it wouldn't mean freedom, it would mean death.

Next was Megan, a twelve-year-old personality, who had never met Dr. Sandler. Barbara introduced them over the phone and Megan talked for forty minutes. She was a very bright, serious girl, a musician and voracious reader, who was quite responsible, a kind of little mother to the young personalities. Dr. Sandler welcomed the chance to get to know her. Megan had a great deal of insight into how the multiple system worked when functioning well. She explained that the key personality was Abigail, an adult who was pretty, self-assured, and the most intelligent of all. Abigail was the personality who controlled the switching. She determined who needed to come out and when. Something had happened to Abigail—she seemed to have disappeared —and now there was internal chaos and rapid switching. Dr. Sandler asked Megan if she'd go inside and play music to calm the others, which she did.

At 3:15, Julie returned. Barbara told her about Tess wanting to cut everyone free, appealed to the older ones in the system to take care of the younger ones, and urged Julie to get them all home safely.

The next day Julie went through class with no apparent difficulty, then asked to see Barbara before leaving. "Can I give you something?" she said. They went into the office and closed the door. "I found this in my bag," she said, handing over a large chopping knife, eight inches long and four inches wide at the base. Barbara thanked her and reported it to Dr. Sandler after Julie left. Dr. Sandler assured the counselor that multiples are survivors. The ability to form the personalities in the first place is a remarkable survival response to childhood brutality; Dr. Sandler had known multiples with several suicidal personalities, but there was always a rescuer who took over in the nick of time.

THEY WERE hoping to keep Julie out of the hospital. Dr. Sandler wouldn't have visiting rights and Julie would sit there for days with no useful therapy, answering questions about hearing voices.

In a session over the weekend Dr. Sandler talked with the younger personalities about staying inside during training and work, emphasizing that these were Julie's special places.

But on Monday morning Julie arrived at Barbara Green's dressed in two pairs of pants, the top pair inside-out.

One of the children had dressed her. There was no adult personality in charge. They spent the day at emergency. It was after dark when she was finally admitted to Franklin Hospital Medical Center in Valley Stream, the nearest facility with a bed. The community hospital had a small psychiatric wing and the care was about what you'd expect.

The associate director of psychiatry, Dr. Kishore Saraf, did not want Dr. Sandler seeing Julie even during visiting hours, saying it would intefere with his treatment. Dr. Saraf spoke with the group home, explaining to Maureen Coley that he did not believe Julie was a multiple and was concerned about the care she was receiving from Dr. Sandler. He felt Julie had a "character disorder" and was a "sociopath." Maureen could not believe what she was hearing and made an angry note about it in the group home record. For years one of the few things that doctors at the best facilities in the area had agreed on was that Julie was *not* antisocial. They couldn't make up their minds if she was depressed, borderline, schizophrenic, or multiple, but they'd always explicitly ruled out antisocial traits. Now this man who'd known her a day said she was antisocial.

Dr. Saraf did not elaborate at the time, but when questioned later, he explained that he does not believe that multiple personality disorder exists. "When someone tells me they have multiple personalities, I say to them, 'I am a husband to my wife, and a lover to my wife, and a teacher and educator to her. I am a father to my children. And a brother. A son to my parents. These are all different parts of me and different personalities. I'd say these are my other personalities. They're all independent, functional personalities. So you see, I have multiple personalities, too. To my mind, everybody has multiple personalities.' "

He was not swayed just because the American Psychiatric Association recognizes the multiple personality diagnosis. "These disorders go in and out of fashion," he said. (He also said he would never call someone a sociopath based on such limited observation, although both Julie and Maureen clearly remember his use of the term.)

Dr. Saraf told Maureen he had no treatment plan yet but would be in touch. He wanted to keep Julie at the hospital at least two weeks. He questioned whether she was doing this to get attention.

Dr. Sandler was concerned about her therapy being interrupted, and Maureen tried to arrange a transfer to Glen Cove Hospital, thinking staff there would be more receptive since they knew Julie, but Glen Cove did not want to extend privileges to a private therapist either. Julie was released after a week.

AND THEN things began to turn her way. The state Office of Mental Health finally came through with funding for the new supported apartment program, and she was one of the first to get one. For a time there was disagreement within the Melillo agency over whether Julie was capable of living alone. The agency director, Dr. Vogrin, and members of the clinic committee argued against it. If Julie could not do well in a twenty-four-hour supervised group home, how would she manage by herself? They viewed community mental health more rigidly, as a linear progression: When you are well enough, you leave the hospital and move to a group home; master that and move to a supervised apartment visited daily by a counselor; master that, and you're ready for your own apartment with a caseworker you can call on. Maureen and Linda Slezak worked more directly with residents and saw their varying needs and capabilities close up. They consulted with Dr. Sandler, who felt it was crucial for Julie to have privacy for the personalities. Julie was enormously capable, she would find a way to cope, but it was hard enough to adapt to a day full of blackouts without having to conform with extra rules in a supervised program.

The supported apartment program was a simple idea, modeled on a federal Section 8 subsidized housing grant. (In fact, if the federal government hadn't made such deep cuts in Section 8 housing under Presidents Reagan and Bush, those subsidies would have been perfect for Julie and tens of thousands of others with mental illness.) Your share of the rent was calculated on a sliding scale, depending on your income. The program administrator found Julie a private apartment that rented for $550. Because she wasn't working at the time she'd pay just $145 (which came from her monthly Social Security disability), and the state would make up the difference with a housing grant. She'd be living in a studio apartment in a complex in one of the poorer sections of the county, but at least she'd be alone. She was assigned an intensive case manager to call if she needed help, although the person would not visit unless Julie requested assistance.

Julie first saw the place on a blistering summer's day. There was no lock on the door, an unplugged refrigerator in the center of the room, windows on just one wall with no air conditioner, the stove didn't work, there were cockroaches, and the bathroom wallpaper featured a blue fern motif set against a silver metallic background. Julie was not the prejudiced type, but she did feel conspicuous as one of the few whites in a complex made up mainly of black working-class families.

Making the apartment habitable was no easy matter. She had to take three buses from Glen Cove to the complex, a two-hour commute (which you could drive in twenty-five minutes). There were times she'd arrive and the building superintendent would not show for their appointment.

But she persevered, making sure the place was clean, fumigated, and suitable before moving out of the group home in mid-September of 1990. In typical Julie fashion, she'd amassed bags and bags of clothes, mainly hand-me-downs from staff who'd befriended her at various programs. There were business suits, skin-tight jeans, girlie dresses—each personality had her own style.

From the stock of furniture allotted the program, Julie selected a couple of kitchen chairs, a butcher-block table, bureau, and black-and-white TV, and managed to lug most of it up two flights herself. She shopped for days at the malls before making the first major acquisition in her life on her own, a large peach futon with a heavy wood frame that would serve as both sofa and bed. Slowly she added to the room as she had money, sticking to her color scheme. She bought peach place mats, a peach sponge. Peach-colored blinds cost a little extra at Pergament, but they were worth it. She went to Curtains & Homes, an upscale furnishing store, saw a set of window dressings she loved but couldn't afford. So she just bought the two valances, in peach.

All around the room she added little touches: a watercolor boat scene she'd picked up for fifteen dollars at a Glen Cove diner; track lighting from a nurse at Glen Cove Hospital who was moving away; a candy dish from the group home and the typewriter that her counselor friend had told her to keep; bunny slippers that were a gift from staff on the hospital borderline unit.

TO AVOID Didi's surprise visits at the vocational training program, Dr. Sandler suggested Julie stop seeing Barbara Green and spend five days a week at a job placement. Di had decided Barbara was her friend, and voc rehab their playground. The younger personalities did seem to understand they were not to come out at work. ("Dr. Sandler says it's just not 'propriate," Didi once explained.)

Julie did so well, within months she was offered a part-time, paying secretarial job, three days a week. She was beginning to realize that the busier she kept her days, the fewer surprise visits she'd have. She took on two other part-time jobs, as an office manager for a small recreation firm and as an aide at a day care center.

She bought a junker for a few hundred dollars. It overheated so often, she kept a jug of water in the trunk.

Nights were still crazy as ever. The way the apartment program was conceived, Julie should have had help from her intensive case manager. The Office of Mental Health had promised that these super social workers would have smaller caseloads, be better paid, and available twenty-four hours a day to keep the most difficult, chronic people out of hospitals and off the streets. But the twenty-four-hour idea died quickly, the victim of union and individual resistance. In practice, many of these caseworkers were not accustomed to community mental health. Many had spent long careers behind desks, with set hours at state institutions, and reluctantly transferred to these new caseworker positions because cutbacks at the state hospitals were inevitable. When the intensive case manager gave Julie a business card, there was a number to call for any crisis after 5 P.M.—the county hospital's emergency room.

Julie asked the caseworker for help once, with cutting the system's red tape. The two went together to the county welfare office and Julie quickly realized she knew more than the case manager. Julie did not bother with the woman again.

HER THERAPIST was her lifeline. Dr. Sandler saw Julie three times a week for an hour and a half per session. Several times, in this period, after particularly difficult sessions with other personalities, Dr. Sandler drove her home and spent the night sitting up at the apartment, helping and observing the various personalities. When Julie emerged again, she was amazed—and embarrassed—to find the therapist. "It's all right," Dr. Sandler would say, "I knew it would be like this." The therapist was with her when she got the key to the new apartment. Julie introduced Dr. Sandler to the building superintendent and it made the younger woman feel good to show the man that she had this kind of person for a friend.

For the three years Julie had been misdiagnosed as a borderline personality, the treatment approach used on her was rigid and inflexible. Letting the patient take a minute overtime in therapy was considered giving in to her manipulations. So was fraternizing outside of therapy. The whole tone of therapy was intentionally confrontational.

This misdiagnosis colored even basic fact-gathering about her condition. Almost every night when she'd been hospitalized on the prestigious borderline unit, in 1987–88, Julie had outbursts and was confined to the ward's "quiet room." In retrospect it was clearly one of the tormented young personalities. Right to the end, even as the hospital reports described Julie as responding well to borderline treatment, she was being sent nightly to the quiet room. And yet no mention of these nightly confinements appears on her records that were sent out to therapists, hospitals, group homes. They weren't part of a borderline pattern. Facts that didn't fit the diagnosis became inconsequential. Important clues were buried.

Therapy for Julie as a multiple was exactly the opposite of borderline treatment—supportive, flexible, almost a friendship at times. Dr. Sandler's office was in her home and she would tour Julie—or Didi or Megan—around the house to show how she lived, get her a drink of orange juice from the refrigerator, point out pictures of her family. Julie had found little to trust in the world up to this point, and now Dr. Sandler was asking that from her and the others.

MOST OF HER free time was spent alone. They were difficult months, full of nighttime horrors; and yet there was beauty, too. Christmas of 1990 was her first in five years outside a hospital, and she was determined to make it festive, even if she was alone.

Every dollar counted, but she bought a real tree that was as big as she was, and for fifteen dollars more, an ornamental angel to sit on top. She considered the angel carefully before buying, asking to plug her in at the store to get the full effect. The angel was eight inches tall, with a dress of lace and cloth. She was blond, like the angels in books, and her face was of porcelain. In each hand the angel held a candle topped by a small bulb. Julie adjusted the angel so the lights in the little fists would shine steadily, while the rest of the tree blinked dark red, blue, and yellow.

She hung the stocking she'd made on 3-West the previous Christmas, filling it from a vending machine, using a roll of quarters to buy a few dozen small, round, clear plastic holders with tiny toys inside.

She bought lots of Christmas paper, even though she had almost no one to give gifts to and was left with six unused rolls. A few days before Christmas, she rode a bus to Roosevelt Field, blacked out in the middle of the mall, and when she came to discovered she'd purchased a stylish bucket filled with colorfully wrapped candy. Though this wasn't in the budget, she knew to keep it. Someone inside was plainly excited about the holiday and making her own plans.

The tree was positioned in the apartment so it faced the futon and she could stare at it as she lay in bed. It gave her a very spiritual feeling. She left the tree's lights on all night, which was a splurge, in terms of electricity.

A friend in program said there'd never been anyone so excited about Christmas as Julie. She couldn't wait for nightfall, to watch the blinking tree in the darkened apartment.

She probably could've had herself invited somewhere Christmas Day, but didn't want to infringe on anyone else's holiday. She did not want to spend another Christmas feeling like some charity case.

As had been true for many years, she did not remember Christmas Eve or Christmas Day.

But Didi did. There is no one on earth who believes in Christmas like a four-year-old personality. "I left the lights on all the whole night," Didi explained later. "What's the sense of wasting all that electricity if you aren't going to look at the Christmas tree, right? It was the most beautifulest tree.

"But you know what? I was waiting, waiting, waiting all night for Santa Claus and he didn't come. Maybe 'cause I stayed up. Santa doesn't like anyone seeing him.

"He didn't bring me one single present. I was a little sad. I think maybe he didn't know where I lived."

FINANCIALLY the smart thing would have been to stay in the subsidized apartment as long as possible. The state wisely set no time limit on this program, and the expectation was that for some, these apartments would become their homes.

Not Julie. She was set on leaving the mental health system, even though this program really required no involvement—except for taking the state's money. She did not want to be on any client list or even a mailing list. Julie craved an ordinary life. "There was this drive in me to get out of the system," she said later. "I don't want this to be my life."

That spring of 1991, she'd done so well in her part-time office job she was hired as a full-time secretary, at twenty-seven thousand dollars a year. Life was still far from easy. She didn't sleep for days at a stretch, as one personality after another came out to claim a piece of the night. The young personalities had a horrendous night and she was hospitalized three days during these months. But it was over a holiday weekend, and no one, except Dr. Sandler, even knew. At another point Marlena refused to go to therapy (Marlena had no intention of being "killed off" through integration with other personalities)—and threatened to run away to North Carolina if any of them met with Dr. Sandler. For several weeks, Julie's only contact with the therapist was over the phone, but this passed too.

Summer was always a good time for her. She loved the beach and sunning and the heat, and that summer of 1991 she felt strong enough to find a place of her own. She answered an ad in *Newsday* for an upstairs apartment in a private residence on a quiet suburban street. When she went to look at it, a downstairs neighbor was barbecuing in the yard. The living room was huge, the bathroom new, the closets roomy. There were lots of windows looking out onto a couple of large maples. Julie kept thinking, Yes, yes, all right! The landlords, a young couple who'd fixed it up themselves, were apologetic about asking for two months' security, but Julie said, "No problem, you want a check or cash?" She'd been saving every penny from her job just for this.

Another nice thing—she wasn't so alone anymore. For her move to this place of her own, she had three friends to help with the heavy lifting, including a new boyfriend, her first ever, who got along quite well with most of the personalities.

chapter 13

SUMMER 1991,
AWAITING MIRACLES

"GOOD MORNING, community residence," senior counselor JoAnn Mendrina answered the phone. First call of the day,
Wednesday, June 19, 1991, and she was already rolling her eyes. Yet
another county caseworker needed more information. This time the
county was trying to decide whether to issue funds for a reinforced bed
that would not collapse like Jasper's last two. JoAnn had been trying
to get Jasper off the floor since the summer of 1990 and had never
imagined that on this, her last day at the group home, she'd still be
negotiating this same damn bed. "You'd think we were asking for the
Taj Mahal, to get this kid a bed," said JoAnn. Jasper's twenty-eighth
birthday was the previous weekend. They'd raided the miscellaneous
cash fund and bought him a blue sweatsuit and his annual lobster—a
two-pounder—which JoAnn cooked for him. "You made that special
for me?" Jasper said. "That's nice." His mother had forgotten him
again.

"Good morning, community residence." A counselor calling in
sick. JoAnn had to find someone to fill the noon-to-eight shift tomor-

row. She walked out of the office and turned off the box air conditioners in the living room and dining room. A dry morning heat was building, but she wouldn't put them back on until a little before four, when residents returned from programs. JoAnn was the original watt-watcher.

"Good morning, community residence." A doctor's office reminding Heather about her appointment to have a polyp removed.

"Good morning, community residence"—it was so ingrained, JoAnn often answered her home phone that way. Her adult kids teased, "Come on Ma, separate," and JoAnn would shoot back, "Pipe down, brats."

She was going to miss the place. Telling Anthony was hardest. He'd come bounding in as usual a couple of weeks ago, yelling "JoAnn, I'm home," and she'd sat him down and laid it out. She was moving to Vermont, her husband was retiring. "I'm tired, I need a rest," she'd explained.

"You're not that old," Anthony answered. She hadn't told them that her long "vacation" at the start of the year was actually cancer treatment, reasoning, "People have enough on their minds."

"You run around this house all day long," Anthony said. "You're a wonder woman, JoAnn." Anthony suggested she commute. "I know you don't like it, but you're like a mother to me," he said, the words JoAnn was dreading. This was just what Anthony needed, being abandoned by another mother figure. JoAnn had not expected this. She had felt certain he'd be in his own apartment by now. For years she'd worked with retarded adults. It was hard teaching them independent living skills, but once you did, they had it for life. Anthony, on the other hand, made great strides until his schizophrenia flared, and then she'd have to start from scratch, reassuring him that his father's voice was not in his head.

Even people who resented her bossy streak were unsettled by the news of her departure. They were used to younger counselors taking better jobs or leaving to get married. But JoAnn? What would 9 Highland be without JoAnn puffing on a long brown More cigarette and asking if you'd cleaned the blue bathroom yet?

. . .

MORNING SLIPPED into afternoon and JoAnn finished her paperwork. "I'm pretty squared away," she announced.

"Good afternoon, community residence." It was Stephen DeRosa calling from the hospital pay phone. He was starting his third month on 3-West and finally had been put on clozapine, the latest wonder drug for schizophrenia. Stephen was supposed to visit the house that evening on a pass, but said he wasn't feeling well. JoAnn believed he was withdrawing and went to work on him. After hanging up, she said, "He'll be here. I told him we were having sausage and peppers for dinner—his favorite."

"Good afternoon, community residence." Melillo's East Hills house had veal parmesan on the supper menu and a twenty-one-year-old counselor needed JoAnn's recipe.

Maureen was leaving early for a meeting. The two women hugged and JoAnn formally turned in her house keys. "It's the original key chain that came with the house," JoAnn said. "Kind of historic." Maureen started to say something, but JoAnn interrupted: "Get your butt the hell out of here," and that was their good-bye.

A little before four, the watt watcher turned the air conditioners downstairs back on and closed the front door. Their labored clanking drowned out the cicadas in the backyard hedge.

People were returning home. From the office, JoAnn listened, and when she didn't hear the door click, called out, "Please shut it. The air conditioners are on. Thank you."

A female resident was going to a job interview and asked JoAnn how much she should say about her illness. "I wouldn't tell them a thing," JoAnn said.

"Jasper! The door," JoAnn yelled.

Anthony stuck his head in. He was fidgety, bobbing and weaving in and out of the office. "I closed the door," he said.

"I heard," said JoAnn.

"I guess this is your last day . . . I'll miss you . . . See you around . . . I guess I won't." JoAnn promised to say good-bye before leaving.

"I'll be in my room," said Anthony.

Heather poked her head in. She wanted a lesson in cleaning her room air-conditioner filter before JoAnn left.

Anthony walked by. "I had a soda. It was good."

The afternoon sun was slanting through the living room blinds. Heather was describing to several of them how the doctor had yanked the polyp from her throat. JoAnn folded a basket of laundered bath mats. About five, a woman who'd graduated the house the year before stopped by with two pink roses for JoAnn. The young woman was living in her own apartment and finishing college. "You'll be proud of me," she said. "I have all my fingernails and toenails." She was wearing a skimpy, summery lime dress, cut short. JoAnn did up the top button. "If you're going to wear a one-piece, you keep it all buttoned, kiddo," JoAnn said.

She supposed it was time to go upstairs and say 'bye to Anthony. When she returned, she said, "He was cleaning his room. I've been asking him to do it for two years."

Several were watching *Neighbors*, an absolutely awful Australian sitcom that they all hated, but no one was motivated to get up and change it. Paula Marsters was preparing the barbecue for the sausages. "I need a man out here," she called. She couldn't get the propane valve opened.

JoAnn opened it, then kissed several of them good-bye and walked out the front door, closing it carefully behind her. She unlocked her 1985 Nissan Centra and climbed in, feeling the afternoon heat sweep over her.

On the radio Julia Roberts' manager was saying he was sure Julia would survive her canceled marriage to Kiefer Sutherland and all the publicity. "Julia's a very strong person," the man was saying.

DESPITE ALL the resolutions to clean up Jasper that summer, he continued to smell. JoAnn's departure didn't help. Just before she left, she caught him wearing his red-and-white-stripe jersey two days in a row and suggested he be given a schedule of what outfit to wear each day. But no one followed through. Jasper's counselor Robert Kouril pressed him to shower before leaving the house mornings and was generally successful. But when they tried to actually watch him showering to make sure he was getting himself clean, Jasper locked the door. He wanted his privacy and was entitled.

Jasper was such an obvious mess to the naked eye, each agency that had a piece of responsibility for overseeing his care blamed the others for failing him. A couple of times that summer a counselor from Progress House, a state-run therapy-oriented day program, called the group home and complained about Jasper smelling. Each time, Jasper had showered that morning. But the ride to program was an hour in a yellow social service minibus that had no air-conditioning and was built for children, not a 350-pound man.

He spent a weekend in July laughing to himself, and at times was even mean—not like Jasper. After a dinner, a counselor told him he wasn't getting the pots clean enough, and he banged them down, saying "Fuck this," and stormed into his room.

Maureen continued to be his biggest defender. "If all this is going on inside, the last thing he needs is more demands on him," she told her staff. "If there's a chore like cleaning pots, someone needs to be with him at all times." The office was quiet. Maureen had lost her biggest Jasper ally when JoAnn left. The younger counselors weren't as sympathetic. They were Jasper's age and felt he could try harder.

"This has been going on for two years," said Robert.

"But if we stay on him, he seems to do better," said Maureen. "More alert, laughing less."

The one time that summer he seemed really focused was at Melillo's annual outing to Great Adventure Amusement Park in New Jersey. He was particularly fond of the American Dream Machine roller-coaster (featuring seven upside-down loops) and Shock Wave, which he rode several times, usually alone.

His fellow residents worked at keeping him away. After the toilet paper holder in the small bathroom beside the kitchen was broken for the fourth time, counselors realized it must be Jasper, snapping it off accidentally because he didn't have room to maneuver his huge body in there. They suggested he shower upstairs in the roomier blue bathroom.

"Can't," said Jasper. Upstairs residents had told him if you live downstairs, you have to shower downstairs.

There was no such rule.

"What will I tell them?" said Jasper.

Maureen told them.

She took out her frustration on his day program, Progress House, and the psychiatrist there for not doing more about Jasper's worsening hallucinations. Maureen discussed it with Linda Slezak and the other group home managers at a July 15 staff meeting. "I talked to his social worker at Progress House about his deterioration. She said, 'Is he violent?' As if that's the point. Do we have to wait until he hurts someone or himself?" Maureen tried to get the Progress House psychiatrist to reevaluate Jasper, but the doctor kept putting it off. "I said to her, 'He was laughing the whole weekend.' She said, 'Maybe he's thinking of something funny.'"

So Maureen visited Progress House to pressure the staff. "I told them, 'We've had Jasper two years, but this is a dramatic change and this is a real backslide.' They seemed to grasp it when I was there in the room. They told me Jasper sleeps through the groups; they're very matter-of-fact about it. He's been telling the Progress House staff they're all possessed.

"He doesn't cause problems for anybody, so they don't care if he's staring at the ceiling. One time I called. 'Oh yeah, he's sitting in the parking lot.'"

Linda Slezak knew Progress House could do better. It was not one of her favorite programs and state budget cuts were undermining it more. When there were layoffs in the unionized state system, workers with more seniority bumped those with less. So while Progress House's budget was not being cut, its staff was being decimated; social workers were bumped out of their jobs and replaced with more senior workers from state hospitals who may never have worked in a community program.

Even so, Linda had the feeling that the entire National Institute of Mental Health would not be able to keep Jasper awake in group.

"Would you recommend a program change?" Linda asked.

"I would," said Maureen. "This is the last straw."

They decided to try Sara Center, the crafts-oriented program that had been so supportive with Anthony. It was run by a nonprofit agency rather than the state, and the director, Jeanne McMorrow, was another Linda Slezak, a person who would do the best that could be hoped for.

"Any news on Jasper's bed?" asked Linda.

"We're in the second year," said Maureen, "but they say just two more weeks now. He's already gone through two."

"Two beds, two bathrooms, he's wearing everything out," said Linda.

"And the couch," said Maureen.

Maureen went back to the house and gave her staff a pep talk on Jasper. She reminded them of what had happened when counselors at the apartment program did not pay enough attention to the voices Stan Gunter heard. "We have to ask, 'Are you hearing things? Are you seeing things? Is something bothering you?' We have to let him know we care and we notice. He's not just a lump in the corner."

"His mother missed his birthday," Maureen reminded them. "JoAnn, a mother figure, left him. His counselor left Progress House because of the state cuts. This may be Jasper's way of responding. It may be healthy." Maureen looked around. Her counselors were staring at the floor.

THAT SUMMER the state Office of Mental Health informed the group home that residents were no longer "residents," they were "consumers," and the department's new philosophy was "empowerment." "All in OMH is now being driven by the consumer," Karen Mankin, an administrator in the state's regional office, announced at one of many meetings held that spring and summer. There were empowerment conferences and empowerment seminars and for a while it sounded like the Students for a Democratic Society had landed in

Albany and were running the state Office of Mental Health. Of course, these were really just the fashionable academic words of the moment —spun out by a team of consultants the commissioner had hired from Boston University—and had little to do with reality.

At the same time New York's mentally ill consumers were being empowered, the state and counties cut aid to mental health clinics by 17 percent, meaning it was harder for the empowered consumers at 9 Highland to get a therapist; closed the Glen Cove consumers' favorite extracurricular activity, a weekend recreation club; and retreated in the face of neighborhood protests against proposed group homes in New Hyde Park and Garden City, Long Island, declaring a temporary moratorium on new group home development.

To empower consumers, the commissioner had created intensive case managers—super social workers with reduced caseloads—who were supposed to respond flexibly. In the early days of the program, these caseworkers had general funds available for a consumer's specific problems. Julie's junker was constantly breaking down. She was afraid it might jeopardize her job, but she hadn't been working long enough to qualify for a car loan. So she called her intensive case manager and asked if the state could help her secure a car loan. "What could be more necessary than needing a car on Long Island to get to work?" Julie asked.

"Sorry," was the case manager's answer. "Budget cuts."

NEW YORK'S Office of Mental Health was the last place you'd expect to be leading an empowerment charge. Historically, it had little to be proud of. At one point, the state's mental illness and mental retardation departments were lumped together in a single state Department of Hygiene. But that changed in the mid-1970s, when a federal judge ordered New York to empty the infamous Willowbrook institution for the retarded and move fifty-four hundred residents into group homes and apartments. At the time, Governor Hugh Carey's administration split the retardation and mental illness sections into two departments. State workers who were passionate about building housing in the community went to work for the new Office of Retardation. During the 1980s that office became a national leader in opening group homes and apartments, humanely shifting retarded adults from institutions to the community.

The Office of Mental Health, on the other hand, remained a dinosaur, presiding over the dumping of mental patients from hospitals into the streets. Governor Carey's budget director, Peter Goldmark, recalls that in the 1970s the administration urged a group home movement for the mentally ill too, but the Albany bureaucrats were still wedded to the medical model dominated by state mental hospitals.

By the late 1980s, the state Office of Mental Health's most visible legacy was ten thousand untreated sick, homeless people wandering New York City. In tight budget times you'd think that at the very least, state officials would have felt a responsibility to make every penny count. But, incredibly, New York had more state mental hospitals in 1990—twenty-two for twelve thousand patients—than it had in the 1950s—eighteen for ninety-three thousand patients. In 1990 the state was still spending over two-thirds of its mental health budget on hospitals, even though the vast majority of mentally ill were living—or trying to live—in the community.

To his credit, the commissioner of mental health, Dr. Richard Surles, who took over in 1987, recognized the problem, understood community care, had a vision of what was needed, and headed off in the right direction. But too often his first-rate ideas did not translate into first-rate action. This may have been because the office's career bureaucrats did not get it, or had seen too many revolutionary changes in their time that were not accompanied by funding. The commissioner's boss, Governor Mario Cuomo, spoke eloquently for the little people and in many respects was a progressive leader, yet during his decade in office he never made the mentally ill homeless a top priority. (Building group homes was certainly nowhere near as high on his list as building prisons, which he did at a record clip in New York State.) For whatever reason, by the time the commissioner's right-minded speeches reached from Albany to the southeastern tip of the state, the message was garbled, the implementation positively bizarre. Long

Island's regional administrators latched onto the radical phrases, but underneath it all, they were still the Flintstones.

To kick off the state's new empowerment policy, over one hundred group home residents (including several from the three Melillo houses) were transported to the state office's regional headquarters in Brentwood, Long Island. The meeting happened to be convened on a day when the electricity was shut off for a repair project, so the newly empowered consumers sat in a shadowy, unlighted meeting room trying to hear speeches without the aid of microphones. The main consumer participation was two group home residents who stood shyly for thirty seconds each, reading something inaudible right off note cards. State officials explained that there would now be countywide consumer meetings and local consumer meetings within each agency to guarantee empowerment. Most of the meeting was devoted to handing out and explaining a new thirty-three-question survey—The Consumer Housing Empowerment Survey—that people were to use to critique the group home where they lived. The surveys were to be taken back to the group homes and filled out by all residents, then placed in a sealed envelope, which was to be secured in a second large sealed manila envelope and mailed back to the regional office. This was to guarantee confidentiality so there'd be no retribution for criticizing your group home. The information would serve as a basis for designing new housing programs. "We want to see what kind of housing you want," state officials kept saying.

Maureen was deeply skeptical about all this. In her experience the most capable people, the ones who'd make hell-raising consumers— Julie, Stan, Heather—were using all their energy to build lives of their own away from the system. When you don't have much money and have to get around a suburban county by bus, and are trying to hold a job as you fend off your illness—there isn't much of you left for anything else. They were hell-bent on escaping, not remaking the system. You don't want to be pounding a podium; you're striving to become part of the invisible "normal" masses. As Julie once said, "It makes me feel much more healthy not to be involved in the mental health system. It's like people should have hopes and dreams of being normal." Activism? The few times Maureen circulated petitions at the house to protest state budget cuts, there would always be several who wouldn't sign even though they were sympathetic; they were fearful of publicly identifying themselves as mentally ill. Stephen DeRosa didn't even like to sit in front of the house, he was so concerned about being tagged mentally ill. As for people destined to spend their lives in the system, they were vulnerable to cynical manipulation because they were often limited by the illnesses.

Still, Maureen pestered the consumers of 9 Highland to fill out the questionnaires. Every time she asked, Fred Grasso said it was in his room; one woman couldn't find hers; Eve felt it was vague and wasn't interested; Jasper could not understand why you'd do something like this if you weren't being paid for it.

After a couple of weeks, Maureen got most of them to fill out the surveys and mail them off in all the confidential double-sealed envelopes provided by the state.

And that was the last that most of them ever heard of the empowerment survey. A year and a half later the survey still had not been made public.

Heather, for one, tried the local consumer meetings. "These meetings were just bullshit," she said. "We spent all our time talking about how we'd get more people to come to the next meeting. For what? Personally, I've had enough." Her consumer career ended after two meetings.

The countywide consumer meetings lasted a few months, before they too died. "We haven't had one in a while," the state's Karen Mankin said five months after the landmark meeting in the dark. "It was an interesting phenomenon. We'd send out personal letters to everyone who came to the previous meeting, but then we'd never get the same people. There was no continuity. We asked people when the best time was and they said at night. But then it was impossible to get busses. Plus they had other things to do."

Was the state's consumer empowerment movement now dead on Long Island? "We did get a lot out of it," said Mankin. "We used what they told us. We didn't say we were going to have another meeting and we didn't say we weren't going to have one." She'd discussed it with Paule Pachter, Nassau County's deputy commissioner of mental health. "Check with Paule," she said. "If he feels we need one, we'll schedule it. It's fine with me. I'd certainly go." The empowerment movement was precisely as effective as you would expect a consumer movement founded and nurtured by a government bureaucracy to be.

There was a genuine consumer movement for the mentally ill. The real consumer movement was spearheaded by the National Alliance for the Mentally Ill, which was made up of some mentally ill people, but mainly their parents and siblings, people like Anthony's father, Dom Constantine, and Fred's parents, the Grassos, and Arnold and Pearl Gould, who had a son at Melillo's Glen Head house. The National Alliance had chapters with paid staff all over the country. They were independent. They worked with the state commissioner when they could, pressuring the legislature and governor to appropriate more money for the mental health budget. And when they couldn't work with the state, they sued—for example, forcing New York to make clozapine available at its state hospitals. If they saw the state doing wrong or being cowardly, they called reporters and were quoted by name in the press. They had information, money, votes, a few important friends, telephones, copy machines, faxes—the traditional American tools of empowerment. They did not need to be empowered by the state commissioner of mental health and his university consultants.

And the commissioner returned their calls and worked with them because he respected them, needed them, feared them.

WHILE THE STATE was pushing empowerment, Maureen was trying to get residents to pick up wet bath mats after they showered. The issue dominated the Tuesday community meetings in June and July. From the beginning, they'd had problems with the blue bathroom upstairs leaking and damaging the living room ceiling. They had the shower, toilet, and sink repaired several times but nothing seemed to end the leaks for more than a few weeks. (One plumber had told Maureen, "I see things here I've never seen anyplace else.")

Twelve adults put a lot of wear and tear on an ordinary residential house. Maureen felt part of the problem was water being slopped onto the floor, undermining the grouting. She made regular appeals for residents to pick up soggy mats after they showered and bring them down to the laundry room, so staff could clean them. "It's just laziness," said Maureen. "The ceiling is collapsing. That's an avoidable cost."

"It's a problem, taking a wet, sopping bath mat, dripping downstairs," said Joe. "It's a big problem."

"Wring it out first," said Maureen.

"I can do it," said Joe. "I'm not talking about myself. But I can't police the world. I'm not going to be the world's policeman."

"What do you think, Fred?" said Maureen.

"Yeah," said Fred.

"The bath mat," said Maureen.

"I think you're supposed to leave it there."

"We've been talking about this for how long?" said Joe. Jasper was absentmindedly flicking the light in the dining room off and on.

"Jasper, please stop," said Maureen. "What do you do? With the bath mats?"

"Leave it there," said Jasper.

"Have you been listening?" Maureen asked.

"I couldn't hear," said Jasper. (He probably couldn't, with all the voices in his head.)

"We'll all do it, right, Fred?" said Maureen.

"Use soap when you take a shower?" said Fred.

Sure enough, the very next Tuesday, Heather began the meeting by saying, "People are still leaving the mats on the floor of the bathroom soaking wet. At least four times I've picked them up."

"I don't know what else I can say," Maureen said. "Fred, when you're done using them what do you do?"

"I leave them there," said Fred.

Eventually they just cut a hole in the living room ceiling and covered it with a grate, so when the upstairs bathroom leaked, instead of destroying the downstairs ceiling, the water dripped down from the second floor through the grate onto the living room floor and could be conveniently mopped up.

FOR SIX WEEKS that summer Marcy, a schizophrenic woman in her twenties, lived at the house. It was without question the most bizarre stay anyone there had experienced. She'd been in a supervised apartment program, stopped taking her antipsychotic medication, was hospitalized four months, and now was supposedly ready to live in the community. Maureen could not imagine what the hospital staff was thinking in discharging her. Marcy made Jasper look like the chairman of the board of General Motors.

Her first several days at the house she would not come out of her room, take a shower, or change clothes. The first words she said to Heather were, "Did you have a nose job?"

People walked past her door on the way to the living room and with no prompting, Marcy would stick her head out and say, "I am not vomiting in here."

Joe caught her hanging up the pay phone when calls weren't for her. She warned one of the most timid residents, "Get out of here if you want to live a long life." Eve put up with weeks of Stephen DeRosa's paranoia but quickly lost it with Marcy, yelling, "Why are you so weird?"

"Did you call me a rabbit?" Marcy asked.

She threatened to report senior counselor Jodie Schwartz to Melillo for making her do a state-mandated fire drill.

Maureen was convinced she was not taking her medication. "We have to make sure she's swallowing," said Maureen. "There's no way she's behaving the way she's behaving and taking it. She has a long history."

"Even when you're watching it's hard to see," said counselor Lauryn Schelfo.

Maureen had seen people palm their meds, hide them under their tongue, spit them down the toilet. She wanted Marcy on a liquid dosage so they could better monitor her, but Marcy refused.

"Fred keeps calling Marcy crazy," said counselor Charles Winslow.

"Fred has good assessment skills," said Maureen.

At a Monday staff meeting Linda Slezak asked, "She's resisting?"

"Everything," said Mauren.

Under pressure from Maureen, Marcy returned to the hospital, voluntarily.

MUCH OF THAT summer was lost to Stephen DeRosa, spent in a medicated fog on 3-West. You'd call about visiting him and he'd say, "What day is it?" Try to bring up a pleasant memory, like the evening Heather played with him on the park swings weeks before, and he'd forgotten it. ("No, I didn't do that. No.") There was a black therapy aide on the ward he was sure was snubbing him. So were several beautiful fat girl patients. He complained that the hospital food was awful, but when another patient said it was good, Stephen looked unsure. "Unless they're doing something special to my food." Nor could he think of anything he missed about the outside world. Not church. "I get communion here." Not the group home. "I don't like that place." Certainly not his roommate Jasper. "Are they ever going to get rid of that guy?"

The hospital psychiatrist, Dr. Melamed, was waiting to see if the clozapine would take effect. In early June 1991, Stephen had become the first patient to be tried on it at Glen Cove Hospital. (He took this in combination with Prozac, an antidepressant.) In a very few cases, clozapine caused a rapid drop in white blood cell count and even death, so weekly blood work was required. Hospital staff proceeded cautiously; they didn't want Stephen to leave until they were sure he was stable.

Everyone in the mental health system had heard the stories of the remarkable "awakening" clozapine produced in certain patients—the overnight disappearance of tormenting voices and hallucinations that had plagued people for years. In some cases improvement was reported within days of beginning the dosage; other times it could be months. Dr. John Katz, of Long Island Jewish Hospital, where much of the pioneering work was done, believed a patient should be given at least a three-month trial. Dr. Jean-Pierre Lindenmayer at Bronx State Hospital gave his patients six months.

These weeks, when Stephen visited the group home on day passes, counselors looked for signs of his awakening.

"HOW DO MY eyes look?" Stephen asked Maureen, Heather, and anyone else who would listen during a July 15 pass to the house. "Do they look all right?" He was afraid they had turned an evil black.

"Brown with a tinge of green," said Heather after taking a close look. It was a hot, still night and the two were sitting out front, talking. Stephen kept saying what a bad person he was. At one point he took Heather's hand and prayed out loud.

"I've been praying, but it's not from the inside," Stephen said. He would dig into himself deeper for a holy feeling, and hold it awhile, but the evil kept edging back. "I abuse God," he said. "I'll go down and then I'll feel better, but like an asshole I'll blow the whole thing. I'm a real jerk."

He kept patting Heather on the knee and thigh. "Am I sitting too close to you?" he asked. He could be wrong, but she seemed to be gaining weight. It made him feel zesty inside.

Heather persuaded him to come for a ride into town to get ice cream. In the car, Stephen kept glancing out the window to see if anyone was staring at him. "I've been defaming God," he said. "It's not my sickness. You think that, but it's not. I have the power to stop it . . . I'm going down, down, down. The other day I was on the abyss of Hell—" He interrupted himself to order a half-pint of vanilla with butterscotch topping at Cove Ice Cream. Heather got hers, then went out in the parking lot to join him. "Where's Stephen?" she asked.

He was standing in the back of the lot, behind a wall.

Heather couldn't figure why a just God would want to punish Stephen. Certainly actions should be more important than thoughts. Stephen volunteered at church bingo, took communion several times a week, did his chores, worked hard at the sheltered workshop and his part-time job.

"I think you can sin with your mind," replied Stephen. "I brought it on myself. I said, 'Fuck you, God.' Then I'd say 'Praise you, Jesus' and 'Thank you, Jesus,' over and over until I thought it would melt away. It helps, but it's not enough." He'd been checking himself a lot in the mirror lately. He was nearly fifty. "I don't see sweetness in my eyes. I see a neutral dead sight, not a real glowing from Christ that other people have. I notice people don't believe me as much anymore . . . People don't notice me."

Stephen liked the idea of taking a drive up to Morgan Park on Long Island Sound before heading back to the hospital. The sun was setting, turning the sky a fiery orange and red above the water. Sailboats tied to buoys bobbed in the harbor, their ropes softly clanging against their masts. These were the waters that F. Scott Fitzgerald's characters had gazed upon in *The Great Gatsby*. The smells of this midsummer eve at a public park in 1991 were the same Fitzgerald had described seventy years before: "the sparkling odor of jonquils, and the frothy odor of hawthorn and plum blossoms and the pale gold odor of kiss-me-kate-at the gate."

Stephen was quite moved, sitting there in the car. "I'm getting feedback from Jesus Christ. Now God is filling me and overcoming that smothering feeling." He wasn't hearing God's voice, but he could see Him coming into his soul through the window of the '84 Honda.

"Please close the window," Stephen said. He wanted to try to hold the feeling in the car as long as possible. He gazed down and prayed: "Help me to always believe in Christ. There's definitely a Christ who is a sole person to believe in salvation. Don't let me go to Hell. You don't want another soul in Hell."

He relaxed. "This other feeling is coming over me, a comforting, soothing atmosphere. Praise you Jesus. Thank you Jesus." His eyes were closed and he was smiling.

A few minutes before nine, the sun set behind Little Neck, Queens.

Stephen was due back at the hospital. As the car drove up the hill, away from the dark waters, Stephen was grateful. "Well, I said, 'Fuck you Jesus Christ' twice, but now all I can say is 'Praise you Jesus, thank you for mercy, for constantly filling in the hole I dig. Praise you in the name of Jesus Christ.' "

The moon was nearly full. Normally he hated a full moon—it was the Devil's work—but tonight he was not going to let it upset him. "I feel good," he said as the car pulled up to Glen Cove Hospital's front entrance. "I still have that feeling I had at the water. God, I could see Him in my soul . . . It was a good feeling. Boy, I'm going to masturbate good tonight!"

He waved a cheerful farewell and, head down, pushed against the hospital's revolving glass door and disappeared into the lobby.

HEATHER TALKED about killing herself most of the summer. It drove the counselors crazy. Donna Rubin would get off at eight, and be rushing out to a night job as a bookkeeper at Roy Rogers hamburgers in Queens, when Heather would stop at the door to say good-bye. Looking very much in pain, Heather would tell Donna, "It's OK, you have to go. Don't worry about me. Nothing really matters. You're off now." Heather knew just whom to pick. Donna is a soft touch. She'd ask if Heather felt suicidal and get answers like, "I don't have any immediate plans," or "I don't know what might happen." It was like dealing with Bette Davis in *All About Eve*, every line had six meanings.

They spent hours talking about it at staff meetings. "This is very tricky stuff," said Maureen. "It's highly manipulative, but . . ." But Heather might kill herself.

Heather's diagnosis was borderline personality disorder and her behavior that summer was straight from a textbook. Everything was to the extreme. Half the residents wanted to kill her because she manipulated so much of the staff's time; and half adored her because she was so kind to them. She used the few thousand dollars she'd inherited from her father's estate to buy things for friends at the house. She bought one of her male friends Double Gulp–size Cokes at the Seven-Eleven and constantly took her best girlfriend at the house to Taco Bell to eat.

Heather and Teresa—another borderline—became inseparable. It is a trait of the disorder, the inability to put normal limits or "boundaries" on a friendship. They'd spend every hour together, make condescending inside jokes about others at the house, and would eat out to get away from group home food as often as possible. Several times they bought a six-pack of Coors and drank in the parking lot behind the CVS pharmacy. If Teresa was going to the July 4 Melillo barbecue, Heather would, too, but if Teresa changed her mind at the last minute, so did Heather. Heather would leave Reese's peanut butter cups on Teresa's pillow at night.

Dr. John Imhof, Heather's therapist, said about her, "Anyone who comes around, she'll give a hand. But she doesn't have bounds. She'll give away her shirt, her shoes, her last penny."

Heather could not set normal limits with other adults because she'd grown up without any. She never learned normal parent-child boundaries—her father started having sex with her when she was four. In the household, the mother's and father's problems were all intertwined with young Heather's. They manipulated the child brutally and sexually for their own ends.

And Heather in turn grew into a manipulative adult. That summer she'd arranged to see two therapists, Dr. Imhof, whom she'd been with for eight years, and Dr. Barris, who'd testified for her at the commitment hearing. She loved all the attention. She'd come back and tell Teresa, "John and I had a good session today. He gave me a hug at the end—I even got lipstick on his shirt."

She constantly complained about her health problems. Her asthma was terrible in the sticky heat. And yet she continued to smoke up to two packs of Marlboro 100s a day even after the polyp was discovered in her throat and she developed a serious lung infection. She'd be puffing on a cigarette in the TV room complaining about how long it was taking the doctors to find what was causing the lung infection. She bought and read several technical books on respiratory illnesses.

When Dr. Imhof went on vacation for two weeks, Heather spent hours telling the counselors she wouldn't be able to make it through without him. Then she spent hours apologizing for taking too much of their time. She talked about getting in her car and driving away. Or going on vacation for a week to make up her mind on "the big question." Two days before Dr. Imhof was due back, she said she felt very suicidal and went to the Glen Cove Hospital emergency room. The hospital would not admit her. Dr. Melamed felt she'd challenged their recommended treatment at the commitment hearing that spring, so she didn't belong there. He suggested she go to the county hospital where Dr. Barris, her advocate at the hearing, practiced.

Heather was outraged. She wanted a private hospital, and if she couldn't get one, said she'd rather just be at the group home.

Dr. Melamed's feeling was "Good. That's exactly where Heather belongs."

MAUREEN HAD warned that if no one took care of Snuffy, the white rabbit would have to go, and after weeks of discussion, the final decision came at the Tuesday, July 23, community meeting. "It's not fair to Snuffy to have her cooped up in a cage and no one paying attention to her or cleaning her," said Maureen.

Joe said, "I just want to be on the record as saying I never promised to help out with that rabbit." Several said they'd like her to stay, but only Fred raised his hand when Maureen asked who would care for her.

"I cleaned the cage once," said Fred.

"Once is not going to make it," said Maureen. (Fred did not say that he'd tried cleaning it other times only to be bullied by another resident, who told Fred, "This is my job, Fred, you're not supposed to be doing it." And then that man rarely did it either.)

"What will happen to the rabbit?" Heather asked.

"Send her to Pilgrim State," said someone.

"We wouldn't even do that to a rabbit," said Maureen. Jodie Schwartz was bringing Snuffy home to live with her.

Fred was taking the minutes of the meeting. He'd summarized the discussion on the rabbit this way: "Also Snuffy the new rabbit might have to be given away because she is a little lonely."

EVERYONE IN the group had to do something during the day. It could be work or schooling, but for most this meant rehabilitative treatment or vocational training programs. A couple dozen of these privately run, government-funded day programs had sprung up throughout Nassau County in the previous decade. Quality varied greatly. One group-home resident used to brag about how many hours he slept on the couch at his prevocational program.

Micrographics in Hicksville, run by Long Island Jewish Hospital, is one of the better programs in the mental health system, training people to microfilm documents. Government offices, businesses, and libraries then hire the graduates as microfilm technicians (for up to eight dollars an hour) to work in record keeping.

Bruce Glick, the director, says that from the program's inception in 1987 to 1991, 350 had enrolled, and 80 were placed in jobs. Training is split into two phases: a classroom setting in the front of the shop where participants learn general office practices like filing, typing, collating; and a back shop, where they learned to photograph documents and develop microfilm. Microfilming takes some skill and independent judgment in sizing and focusing, although most of it is by rote.

The typical stay at the program was less than a year. As of July 1991, Fred Grasso had been at Micrographics one year and eight months.

He was still in the first phase, office skills.

When asked how Fred was doing, Glick said, "Very well. He's made good progress. He went from typing twenty to twenty-five words per minutes to forty on his own. The secretary sometimes gives him memos to type."

Did they think Fred could get a secretarial job?

"I'm not sure about that," said Glick. "An assignment with a lot of steps could get confusing for Fred. I'm not sure he could answer the phones either . . . He's somebody I never thought would get to the point he did. He's come a long way."

As an example of Fred's progress, Glick mentioned "spitting." "It took a while but he doesn't spit anymore," said Glick. One side effect of clozapine is excess saliva. Fred used to rise from his desk several times daily, open the front office door, and spit into the wind. They'd worked on ways to handle the problem more discreetly, like chewing gum.

A traditional office worker occasionally stretches, or goes to the water cooler; Fred made extraneous sounds, like a bird trilling. "Fred was high-fiving people," said Glick. "Not how you'd conduct yourself in the office. He was also poking the secretary in the side and back when he walked past her. Fred was being friendly, but it would ruffle her feathers. It is not something you can do here.

"He could sit for twenty minutes, then would need to wander. He just stood up and leaned against the wall and gazed out into the room. Fred now could probably sit for thirty minutes or thirty-five when he's involved with something, and then needs to get up." You were supposed to let the supervisor know when you were taking a break. Only two at a time could go. "About 40 percent of the time he'll let you know," said Glick. "The rest he'll just sign out and take the break even if two people are already out. You'll say, 'Please tell me when you're going out,' and he'll say OK—Fred's very nice about it—but then he won't and if you ask why, he can't explain.

"Sometimes people are put off by his quietness," Glick added.

For most, the goal was to get that tryout at microfilming in the back shop. "Fred had a project to do on microfilm to see if he could advance to the second phase," said Glick. "He'd developed the film, and to complete it, he has to put it in a plastic jacket. His film sat beside that typewriter six to eight weeks. We'd say, 'Fred would you like to complete it?' 'No.' 'Fred, do you have any interest getting back to this?' 'No.' So we allowed him to continue on typing." Every day he sat in the same corner, typing a business-letter drill.

Nancy Conniff, his counselor, gave him copying to do on this summer day, a five-page article. Most would have said, "Do you want me to collate it too?" Not Fred. He copied it and returned it to Conniff. So she told him to collate.

"He can collate out the wazoo," she said, "but you have to tell him." He completed the project perfectly. Watching Fred, knowing what a bright college student he'd been, made them wonder what exactly the schizophrenia had robbed from him, why he could still type forty words, copy, collate, but couldn't make the jump from copying to collating on his own.

It was as if his thought process had lost its elasticity.

"Have you had enough?" Conniff said to Fred. "OK, why don't you go back to typing?" He returned to his corner. "He just keeps typing and typing and typing," she said. Fred spent three years at the program, but never did get to the second phase.

ON JULY 25, 1991, at 4 P.M. at Glen Cove City Hall, Grace Wallace was married. Grace had lived at 9 Highland a year and a half, graduating from the house earlier that spring. The ceremony was performed by none other than Mayor DeRiggi, who did about a hundred weddings a year. If the Mayor realized that this glowing bride was an alumna of the group home he had worked so industriously to kill, he did not let on. Grace didn't care—she just needed someone official.

Only Maureen grasped the beautiful irony of it, hooting with delight when she heard. In three years the Mayor had progressed from trying to railroad them out of town to marrying them off.

ON AUGUST 9 Stephen DeRosa left Glen Cove Hospital after a four-month stay. He'd been on clozapine exactly two months and still was not doing particularly well. When a friend at the house heard, he said, "Turn down the stereo, no more MTV, everyone on tiptoes, Stephen's back." Stephen continued to be obsessive about religion and was acting paranoid. Maureen told her staff, "We're just going to have to work with him and hope he improves."

"He needs to hear he's not going to hell," said Paula Marsters.

"Once a day he'll tell you he's going to hell," said Jodie Schwartz.

"Which is why I want him home," said Maureen. "He needs to get past these obsessive thoughts. He gets very comfy in the hospital—after ten years at Pilgrim."

A few days later it hit, the awakening, arriving like a bolt from the heavens. Stephen returned from his family's store, where he cleaned once a week, and announced, "I'm healed." He was beaming, positively ecstatic. "I'm not going to hell! I feel great!"

He had not looked this happy in months. The counselors assumed the clozapine had finally clicked. But that was not how Stephen explained it. "I met this woman at the store, Veronica Healy. As I walked by her I had a guilty feeling so I went back and asked, 'Am I going to be healed?' She told me, 'You will be healed.' So I'm not going to hell."

Those who held onto the notion that mental health was a rational process asked Stephen why this woman's opinion had counted so much. "I checked with my therapist, Ed Tooher. He agreed with what she said, so I had two opinions."

Paula Marsters, Stephen's primary counselor, noticed the change right away. "It just happened," she said at a staff meeting. "I walked in, and there was a 180-degree shift. I couldn't believe it. At dinner tonight he was saying he had the best day at program, the best day." Each counselor had a Stephen DeRosa story. One heard him talking about what a good guy Jasper was. ("I love him, he's great.") Another described Stephen marching through the house in boots and gloves, tackling his bathroom chore with relish again.

"I've never seen him so happy," said Donna Rubin.

"He sat down beside me at dinner," said counselor Charles Winslow. "He says, 'Charles, I'm not going to hell.' "

STEPHEN FELT full of possibilities. At Friendly's that week, he explained he was looking into a sewer cleaning job. Stephen loved unstuffing pipes—he tinkered with the group home toilets constantly. A rotar-rooter outfit had done work at his mother's house and he'd engaged the repairman in a lengthy discussion on snaking technique.

"I asked him how you get into the business. He wrote down a phone number," said Stephen displaying the paper. "The guy said all I'd have to do was call and I'd have the job." That was a year ago. Stephen was ready now.

He smiled at the waitress. "She's such a sweet girl," he said, "No, not our waitress. The fat one there. . . . I'm so spontaneous. I cleaned the kitchen tonight. It felt good. It needed it." The waitress walked by with a chocolate shake. "You're doing a nice job," Stephen told her.

He was enjoying Sunday mass again and his cleaning job at the family store. "I get behind the toilet, really scrub good. I take off the cover, flush and bring the water up to the top. When it's ready to go over, I let it out, it goes down and cleans it good. I hate people when they clean—they do just any fucking thing."

On the way out, Stephen nodded to the large waitress. "Keep up the good work," he said.

Strolling up the driveway at the house he commented on the moon's splendor. "It looks like a girl sitting on her side," he said. Was ever a man so chipper? "I'm glad I like fat girls. I like being different. Everyone in this country is the same. They like the skinny little girls. So predictable." At 10:30 Stephen decided to call a new girl he'd met on the yellow bus. "She said, call her. She used to be just a little plump and I wasn't interested. But she's got really fat. She looks beautiful." He phoned her group home, but she'd gone to bed.

THE PSYCHIATRIST who'd treated Stephen at Glen Cove Hospital called the house on August 18. The doctor was going on vacation for two weeks. At that point he was the only psychiatrist authorized by the hospital to oversee clozapine treatment. (They were still being cautious about side effects and liability.) The doctor told Maureen that during his vacation, Stephen would be taken off clozapine and put on a traditional antipsychotic, Thorazine. The doctor noted that during Stephen's hospitalization, his blood pressure had gone up on clozapine a few times—another troublesome side effect.

Maureen wasn't happy. Just as the drug was finally working, they were taking him off? Couldn't they find someone else to oversee him for two weeks? Fred Grasso had been on it without incident for six years. Ed Tooher, Stephen's therapist, felt the same way and made a rare call to the group home to express his dismay.

Only Stephen remained unfazed. "Maybe this is the message from God that I don't need it," he said. "I'm not trying to press it. I don't want to go off the deep end. I don't want to explode." (He'd let them do what they wanted; he was quite sure Veronica Healy deserved the credit.)

When the hospital psychiatrist returned from vacation, he saw no need to switch back to clozapine since Stephen still seemed fine. It drove Maureen nuts. Even with a caring, supervised environment—a group home plus a good community hospital—the sort of scientific controls you'd expect in medical treatment did not prevail. Weeks after Stephen stopped taking clozapine, the medication could still be in his system. Maybe his continued high spirits were the lingering effects of the clozapine. How would they ever know if they didn't stick with one thing, give it a full test run, then step back and analyze the results?

This was the funny thing, though: Stephen continued in high spirits for months, long after the clozapine would have been out of his system. Who knew? Not Maureen. Maybe it wasn't the clozapine—or the thorazine. She'd known him for two years now and he seemed to be fine for a stretch, then bizarre for a stretch, independent of daily circumstance. Maybe these drugs just made Stephen's illness more manageable until the schizophrenia went through some necessary cycle of its own—some electrical or chemical roulette deep within the brain, still far from contemporary medicine's reach.

BY MID-AUGUST Heather was worse. She suddenly paid up her bill to Dr. Barris. She made plans to leave Teresa her few belongings. She tried to cancel her August 16 appointment with Dr. Imhof, and after agreeing to come in, barely talked. He wanted her to go to the emergency room. She resisted, relenting when he threatened her with involuntary commitment.

They sat together in North Shore University Hospital emergency for a while, joined by Teresa and a security guard. Then Dr. Imhof had to leave.

Heather was mad. She felt deserted. He couldn't even wait until she was examined? Didn't their eight years together mean anything to him? She went into the woman's room, slipped into a stall and pulled a razor blade from her pocketbook.

Teresa was curious about what was taking so long. She stuck her head in and there was Heather, squeezing blood from her wrists.

"Why'd you do it?" Teresa screamed.

"It felt good," said Heather, "I'm glad I did it. You know darn well how it feels."

The cuts were not deep—no stitches were needed. Asked later why she hadn't cut deeper, Heather said, "What was the point? I knew I wasn't going to be able to kill myself. I was right in the emergency room. I was just angry."

She'd expected to be committed at North Shore. It had a big, modern psychiatric ward, much to Heather's liking. She'd been there for much of 1990.

But it was full. She wound up committed at Central General Hospital in Plainview, an old community hospital with a small psychiatric ward that does not allow smoking. Heather was furious; she wasn't even going to be able to get a decent hospitalization out of this.

ON A LAZY Friday afternoon in mid-August, residents from the three Melillo group homes took their annual fluke-fishing trip on the charter boat Miss Freeport. Several caught fluke. For the squeamish, Linda Slezak removed the fish from their hooks.

Stephen DeRosa chose not to fish. Instead he leaned against the cabin, his head tilted toward the sun, taking in the soft ocean breeze and the scent of the salt marshes. He had a faraway, dreamy smile and when a friend asked what was on his mind, he said, "I'm listening to Rachmaninoff's third concerto. I can hear every note." (In *The Man Who Mistook His Wife for a Hat*, the neurologist Oliver Sacks describes patients with physiological damage to their temporal lobes through strokes or seizures, who hear songs playing so distinctly in their brains, they assume the music is coming from a radio.)

Stephen shut his eyes and beamed, a man on calm seas, at peace with the world. "I'm right at the part where I turn the record over," he said.

ANTHONY REGISTERED early for the fall semester, choosing two psychology courses at Nassau Community College. He and his dad talked about minimizing the pressure this time and decided Anthony would buy the textbook and read it during the summer, getting a jump on classwork. When they went to the college bookstore, there were two basic texts for introductory psych. Anthony wouldn't know which his instructor would choose until class assignments in September. So Dom and Anthony agonized, debated, then gambled, laying out twenty-eight dollars for one of them.

Every night that summer, Anthony went to his room after supper to study. When you'd see him, he'd report, "I just read 28 more pages, I'm up to 287."

He was up and down all summer, at times bullying people he thought he could safely pick on. "Fred the great," Anthony kept saying meanly one evening. "Fred, you're quite a specimen. Can you move?"

Fred sat on the couch, his usual sphinx self, until it became embarrassing not to respond and then he looked right at Anthony and said, "You ever make the Dean's list in college?" he said. (Fred had.)

Anthony had several bad days of hearing his father's voice, though he tried to hide it, because he had tickets to see Bob Dylan in concert at Jones Beach and was afraid they wouldn't let him go. On the same night that he smashed a Barbra Streisand tape against the wall of his bedroom to punish his father, he later announced, "I've changed in the last 15 minutes. I'm a new person." He'd called his father, talked over "family business." "It was an amazing talk. I can't say anything about it. Everything is straightened out."

He wanted to go down the hill for ice cream. "Before I was like in a block of concrete. Now it's like the blood in my skin is being transfused with nature. I feel great." He was practically skipping. He stood at the corner of School Street and was so involved talking about his new status, he missed the light changing twice.

"I'm cured. This is the first day I'm starting a new life," he said. He gestured toward the customers at Avanti Pizza and Subway Deli. "I used to think all those people could see inside of me and read my thoughts." In line at Brigham's he flirted with the counterwoman. She smiled at his sweet teasing and seemed pleased to be noticed. He was planning on getting a dish of chocolate with hot fudge on top. Then he heard someone in line a few people ahead of him order hot fudge on her ice cream. Anthony's face froze. "Was that from me?" he said.

His sharp mood swings worried Maureen, who contacted his psychiatrist, Dr. Jeffrey Ordover. The doctor didn't have much to suggest. He'd pushed up Anthony's antipsychotic Prolixin about as high as he could, to fifty milligrams daily. More would leave Anthony doped and dozy. He'd been tried on most of the antipsychotics and the only thing Dr. Ordover could suggest now was giving clozapine a shot. Anthony was receptive but they decided to wait to see how he did at college that fall.

On August 19, Anthony said, "I've read 350 pages in my psychology text. I spent 2½ hours at the library and sat in the smart section near reference books. That's where the top people sit. They were all adults. One asked me what I'm reading. I said, 'I'm not that smart.' He said, 'The people who do the best often aren't the smartest. They're the ones who plug away.' "

On August 20, Anthony said, "I don't want to say too much about the voices, they may come back but I really feel like my brain is getting better."

On August 23, he said, "I'm past 400 in my psychology book. I'm reading the best ever. I'm letting the book talk to me."

On August 28 he came back from the Glen Cove library after working on the computerized system that had replaced the Reader's Guide to Periodicals, and said, "I tried to use the computer and couldn't follow the directions. I wasn't in a rush. I wasn't nervous. I could read the words but I couldn't understand what they meant."

HEATHER THOUGHT she'd go mad. The Central General psychiatrist came onto the ward each morning and if you wanted to see him, you stood in line and waited for your five minutes. For what? To start telling your life story in 50,000 five-minute installments? Give off another revelation you'd already repeated 100 times? Heather tried to reach Dr. Barris and Dr. Imhof, but they did not immediately respond to her calls. When she did get them they were not very sympathetic. They made it clear her behavior was growing old.

"This hospital stay's not going to help me," she complained.

They agreed.

"Then why am I here?" she said.

"Good question," they replied, "why are you?"

She talked about requesting a hearing to get out. She'd have to do it herself this time, they said. No more rescue missions. They felt she'd be better off convincing the hospital staff she was well.

Dr. Imhof did not tell Heather, but he had called Central General about coordinating her medication. His calls were not returned. He was amazed when they quickly changed her antidepressant from Tolferal to Ludermal without consulting the therapist who'd overseen her care for eight years. (As Dr. Imhof would later say, "It's what fascinates me about the mental health system.")

Visitation was held in the ward's recreation room. On the night of Monday, August 26, there were two TV's going, both turned to "Jeopardy," a radio blasting, and small worried knots of family members spread throughout the room trying to speak over the racket. (If you didn't know better you'd assume the hospital was trying to drum up business by inducing fresh nervous breakdowns.) Heather asked if there was someplace she could take a guest to talk quietly and a staff aide let her use the isolation room, where patients were held if they became violent.

Heather had been in ten days and played the game this time to get out. Both Dr. Barris and Dr. Imhof had guided her on how to answer the hospital staff's questions. She'd be returning to the group home at the end of the week.

She'd resolved to never let this happen again. She'd only been able to sneak a few cigarettes and was colossally bored. It had finally dawned on her what a waste of time these hospitalizations were. She knew she needed to get at her problem through therapy with John Imhof, but they were stuck.

"I can't talk to John about incest," she said, staring down at the gleaming linoleum in isolation. "He'll think I'm horrible.

"If I finally do go into the incest with him and don't get better, I'd completely fail him. I've been trying so many years, I don't have trust in myself to make progress. For years in therapy I never talked about it. John asked me directly at one point, 'Did it happen?' I said no. I went home and it bothered me so much I called him and said 'I want you to know, I lied to you.' "

"As a youngster I didn't know right away what was going on, that it wasn't supposed to happen—except it physically hurt me. Then I got a further idea something was wrong when my mother took me to a doctor because my father had hurt me and she lied to the doctor about it.

"The terror goes from being frightened and saying, 'I pray he won't come tonight,' to the point, 'Can I just get this over with?' It's like numbing your body so you don't feel it, just, 'Let it be over.'

"And then there's the part when you're little and don't know better. It makes you feel special and important. You're pleasing your father. I know I meant more to my father than my mother did. And my mother was being mean to me and I didn't understand why. If I did something wrong—it didn't matter what, like messing up the playroom—she'd lock me in the closet up to four hours.

"It made me feel good to be more special to my father, to be spiting her, to be doing this. So by doing this with my father, I was spiting my mother and I enjoyed spiting my mother. I enjoyed it."

Heather grew quiet. It wasn't something she'd said before. Down the hallway the Final Jeopardy round had just concluded and an aide was shouting, "Attention, visiting hours are now over. Attention . . ."

ON THE 29th, Dr. Imhof met with Maureen and Paula Marsters to plan Heather's return to the group home. Maureen was weary of being on suicide watch but the therapist assured her Heather was not suicidal. "I can't tell you the incredible job you've done," said Dr. Imhof. "I'd vote 100 percent she remain here for the time being. Heather gives out cries for help. The thing is to teach her how to do it without hurting herself."

Heather had called him from the hospital and said she was ready to talk about the incest. "Part of Heather is self-destructive," Dr. Imhof explained to the two group home counselors. "She feels she deserves to be punished for the incest and being such a bad person. She feels she should have stopped this as an 8- or 10- or 12-year-old. She should have gone to the police in some way and stopped it. She's lived with guilt for years. She sees herself as responsible for causing her father's attention to her.

"The other part of Heather is very much a survivor trying to help others. Inside of Heather is a very bright individual. She's probably read more books than all of us combined. She has rooms of books in her brother's house. I believe Heather's going to make a major contribution some day, either by helping others with these problems or through her own family."

He'd signed her up for an incest-survivor's group that met weekly in Port Washington, though she wouldn't be going for a while; the waiting list was quite long.

. . .

ONE PERFECT starry night near the end of summer, several of them were sitting out front. The train whistled every hour, the firehouse horn wailed from time to time and for a few hours, Glen Cove felt like Grover's Corners, New Hampshire. Joe said, "I know what I love about this place, a group of people sitting talking."

Joe had been living there a year and a half and would be leaving soon. Someone said they thought he would do great in his new apartment. "I take it one day at a time, that's all I can do," Joe said. "You think I want to be this way? I'd give up everything in the world, for five good years, just to be like everyone else. I could make money, start a family, five years would be enough to get it all started."

The conversation drifted to what had helped them make it through their depressions. "I could look up 'depression' in my textbook," Anthony said. That wasn't what they meant.

"You mean from my life story?" Anthony said. "When I was in the hospital, really alone and my Dad held my hand and told me the family loved me."

Teresa said she'd been so depressed once she was practically paralyzed and her mother came from Oregon. "We didn't have one conversation. I couldn't talk, but just that she was there and I knew she loved me. It doesn't matter so much what you say because you can't believe what's being said, just saying it."

They were all quiet then for a while, their cigarettes glowing red in the dark. "Look," Joe whispered.

"I see it," said Teresa.

A mother and a half dozen baby raccoons scooted across the lawn to the driveway, disappearing around the corner of the house.

FRIDAY, AUGUST 30, was hazy and 96 degrees, one of the last brutal days of that unbearably hot summer. Paula Marsters—who weighed 100 pounds—lugged Heather's tan vinyl suitcase up to Central General's third floor locked ward. Even empty it weighed a ton. She buzzed and waited to be let in. Through the meshed window of the steel door, she could see Heather's eyes, searching.

Heather gave Paula a monstrous hug. "God am I glad to see you," she said. "I can't wait to get home." She was going to get herself a carton of Marlboros, a Big Gulp Coke from 7-11, and park in front of the TV. Heather took the suitcase and went to pack her clothes.

A patient on the ward saw Paula, all tanned in a flowery, low-cut pantsuit and said, "You're being discharged? You just got here five minutes ago." An aide handed Paula a pink card, which had to be taken down to the hospital cashier, where she would be issued a white card, which had to be brought back up to the ward so Heather could be released. While Heather waited another aide stapled an ID bracelet on her wrist, even though she explained she was being discharged in five minutes.

Paula went around to get the car and Heather sat on a bench in the sun out front of the hospital. She pulled out a Marlboro and was so anxious for a smoke, she dropped her lighter on the sidewalk. It had to be over 100 degrees in the sun, there was no air, the cicadas' buzz was deafening, and Heather looked stronger and happier with each drag. "I really put on a good act to get out of there," she said.

Paula pulled up in her tiny yellow Ford hatchback and they hoisted the suitcase into the trunk on top of a beach chair. As they drove off, Paula had something loud playing on the radio and Heather was hanging out the window taking one puff after another. To all the world, they looked like two friends on their way to Jones Beach to get an early start on the Labor Day weekend.

And that was Heather's last stay at a mental hospital.

IN THE WEEKS before Joe moved out to an apartment program, he alienated practically everyone at the group home. He'd get in arguments with residents, bark at the counselors. "He's scared to death," Maureen told her counselors at a Tuesday night meeting, urging them to have patience. "By creating all these problems it's easier to go. It's like he has no choice. It's easier than saying, 'I'm going to miss it.'"

On Friday night, August 30, Joe came charging downstairs about

11:30 and banged on the office door. "We've got a big problem!" Joe told Lauryn Schelfo, a new counselor. "You got to go upstairs. Anthony is masturbating and he's smelling up the room."

Joe had finished watching the late news and was ready for bed. He walked into their shared bedroom and noticed Anthony. "Holy cripes," Joe said. "Don't do that in here. You're supposed to do that in the bathroom. That's the proper place." Anthony felt if he ignored him, Joe just might have the brains to go away discreetly.

"This is your job," Joe told the twenty-two-year-old counselor. "You have to do something." Lauryn suggested it wasn't that big a deal, and Joe ought to try to work it out with Anthony.

Joe marched upstairs. People were peeking out of their rooms to see what the commotion was. Joe made sure everyone knew. "Right in the bedroom," he said. "I don't know how I'm going to handle this—I guess I'll just have to tell Anthony's father. Get his dad to put a stop to this."

At the mention of his dad, Anthony charged out of the room and punched Joe in the chest. Joe and Anthony are solidly built men, about the same size—five feet nine and maybe 190 pounds. Of the two, Joe, a former marathoner, is the stronger from his years of running and long-distance biking.

Joe immediately turned and ran away, racing downstairs, shouting, "Call the police. Anthony punched me. He hit me. It's assault. He is in violation of house rules."

Lauryn calmed Joe. He wasn't injured, simply outraged. "Anthony hit me, he hit Stan Gunter, they should kick him out. He broke the rules."

When she tried to talk to Anthony, he ran back to his room and slammed the door. She peeked in, but he screamed wildly and took a few steps toward her. So Lauryn shut his door, returned to the office and called the emergency beeper. Debbie Dombrowski, manager of the Glen Head house, was on call that weekend.

"Put him on the phone to me," said Debbie. Anthony came down to the office sleepily. "Hi," he said into the phone. "Are you the blond girl from the fishing trip? I remember you." Anthony said he felt terrible, embarrassed, humiliated. He didn't know how he'd face Joe in the morning. "Is it OK if I don't talk about it?" Anthony said. "I just want to go to bed." It was OK.

LABOR DAY is supposed to mark the end of summer and this year, thankfully, the weather obeyed the calendar. Tuesday, September 3, the temperature was in the sixties with a stunning cloudless blue sky and a crisp fresh breeze. After one of the muggiest summers in years, stepping into the front yard that morning felt like putting on a freshly laundered dress shirt.

Joe slept late—one of the good things about moving was they let you skip program for the day. He wished he could find a way to move every day. He piled his clothes into a plastic laundry basket and carried out a few shirts and slacks on hangers.

Then he slipped off with hardly a good-bye. Maureen was right, Joe was one of the ones who wouldn't stay in touch. Before he drove off, he did say, "If you see Anthony, tell him he's a good guy. Tell him I forgive him."

chapter 14

MY ILLNESS IS MANMADE

JULIE WAS the kind of secretary supervisors cherish while they have her, because Julie plainly wasn't going to be a secretary very long. There was a gleam there; you knew she'd be running something someday. She had great powers of concentration and would do whatever was handed her. There was a day she typed fourteen letters, a fifteen-page grant proposal, a technical bibliography, and a stack of envelopes. At 5 P.M. she looked up and told a friend, "I don't think I talked today." She was a favorite among customers and sales reps, got along great with the other secretaries in the office, and would often go out with them for a drink or to the beach. But she also was respected by the senior supervisors—men and women—who felt it rare in this day and age to meet a young person so hardworking, purposeful, kind, and hip. Older people were relieved to discover someone in her twenties who shared their values. Everyone in the office sought her out. She convinced one of the shy secretaries to come along for a beauty appointment; she made friends with a janitor and persuaded her boss to write the man a recommendation for a better job listing. Julie was always in the middle of something.

That fall, in the evenings she took a course at a local college to get certified as a child care worker (she was thinking of taking a part-time job at a group home for abused children). She volunteered at a local charity, sewed yarn dolls for her friends' kids, and baked a cake for her therapist's birthday.

Julie was honest. She desperately needed a new car, and a salesman at a dealership agreed to arrange the financing if she lied. She was supposed to say she'd been at her current job two years instead of six months. It was a common practice, but she would not do it. She was afraid someone would call to verify the information with her boss and she'd be caught in a lie at work. Instead she bought a secondhand car with cash, using every last cent of her savings.

Though she'd left the mental health system behind, she did not forget friends from hospitals or the house. She visited 9 Highland every four or five months, playing softball with them, driving Stephen De-Rosa to the hospital to visit when Heather was sick.

Since the start of the year, when she met Jim, a divorced business-man, she'd dated only him, though she'd had offers from far more dashing types. Young professional men constantly asked her out. (During a cruise with some girlfriends on a party boat around Long Island Sound, a stranger approached her and said, "I just want you to know, you're the most beautiful woman here. I'm not trying to pick you up, I'm married, but I just felt like I had to say it.") There was a sense of mystery about Julie, an aura, something elusive, a touch of moonlight in her eyes, a hint of a hidden life. And of course, that was it exactly.

Occasionally this life slipped into the workplace, but no one caught it. In the early days of the job, Didi popped out. Scared, the four-year-old called Jim at his office: "Jim, how you doing? It's Di!"

"Didi! What are you doing out at work?" he asked. "Go back in and get Julie."

"I don't know how to get back in," she said. Jim told her to find the women's room—Julie's refuge from the time she was a little girl—and sure enough, one of the adult personalities, Abigail, came back out and took control.

Julie wasn't always the one who came to work. But it was always an adult personality, and the important thing was that they all had the same skills so there were no lapses. After a while, she stopped worrying about being discovered at the office. As she said, "I've lived in hospitals where they were looking for pathology and couldn't find this." During one stretch that fall—when the young personalities were having horrible trouble at night—Marlena showed up at the office for several days. She did her tasks fine. But Marlena was quite different from Julie when she let herself go—irreverent, sassy, bitchy. She often wore tighter, more suggestive outfits. She carried herself differently. She had a way of cocking her hip, throwing her hair back. Julie and Marlena might put on the same pair of slacks, but when Marlena wore them, you suddenly noticed the panty line underneath. When Marlena got in your car she would, without asking, immediately begin hitting the radio buttons, pounding one after another until she found some rock music that was loud enough. It would not occur to Marlena to ask if you minded. She was a teenager.

A few of the secretaries commented to Julie that she didn't seem to be herself that week. At one point Marlena walked into her boss's office and told him that one of their coworkers should be fired, declaring, "That woman is an occupational hazard." The supervisor howled —it happened to be absolutely true—but coming from his normally politic, reserved secretary, the comment was a stunner. Julie pieced this together later. For weeks after, coworkers privately congratulated her for having the courage to report an occupational hazard when she saw one.

ONLY A FEW knew of the multiple personalities: Jim; Dr. Sandler, her therapist; and a couple of people from the mental health system, like Tim Cook, who'd become a friend after he left the group home job. These people's relationships with Julie were never straightforward. Tim Cook called one night—she typed his graduate school papers for him—and got Didi. They had a nice chat about toys and Raggedy Andy and Tim said it was fine for Di to call him anytime and if he wasn't there, she should leave a message on his machine. "No way Jose, I don't leave messages," said Di. "If you call back, you'll get someone else, and they won't let me out." Tim said good night and then tried Julie again fifteen minutes later.

"Julie?" No. "Marlena?" No. "Di?" No. "Is this Abigail?" Why? "Can you tell Julie I'm calling?"

"No, I can't do that," she said and hung up.

This small group of friends saw the real miracle of Julie because they measured her daytime success against her terrifying nights. Every night some personality relived a piece of the childhood bestiality. There was no break. If Julie was lucky, they stayed indoors.

SLOWLY, through Dr. Sandler, Julie learned about herself. She came to understand what was known about the disorder and what was not. People like Julie had minds with the ability to create alter selves through a mechanism therapists liken to self-hypnosis. How Julie had this particular survival mechanism from a very young age, no one could say. (Why do some sexually abused children become multiples? Some alcoholics? Some obese? Some nationally syndicated talk show hosts?) But there was no mistaking it helped Julie survive. In therapy, Megan, a twelve-year-old personality, had told Dr. Sandler about the "Father person" tying her to the bed for hours at a time. Megan explained to Dr. Sandler that she'd passed those horrifying times with the other personalities inside.

Julie came to understand that just as no two schizophrenics were alike, multiplicity was different in each person. She and the other personalities had to figure how *their* system worked. Through therapy they realized that the immediate mechanism young Julie had used for creating a new personality was dolls in the house. The mother bought dolls as gifts, but then for her own crazy reasons would not let Julie play with them, lest they be broken. So for years, the dolls, wrapped in the original plastic, sat untouched, high on shelves where Julie couldn't reach them. It is not hard to envision how those "safe," aloof dolls held a fascination and a pull for the little girl who never felt safe.

The multiplicity was quite complicated. Each personality had a different range of consciousness, awareness, and memory. Some were locked in the violent past; some knew only the present; some knew both; some knew the other personalities; some were aware only of themselves. They'd all tell you they looked different. Four-year-old Didi described herself as being thin with "long, long brown hair that comes all the way down to my coolie." She liked to wear it in a ponytail and said Abigail would tie it for her. The five-year-old Scared One (she would answer to no other name) was chubby and wore pigtails. Didi's favorite color was pink, her favorite flavor strawberry; the Scared One's favorite color was purple. Di and Julie were ticklish; the Scared One was not.

Jim stored a dozen different flavored ice creams in his freezer to keep everyone happy.

For many of the personalities there was a world inside Julie's head, a land with grass and sky, night and day. If a personality locked in the past, like nine-year-old Betty, came out in the apartment and was afraid that the Father person was about to get her, Jim could sometimes calm her by suggesting she go back inside and lie in the tall grass. "Just look up at the beautiful, blue sky and the big white clouds and no one can see you in the tall grass, you're safe." And then Betty would be gone and the face would go blank and suddenly another personality would pop out. Julie, on the other hand, only knew of this inside world by descriptions from Dr. Sandler or Jim.

To know Julie and the others was to get a peek at the immense complexity of the mind. Though bright, Julie had trouble with reading comprehension. She even had difficulty describing the problem to others—she'd say she couldn't concentrate or she was zoning out or it must have something to do with the other personalities. The twelve-year-old Megan personality was sympathetic: "Julie can't concentrate. There's so much noise in the head. Julie doesn't hear it, but it's very noisy in here. Even with people trying to be quiet, there are just so many people walking around in here." Megan, on the other hand, was a terrific reader. She had emerged as a personality in adolescence, during a very bookish time in Julie's life. Talking to Megan, you could see what a serious, bright, sincere sweetheart of a sixth-grader Julie had been. She'd belonged to the library reading club until the "Mother person" made her quit. Megan said she'd like to go to Harvard, "but I can't get out." When Julie went to a book sale, it was Megan who would pop out and find the obscure classics.

At one point in therapy, Julie was talking to Dr. Sandler about her reading problem and wondering how she'd be able to get through a college course she was taking. "It takes so long and I have to struggle so much just to read a few pages." Dr. Sandler suggested she might have Megan do the reading and take the test. Then Julie had to consider: Was she better off as a twenty-three-year-old with a reading problem? Or no reading problem but only twelve? Did she want to give up that kind of control? If she did, how did she arrange it?

On many matters, there already was a division of labor. Only the adult personalities drove. Occasionally during a ride, Didi would hear a tune she liked on the radio—("Do I hear the theme from *Beauty and the Beast?*")—and pop out. But it was only a matter of moments before the older ones cracked down. "Abigail gets ma—a-a-ad at me," said Di. "She says get back inside now."

To good friends like Tim Cook there was Julie and then all these other personalities. But those who knew her the very best—like Jim and Dr. Sandler—saw Julie as one among sixteen, no more important or dominant than the others.

WHEN TWO personalities were in conflict, tugging the mind in different directions, Julie was in agony. "My head is splitting," she said one Saturday night. "I can't even stand up. I've just been lying here on the couch since seven, too weak to move." The week before, Marlena had seen a late-night TV commercial for beautiful young women interested in a modeling career. She called the number and arranged for a free introductory screening. A few days later she made herself up special, then took the train into New York City for an interview. It turned out Faces International wasn't exactly a modeling agency. It was more of a magazine showcasing aspiring models that also offered training and agency leads.

The modeling business is full of exploitive types ready to take the money of pretty young women and men aching to be stars. A general rule among professionals is that legitimate outfits provide a single service: there are agencies that get models work; there are fashion photographers who do portfolios for a fee; there are schools that provide training. Operations that offer all those services under one roof raise a red flag among consumer groups.

"The woman said she felt Marlena had a lot of talent," Julie explained. "She had Marlena read a short commercial. What came across —Marlena doesn't have a lot of technique and experience." Fortunately Faces International offered a class starting at the end of September with only fifteen slots. "The woman said they're very selective." Once Faces received a check for $350, Marlena's place in the class would be guaranteed.

Julie found out what Marlena was up to by accident several days later. She attempted a bank transaction at an automatic teller machine and found her card was temporarily voided. Marlena had tried to use the card to transfer $350 from savings to checking to cover the Faces fee. Unfortunately, Marlena did not know Julie's identification number, so she made several (incorrect) guesses and at some point, as a security precaution, the system temporarily took the card out of service. Julie asked Jim if he knew what was going on, and, caught between two personalities, he now told her the basics of Marlena's plan.

"The $350 really depresses me," she said. "I have no control. I work so hard for it. I'm fanatical about saving. This is hard-earned money. I could use that money. I can't seem to hold on to a normal situation. I took care of moving, a car, and when things calm down, this happens. Will I ever have a situation of normalcy?

"My head is splitting and that part of me couldn't care less about what it's doing to me. I feel like 'My God, where is this leading?' It's not one of my goals in life to do this. For me this is a relapse. Dr. Sandler doesn't look at it that way. She looks at it as Marlena pursuing a career. I guess Dr. Sandler thinks of me as us. I think of us as me.

"I feel bad. Marlena doesn't like Dr. Sandler. She won't talk to her.

The only one she'll talk to is Jim . . . It's hard. She's completely opposed to things I'm interested in. She wants to be a star."

You could barely hear Julie now. "I don't feel like I can stand up. If I do I'll faint. I feel lifeless. If I'm going to be like this very long, I'll just have to go along with the modeling."

Julie rested and formulated a plan. She asked a friend if it would be possible to do a background check on the company. If it was questionable, she would resist taking the course. If it was impressive, "I'll just have to do it." Marlena deserved her shot, too. In the meantime Julie would cancel the check. Writing another would be no problem in the event of a positive report.

Other personalities had strong feelings about Marlena's modeling career. Megan was against it. It's "exploitive and demeaning to parade in front of cameras." The studious twelve-year-old was quite adamant, and wondered if it would be possible—in case the modeling company had an impressive track record—to lie to Marlena about it. This was a very tricky request. Putting the ethics aside, if you agreed to lie to make Megan feel better, Marlena would likely overhear immediately and (rightfully) be outraged. And if Marlena was mad enough, she could cut you off from all the others. You were dealing with sixteen different people, but you were dealing with sixteen pieces of one person, too. It wasn't like you could put something over on one personality—one way or another, word filtered through the system and the mind.

It turned out that the Better Business Bureau of Metropolitan New York had quite an extensive file on Faces International. The BBB in 1991 contacted fifty of three thousand modeling hopefuls whose photos were published in the Faces publication; "68 per cent alleged high pressure sales tactics; 86 per cent stated they were dissatisfied with their Faces experience.

"In reviewing Faces' claims of being selective, the Bureau analyzed profiles of 66 rejected applications provided by Faces. According to Faces' records, 24 per cent were rejected for being drunk or stoned at the interview; 21 per cent were children with bad grades, unsupportive parents or behavior problems; 21 per cent couldn't read or speak English . . . 8 per cent were totally unemployable; 8 per cent had physical defects.

"Our file experience shows this company has an unsatisfactory record with the Bureau."

Marlena did not contest the findings.

"MY ILLNESS is manmade," Julie often said, and the haunting thing about being her friend was that over time you saw the process firsthand.

You eventually met the little girls who went through the abuse at each stage of her life. You weren't listening to an adult recount it twenty years after the fact; you were seeing the child experience it again. You often couldn't tell exactly what was going on—it undoubtedly will take years of therapy to sort out the worst violences done to Julie—but the terror and cruelty were unmistakable. It was like watching a two-actor play with only one of the characters onstage.

SHE KNEW when nine-year-old Betty had been out. Julie would wake from a blackout and find herself in the closet. It was the only place Betty felt safe.

Betty called one night, sobbing on the phone. "He's going to get me, that man," she said. "I'm going to die. He's going to get me. I feel it. He's after me. I feel it. No! He's here. Yes, it gets me, I feel it, I do, I do, I feel it. He gets me. He does with his knife. I hear the knocking, bang bang bang. I feel him, I do! I do!"

You'd assure her that the Father person couldn't harm her anymore and try to find something to soothe her. Didi liked holding a doll when she was scared. "I have no dolls," said Betty. "I'm not allowed to have any treats. I don't want to get in trouble. I just want to go away. I want to go away to the world with the blue sky and the big tall grass."

Another night in early December she called, crying in a voice barely audible. "He got me," she sobbed. "He made me bleed and he's going to come back. I've been bleeding all day."

Sometimes another personality could help. Was there someone for Betty?

"I don't know."

Marlena?

"Marlena doesn't help."

Abigail?

"Who's Abigail?"

Megan? "Megan helps," Betty said. There was a pause of several seconds and then Megan came on sounding very tired. She was lying in the dark, she said, too weak to get up. "All this switching around tired me out."

Megan knew about the bleeding. "He does it to her," she said, "and when he's done he just goes away and leaves her there bleeding in the bed. And she cries a long time." Megan, always the practical one, asked, "What do you do for the bleeding? . . . Warm water and a facecloth? . . . That helps? . . . Thank you." It was well past midnight. She apologized. "I'm sorry to keep you up so late."

Sometimes Jim would come home from work and find her in his closet; sometimes she'd duck in during the course of an evening home together. Jim would try to coax her out, but she would not budge. During a calmer moment, Betty explained, "I know Jim gets mad at me. He yells, 'Get out, get out.' I met Dr. Sandler just a little bit and she wanted me to get out of the closet, too. I won't. It's better in there. He can't get me. The Mommy person can't hit me with her spoon. At least they can't hit me in the closet."

ONE RAINY night, when it was thundering and lightning and the power was flickering, Megan called. "It's a mess here," she said in a prim voice. This, it turned out, was the Megan personality at seven years old. She was the same serious-minded and bright girl as the twelve-year-old Megan personality, but at a younger stage.

"The little girl wet the bed," young Megan said. It wasn't possible to talk Megan through the steps necessary to change the bed ("I'm too little to lift the mattress," Megan explained). She considered the possibility of taking a clean pillow and blanket and sleeping on the floor. "It might work," she said, "it might not work. It's really bad."

This was not why Megan had called. She was trying to decide whether to divulge the real trouble to someone outside the "family." Megan was a big believer in the personalities' handling their own problems.

"Tess wants to go with Patricia—to heaven," Megan finally said, quite calmly. "She really really wants to go, bad." Megan was explaining that the ten-year-old Tess personality was now suicidal.

Patricia was Julie's young sister who had died in infancy. The reasons were clouded, and this had caused young Julie tremendous distress at the time. The Tess personality was created during that crisis and was haunted by it. On the anniversary of the infant's death, on the dead infant's birthday, and on several more obscure anniversaries, the Tess personality would go running out of the house—scantily clothed even in the dead of winter—and somehow make it to the baby's grave to pray for her soul. Tess fantasized about killing herself and joining Patricia in heaven. Two years earlier, when Julie had been caught in the kitchen of the group home in the middle of the night with the knife to her wrist—it was Tess.

On this night Tess had brought a knife to bed with her. "It would be bad to go with Patricia," said Megan. She meant it was a sin to kill yourself. "Tess's a bad girl to do that. I don't want to get in trouble." Megan did not want to go to Hell.

Megan didn't think she'd be able to dissuade Tess. "I don't know if I can change her mind," said Megan. "She's bigger, she's ten."

"I'm afraid Tess will come back out," said Megan in the calmest, most matter-of-fact voice. "It's such a big knife." It was too big to flush down the toilet, she said. Could she throw it out the window?

"I could try to do that," Megan said. The line went quiet. The seven-year-old was calmer in a crisis than most adults. As a child, Julie was forced to raise herself from a very early age.

The line went dead. Tess answered the call back. She was weepy and kept saying, "I want to go with Patricia. Patricia is the only one who likes me. My life is like—you don't know how bad it is." There was no consoling her. The line went dead again. Fortunately Jim was home. He said he'd work on getting an adult to take control. At 12:50 A.M. the phone rang. "This is Marlena . . . Oh yeah, everything is marvy . . . I wasn't in control but I am now. You can go now. Go take care of your twong." It certainly was Marlena, although there was just a touch of softness in her voice that sounded appreciative.

ONE OF THE last personalities Jim met was Clare. She came out one night, said she was fourteen and wanted to go home. She had no idea where she was, no idea who Jim was, no awareness of the world inside of Julie's mind, no clue that she was one of several personalities. She was convinced it was 1981 and if she didn't get home from school in time, she'd be in terrible trouble. When Jim showed her a newspaper and calendar she looked panicked and cried. All he could figure to do was get her to go to sleep.

Months later they realized why she'd panicked at seeing the date. This personality lived in fear that she was pregnant by the Father person. The calendar would have meant she'd had a baby by now, but she didn't remember having a baby.

Julie once commented, "When people think about incest, they forget the fear of pregnancy. When you have your period it's such a relief and then it happens again and you're in fear all over. I don't know what I would have done if it happened. You're missing your period and part of you is denying it." Julie said she could understand those stories you read about a young woman killing her newborn. "It's the denial. When I was at Glen Cove Hospital I got this new roommate and that day, they took away all the copies of *Newsday*. So naturally we had to find out why. It turned out she had given birth to her child and killed it and then went to work. She was staying on 3-West, waiting to go to court. So everyone on 3-West had it figured out. Some spurned her. One night I said to her, 'I just want you to know, I know. And you don't have to say anything, I understand. But I'm not putting a judgment on you.' She really talked a lot about it after that.

"If I had been pregnant by my father, I would have been finished. My mother would have made me have the baby. She would have kept it and I would have been damned, the immoral daughter, trapped in the house with my father's baby. I wouldn't have made it. I probably would have killed myself.

"People picket against group homes and I haven't hurt anybody. There's no one marching around my parents' house picketing what they did. I'm sitting in a group home and there could be someone on the next block beating the shit out of his kid and yet I'm the one who's labeled, they protest against me."

Once in a while, as a personality faded and went back inside, fourteen-year-old Clare would pop out. And she'd be totally disoriented, worried that she hadn't done her homework, trying to make some sense of being in a strange apartment. She wouldn't touch anything at Jim's place, wouldn't turn on the TV. "I'm not allowed," she said. "It's not my home."

"Is this Easter vacation?" she asked sometimes. "Did I fall asleep? Did I have the baby?" She'd ask questions like, "Would a doctor say you were pregnant by mistake?" Then, finally, she would begin saying —almost chanting—"It's not really real, right? It's not really real. It's not really real . . ." And she'd disappear.

NIGHT AFTER NIGHT, the personality that caused the most turmoil by far was the five-year-old Scared One. Something awful had happened to Julie at five. Di, who was four, effervescent and well adjusted, absolutely refused to celebrate her birthday. She was adamant about not turning five. She would let Jim give her a "special-day party," with special-day hats and a special-day cake, but never a birthday party.

The torment the Scared One went through each night was so horrible, Jim cried the first time he saw it. He was twice her weight, yet he could barely restrain her, she fought so ferociously to escape, ripping at his hair. The only way he could keep her from running out of the house was to sit on her, and sometimes he had to for several hours, until she recognized him. This was the personality who had so worn out Tim Cook on the group home camping trip two years before.

When she was thrashing about, screaming, it was like she was in a dream, and no matter what Jim did he couldn't reach her, couldn't convince her that she was not being attacked by the Father person. He'd grab her hand and run it over his face, telling her over and over, "This is Jim's nose, this is Jim's mouth, this is Jim's eyes," but it could take hours to get through.

At some point the Scared One would come out of this trancelike state, and Jim could comfort her, but then she blamed Jim for not saving her from the horrible man. "Why didn't you help me when I was screaming?" she'd ask in a small, weeping voice.

She tore up his apartment once while he was at work.

If Jim wasn't there to sit on her, she could run out of the apartment in the dead of night. The Scared One would race wildly until she grew weary, then another personality would come out, lost and disoriented. It might be Megan, who'd call you from a pay phone. But if you asked where she was, all she could say was "near some water" or "a big road with a lot of cars." When you tried to get more detail, the personalities switched and the line went dead. If it was Didi who popped out lost, she'd try to reach Dr. Blank, Julie's first therapist, whom Di was quite fond of. Di kept his number "inside, in a special place in a little box, nobody knows where it is." But when Di phoned the hospital, she would get an overnight operator. "Dr. Blank's not available," the operator would say. "Can I take a message."

"This is Didi," she'd say. "D-i, d-i." It frightened and confused Di. "The people at the hospital laugh when I call," she later explained. "They tell me to call back in the day. I was lost and they wouldn't talk to me."

JIM TRIED to build a friendship with the Scared One. For the longest time she wouldn't take anything from him. He knew from Di that purple was her favorite color, and he gave her a purple doll. She would not play with it. She would not wear the purple underwear. He gave her a container of purple tissues, but when he handed her one, she tried stuffing it back in the box.

Eventually he did make some progress. The amount of time he had to sit on her decreased, to about an hour on good nights. And she'd come out more often and do ordinary things with him, like watching the Olympics on TV. She liked a woman skier with a purple helmet. She stopped the toilet from running one night by jiggling the handle, and after Jim made such a big deal of it, she talked about becoming a plumber or skier.

Jim was the first person she'd trusted even a little, a major accomplishment on his part. The Scared One rarely came out at Dr. Sandler's and when she did, things would get wild. "The Scared One was very bad," said Di one evening. "She ran out of Dr. Sandler's office and then all around her house, with Dr. Sandler chasing her. That was bad, bad. She's not supposed to go out of the room. She ran into a bathroom and locked the door. Dr. Sandler tried to get her to come out—Dr. Sandler was banging on the door and the Scared One must've thought it was the bad man. She opened the door, pushed Dr. Sandler away, and went running out of the house and she didn't come back. And you know who she was looking for? Jim, that's who."

THE MOST amazing thing of all was that this went on night after night, and yet every morning Julie would be on time for work, her usual glowing self. Her first year on the job, she did not take a sick day or vacation day.

One night, talking about all the craziness, Megan said, "This sounds terrible, but sometimes I wish I could make other people understand what we've been through, what it's like to go through this every day, to live this pain every day, day after day. I'd just like other people to know.

"Is it bad to want other people to feel this? Not all the time, just for a little while, just so they'd understand. The worst thing was waiting for something to happen, not knowing when it would happen. We had to watch out the window for the Father person to come home. We had to have his slippers ready when he walked in the door. If we were slow, he'd kick us. We'd have to stay near him and we didn't want to be near him, but we had to stay there and we never knew when we'd do something wrong that would set him off. If we came home from school late—we had twenty-two minutes—the Mommy person would beat us and if we came home early she'd beat us and one time the Scared One ran away. She was playing . . . at the playground and she knew the Mommy person was going to beat her . . . When the Scared One got in, the Mommy person started pulling her ponytail. And she hit her with a big salad spoon. And the Scared One got away somehow and ran out the door and ran to a friend, Bonnie's, house. Somehow she found it, I don't know how, it was far away. And she knocked on the door and Bonnie's mother was surprised and said, 'Are you all right?' And the Scared One said, 'Can Bonnie come out and play?' And Bonnie's mother said, "Is everything all right? Can I help you out?' And the Scared One didn't say anything about the Mommy person, she just said, 'Can Bonnie come out and play?' And so Bonnie's mother said, 'I better bring you home, you came a long way.' And she took her home and the Mommy person said, 'Oh, thank you,' and was nice. And then she beat the Scared One and beat her with a spoon and when the Father person got home he tied her up so she'd never run away again and strapped her with the belt all over and she had marks all over.

"And the next day was a field trip at school. And the Mommy person said she couldn't go. And I don't know what the Mommy person said to the teacher, but the teacher asked, 'Is everything OK?' And the Scared One didn't say anything. And the teacher said, 'What you did was very bad.' We don't know what the Mommy person told her. And we had to stay with the second grade while the class went on the field trip.

"The Scared One tried to run away one other time, but she didn't get that far. And after that, she said she wouldn't try until eighteen, then she'd run away, but she never grew up." The Scared One was condemned to a lifetime of being five.

·   ·   ·

WHILE PART of knowing Julie was the tormented "children," there were other personalities who were a delight to be friends with. Megan was twelve going on forty, with a bright adolescent's love for music, books, and ideas. Marlena's sarcasm could be hilarious and deadly—she had Holden Caulfield's clear eye for spotting a phony.

And then there was Didi, the irrepressible Didi, usually happy as a lark. She was always popping out when you were talking to another personality, putting in her two cents. You'd say good-bye to Julie, when . . . "Hey, it's me, Di!" Others accused her of talking too much. "Marlena says I'm a real blabberymouth," Di explained. Di's philosophy about this was "So what!" Di did not give one hoot. She was having too much fun. As she said, "I really am pretty amazing for four, if I do say so."

Di was a peek into the childhood Julie would have had in a healthy family.

Julie says that one of the things that saved her, growing up, was being allowed to watch Channel 13, the educational channel. Didi was quite the expert when it came to these shows. And she had that gift many four-year-olds share—to be able to discuss five hundred topics in a row without a single transition problem. "I like Big Bird," she said during one of her regular late-night calls. "I saw Big Bird's birthday party. It's fun. I know Elmo but I really like Cookie Monster. He likes chocolate chip cookies. And guess what? One time Jim gave me a cookie monster cupcake. Is that the greatest? I couldn't eat it all. I don't have a big stomach like Julie. I'm only four!

"It's not always easy being four. Sometimes there's no strawberry cow's milk in the house. Strawberry is my favorite, favorite, most favorite color.

"I like Ernie and Bert and Mr. Snuffleupagus. He's sad a lot. I like Bob. He sings the best.

"You want to hear something funny about the Grouch? He's just pretend grouchy. It's not nice to be mean.

"I like Mr. Rogers. He tells me I'm special. Nobody else tells me I'm special. I like . . ."

Di loved going to therapy at Dr. Sandler's. She liked having the chance to come out and play. "Dr. Sandler is the greatest in the whole, whole world. She had a little dolly for me. I love my little dolly." (Di would pronounce this "I wuv my wittle dowwy.")

Between visits, Dr. Sandler kept Di's dolls in a closet. This concerned Di. "I said the dolls are very, very sad to be in the closet. So you know what Dr. Sandler did? This is what. She got a little itty bitty rocking chair and put them in it and now I see them all the day. And you know what? Dr. Sandler said nobody else plays with them. Isn't that stupid? I love to play with them. You'd play with them if you was there, right?"

Di wanted Dr. Sandler to read her a book. She told Dr. Sandler that inside, Abigail reads to her, a book "about a little baby, and nobody bothers the little baby." Dr. Sandler promised to get Di a book about multiples. "It's a special book for little children," Di explained later. "She has to get it for you know who—me! Di!"

There was nothing in the world quite like hearing Dr. Sandler's therapy sessions filtered through Di. "You know what Dr. Sandler said?" Di said one evening that fall. "She said there are people inside of other people's heads. I was shocked! She said I'm in someone's head. I said, 'I can't be in someone's head. I walk around on the grass in here. If I was in someone's head, I'd fall out of their nose.' "

During November, when Julie was having a lot of trouble, Di saw Dr. Sandler several times a week. She drew pictures of life inside, including the tall grass. When Dr. Sandler finally got the book on multiples, Didi was disappointed. "A stinky book," said Di, "A sad book. Very, very stinky. Dr. Sandler said she didn't know it was going to be too grown-up for me. It just had a little pictures." Little pictures was not Di's idea of a book. She wanted Dr. Sandler to read her *Cinderella*. "Dr. Sandler showed me a copy of *Beauty and the Beast* she had

from when she was a little girl," said Di. "It had real gold pages. It was
from when Dr. Sandler was little and that's a really, really long time
ago. I can't count that high, that's how I know it's a big number. And
guess what? I can count to 20."

THROUGH Di you could gauge Julie's bad periods, her better
stretches, and the progress she was making. On most days, Di could
control going in and coming out. "You want to speak to Julie?" she'd
ask casually at the end of the conversation, and then out would pop
the Julie personality. But during bad periods when there was something wrong with the switching mechanism, Di would get stuck outside. That was the problem at the vocational program in 1990.

Di would grouse about having to spend so much time inside—it
was her pet peeve—but she had learned the rules Dr. Sandler, Jim, and
the Abigail personality had all laid down to her. "It isn't fair," Di said.
"They go to work in the day and I can't come out." Not that work was
any big deal. If Di were in charge she could have come up with a lot
more interesting things to do than work. Once in a while she would
take a peek out at work. "It's boring," she said. "Julie had to go to the
library today to do some research for her boss. I couldn't even understand the words. There were no pictures in the book. What kind of
book is that?

"I can only come out in the privacy of my home," she said. "And
you know what? I'm not allowed to play outside with other children.
People will laugh at me, right?"

The worst thing about staying in all day was that Di missed her TV
shows.

The good news was that Jim took them places on weekends, and it
was all right to come out. They went to a carnival, and Di popped out
on the Ferris wheel and got to eat a caramel apple. (Marlena also had
to have her own caramel apple).

Jim owned a power boat that they used on summer weekends. "You
know what?" said Di. "I go in the water and I can't touch the ground.
You know what Jim did? He put a little jacket on me. He put a little

string on it so I won't float away. I was laughing and laughing. And if I went too far he pulled me in real fast."

And of course, no one knew how to arrange a special-day party like Jim. "He made me a strawberry special-day cake," said Di. (Strawberry is her very, very favorite.) "And you know what? We had big special-day hats. They was really, really pretty. I had a pink one and the Scared One had a purple one and Jim had a blue one. They was big hats and they held on around my chin. I told Jim I loved it, my special day. I told Jim I love him, he's the best in the west. Yeah, he was laughing. In the whole world he's my very, very favorite. And Jim says I'm a very impressive girl."

Among the personalities, only Megan spoke negatively about Jim. The young ones had become so dependent on him, she was afraid what might happen if they ever split up. She was not going to fall into that trap. Megan rarely talked to Jim, nor would she take anything from him. When he was at work she'd play his classical CD's, but was always careful to put them back exactly the way he'd left them. Jim would have never known she'd touched them, if she hadn't felt morally obliged to inform him.

"We live together on the inside and we don't want or need anyone else," Megan once said. "I think he tries too hard. I don't want him feeling sorry for us. It almost seems masochistic."

But even Megan, stern as a church lady, would concede this much: "He is good with the Scared One. That's good. It keeps us out of the hospital. That's important to everyone. We won't go there anymore."

LATELY THE adult personalities had been thinking it might be nice if they all married Jim, and Di was 100 percent in favor. Di told Jim when she wore the white dress for her wedding, she wanted the song to be "Beauty and the Beast." "We played the tape," said Di, "And Jim dipped me so far down—I didn't think I'd be able to get back up, and you know what? Jim doesn't even know how to dance. He danced like hugging. He doesn't know one hand is supposed to be like a hug and one isn't.

"The Scared One wants to get married on a boat and we all agree. We don't want to invite the Father person and so we can't have any family. And so we can't invite friends, since we can't invite family, so we just want to get married by ourselves on a boat.

"I want to dance but I don't want to dance like Cinderella. That's too fast. I'd be going fast, fast, and my dress would come up and everyone would see my underpants. We don't want that! No way, Jose."

TO FOUR-YEAR-OLD Di, their relationship with Jim was like a fairy tale on the Disney channel, but to Julie and Jim it was much harder. Jim was often exhausted. He'd be up much of the night calming the young personalities, and then have to get up for work. He'd be trying to wake up in the shower when suddenly there'd be a pounding on the stall door and Didi shouting: "Jim! Jim! *Sesame Street* is on. Big Bird! You're missing it."

It was like he suddenly had a family with a ton of kids. He was constantly being called on to referee disputes. Di would be mad at Marlena, claiming Marlena drank her strawberry cow's milk. "Jim bought that special for me, D-i, d-i."

When Julie finally came out again in the morning to go to work, Jim was always amazed. She seemed so rested. It was as if she'd been sleeping all night while he and the other personalities were reliving the horrors.

FOR JULIE'S PART, she felt she didn't get to see enough of Jim. He was a workaholic. But that wasn't all. Julie felt Jim paid too much attention to the young personalities. She was concerned that he liked other personalities better than her. She once asked if the young ones were part of the reason he stayed with her, and he'd answered yes. This worried her—she didn't want to feel like some kind of social work project.

One of Julie's most admirable traits was her ability to confront a problem head-on. Others might let this slide. Not Julie. The solution was obvious to her: If you're having problems with your steady, you get couples counseling. So she went looking for a counselor who'd be comfortable working with her and Jim. She explained she wasn't looking for therapy for being a multiple—she had Dr. Sandler. They needed to talk about their relationship and how the multiplicity complicated things. "What I really need is to get Jim to talk about it. Every time I bring it up, he's too tired or he has to make a phone call. He hates to talk about anything."

Leave it to Julie to find a qualified marriage counselor who was familiar with the disorder. ("It really wasn't that hard," she said.) At the first session Jim told the counselor he'd never felt about a woman the way he felt about Julie. With other women, he said, after a few hours he felt like running out of the room screaming. Never with Julie.

"Really?" Julie said. Jim was always so tight-lipped. She liked hearing things like that.

A S M U C H A S she could, Julie learned to cope. She found that Holliswood Hospital in Queens specialized in disassociative disorders and arranged to be sent there if she got bad. At least if she needed a hospitalization, the time wouldn't be totally wasted. She learned the seasonal pattern of her problems—when Tess would be mourning Patricia—and warned friends. "I just wanted you to know I may disappear," she said one night that fall. "I disappeared about this time last year. You can try calling and if I don't respond, it's not you. One of the other members may be pretending to be me. If they tell you to get lost, it's not me."

But mainly she tried to live her life with as much dignity as possible, given the facts.

That fall her office was reorganizing and the secretaries were swamped. Julie had the idea to call the vocational program that had trained her and see if there was someone who was ready to volunteer in the office. Her old counselor, Barbara Green, had a woman in mind but she warned Julie, "Be very gentle with her, she's very fragile."

"Come on," Julie said, "You know me."

Barbara Green actually walked the new woman over to be sure she'd get there.

Julie made the new woman her project. She was neatly dressed, but what Julie noticed was how she carried herself. Very meek and second-class. She clearly suffered from some depressive disorder.

Remembering her own experience, Julie was explicit about everything. "We need you to do filing," she said. "Don't worry about speed. I don't care how slow you go, the big thing, it has to be right. I don't want you to get mixed up by saying, 'I'm working too slow.' At the start of a job you always feel, 'Oh my God, I'm so slow.' "

The woman was nervous, tense, mousy.

She did great.

When Julie was new at the job, she was so interested in making a good impression, she felt she shouldn't take her breaks or lunch. "I want you to know you have two 15-minute breaks and an hour for lunch and you're required to take it," Julie told her. "If someone gives you work just before lunch, it doesn't mean it has to be done that second. You go, and come back to it." Julie felt the most important thing to learn in a new job was not being stepped on.

Through the weeks, Julie kept an eye out. She told the woman, "You really can use this experience as a tool to get a job. You can use it on your résumé, you can use people in the office for a recommendation." Julie did not say that's what she had done; she didn't want anyone in the office knowing her past.

The new woman was a big help and Julie talked her up to the other secretaries. "She was monumental in moving our records around, wasn't she?" said Julie. Julie gave her extra jobs, to build her confidence. After a month, she was started on answering the phones. Nothing too intimidating—just asking callers to hold until a secretary picked up. Julie showed her how to type index cards for the filing system.

"You're so fast," the woman said.

"I have to be," said Julie. "I talk so much."

After several weeks, the woman got the confidence to say to Julie, "You want to come to lunch with me?"

. . .

ONE EVENING in October, Julie stopped off at a drop-in center run by the mental health system. She still visited this program occasionally, though she couldn't say exactly why. Julie saw some old friends and felt the progress she was making. It seemed to help her confidence.

And there in a chair in the lobby was her little office helper, crying. When the woman saw Julie she wiped her eyes and said, "Hi," in an apologetic way."What are you doing here?"

"I come here once in a while," said Julie, hesitating. "I've had problems in the past. I was in the vocational program you're in now."

"Really?" said the woman. "You?"

"It helped me a lot," said Julie.

"You?" the woman said.

"Just nine months ago," said Julie.

"My God," said the woman, "You run that office."

chapter 15

MENTAL PATIENTS, AWAKEN!

STAN GUNTER was returning to the group home. The staff had been unsure if it was a good idea at first. Success stories weren't supposed to reappear. A different group home where he had no history might be easier.

But Stan wanted 9 Highland. During his recuperation, when he needed someone to talk to, he'd call the counselors. When Linda and Maureen had visited him at Brunswick Rehabilitation Center a few weeks earlier, he told them, "I appreciate you have an understanding of the phenomena of the voices. If no one understood this phenomena, I'd be in trouble."

It was important to Stan that people saw he hadn't jumped because he was depressed; he'd jumped because the voices told him to.

His physical progress continued to be remarkable. In July he'd needed two nurses to help him go to the bathroom at the hospital; in August he got around in a wheelchair. Now he was driving his car again and walking with the aid of a three-footed cane. He was given a battery of tests to determine whether he'd suffered brain damage, and scored 100 on all of them.

Stan was ready to move out of his parents' place. Since the incident they watched him too much. They wouldn't let him drink coffee or smoke cigarettes, two of his great joys. They wanted him to eat something for breakfast, and he wasn't a breakfast man. He preferred a ham sandwich around 10:30.

They treated him like he was going to jump off another building.

TOWARD THE END of September, just as he was supposed to begin a three-day trial stay at the house, Stan's father called Maureen to say they'd changed their minds. "Stan will not be coming for a visit," Mr. Gunter said. "It's too much, he's not up to it. Maybe in January."

Maureen said there might not be an opening in January. Her guess was that Mr. Gunter was scared to death to trust Stan with anyone.

She knew the Gunters well. They'd visited Stan every day during his three months at the hospital and rehab center and threw a big barbecue for him when he'd moved back home. The first time they met with Stan's psychiatrist after the jump, Mr. Gunter wept.

But Maureen also was aware how hard it was for Stan to be around his father. "He almost considers himself a doctor," Stan once told her. "He thinks he can find the perfect medication to make me better. He's always been angry about my illness." Stan's schizophrenia had been one of the few problems his engineer father had not solved.

Mr. Gunter was a charming, cosmopolitan man, but there was a hardness and directness to him that devastated Stan. One sunny afternoon in mid-September, Stan and his parents were sitting around the Gunters' glassed-in den that overlooked their wooded backyard, discussing Stan's recovery with a guest. Mr. Gunter was describing how Stan had tried to help his girlfriend Jenny—who also suffered schizophrenia—cope with her problems.

"It was like the blind leading the blind," said Mr. Gunter. It took Stan ten seconds, but finally, in a controlled voice, he got the words out: "I'm not blind."

Maureen did not back down to Mr. Gunter. She got him to agree to let Stan make the trial visit, assuring him that it did not imply a commitment. She knew once she got Stan in the house, it would be hard to pry him loose.

ON SEPTEMBER 23, Stan drove up in his car with a little suitcase his mom had packed him. He limped in and was greeted like a returning hero.

"I'm just so happy to be alive," he told them. "It's a miracle. And I'm happy to be free. I can't believe I'm here." In the late afternoon he sat at the piano and played several songs—"The Rose," Beethoven's "Ode to Joy," "Amazing Grace," "Let It Be"—and then as a reward to himself, smoked half a cigarette.

He seemed so lively and healthy, a new woman at the house asked why he needed a cane.

He was nervous about returning to his haunts, but his girlfriend insisted they go for dinner at Avanti Pizza. "They love you," she said, "they miss you," and indeed it was the hero's welcome all over. Stan and the owner talked in Italian and the man refused to let Stan pay for dinner. "Miracoloso" the owner kept saying.

Maureen was right—once Stan visited, he stayed. He liked living with others who had the same problems. He felt less conspicuous.

He developed a routine. After dinner, he drove over to visit Jenny at her supervised apartment in Glen Cove, greeting her with his usual "I'm ready for my hug." She'd make him coffee and served Sunshine chocolate Dinosauris cookies.

He was rooming with Jasper now, which was working out fine. They'd known each other two years. He could practice his Spanish on Jasper. They were always *hola*-ing and high-fiving. "Jasper is a good guy," Stan said.

Stan had never noticed that Jasper smelled bad.

.   .   .

ONE IN FOUR people with schizophrenia attempts suicide; one in ten succeeds. Because Stan had survived such a close call, because he was so bright, his situation seemed to offer a peek at what goes wrong.

Why did Stan jump?

Stan's answer was the voices. But why did the voices tell him to harm himself this time? He had heard voices on and off for years; when he was in Denmark in the early 1980s, they spoke Danish to him. Why did he obey them this time?

Stan insisted that he had not been depressed before the jump. He talked about the voices like they were independent agents, unrelated to anything going on in his mind or his life.

But there were indications that this might not be so. The first time the tube was taken out of his throat after the jump, Stan told his father that he'd been upset about his relationship with Jenny. He mentioned they'd been going out four years and were in a rut; he had a crush on counselor Paula Marsters, who still treated him like a group home resident; and he felt guilty that Jenny liked him more than he now cared for her—especially since she kept talking about marriage. Stan told his father, "Part of why the accident happened subconsciously was because I had this dilemma."

Stan now had no recollection of telling his father any of that.

Mr. and Mrs. Gunter had another theory. They believed Stan was depressed about his lack of progress, and that had set off the harmful voices. Stan was thirty-nine. He'd recently told Mr. Gunter, "Look how much you'd done by forty, and look at me."

Said Mr. Gunter: "I think he looked at his life and realized he hasn't accomplished a damn thing."

In recent months Stan had resumed seeing his longtime psychiatrist, Dr. Rieben. She had another theory. She believed the vision of God and Jesus battling was really about Stan and his father. She saw the God that had goaded Stan into jumping as the father figure, large and frightening. And Jesus was Stan, the angry, fearful son.

Stan had spent much of his adult life dependent on his father's financial support, though what he'd wanted was an independent career in music. The father was skeptical and Stan ached to show him he could do it, but he never could. His first breakdown had come while he was pursuing a graduate degree in music. In recent years he hadn't even been able to give people lessons.

When Stan's father talked about his son's love for music, he'd shake his head and say, "This is not real."

In the vision, when Stan was not able to finish playing his song, God grew enraged.

Mr. Gunter was the most important person in Stan's life, Dr. Rieben felt. Stan wanted his approval yet no longer believed it would happen. It was never all right between the two, Dr. Rieben reasoned, and Stan had jumped to make things all right, to at last end the epic conflict between these two forces before they destroyed everything around them. To avert nuclear war.

Maureen had heard the theories and believed the voices were set off by a depression, but couldn't nail it down more. She tried talking to Stan. After he first moved back to the house she was discussing his meds with him. He'd been put on Wellbutrin, an antidepressant, in August. Was it helping? she asked. Was he depressed?

Stan told her: "My parents say I'm doing better. I'm not completely aware myself." The star witness had lived to testify, but his long suit wasn't motive.

What Maureen did know was that the jump was always on Stan's mind now. He blamed himself for having been suckered by the voices. He'd say to Maureen, "I thought I was saving this world, but it really was for nothing. It was such a waste."

He was quiet and private, and you got no sense of the depth of his despair unless you caught the rare moment when it surfaced. His left arm was so badly broken in the jump, the flexibility in the elbow was now gone, and he couldn't make the stretches to form guitar chords anymore. In many ways he'd liked the guitar better than the piano. He'd composed two dozen guitar pieces and enjoyed playing at parties, cafés, and for friends. The guitar traveled where the piano could not. One night that fall, he was listening to a tape of his original guitar music at Jenny's. "I wasn't a bad guitar player, was I?" he said. Tears were rolling down his cheeks and he whispered, "Damn, I miss it."

STAN'S MUSIC did his talking. The night of the staff meeting Tuesday, October 8, he performed a string of Spanish flamenco pieces.

"We're being serenaded," Maureen smiled. The piano was just ten feet from the closed office door. While Stan performed song after song from memory, this is what the staff discussed:

"Stan hasn't been taking showers since he's been here," said Maureen.

"He's sleeping in his clothes," said counselor Sandra Ford.

"It's the same thing that happened his first time here," said Maureen. "He's not brushing his teeth, either."

Outside, Stan was playing "Maria" from *West Side Story*. The new female resident, Marie, had asked for it the week before; Stan didn't know the music, so he'd learned it.

"I know Stan's going to sleep early," said Maureen. Most nights he was in bed by nine o'clock. "I think we're going to have to say he doesn't get his meds until he puts on his pajamas."

He was also skipping his rehabilitation program, saying he didn't feel well. Then counselors would discover he was well enough to go to Radio Shack to buy a part for his ham radio.

"We can't let him withdraw," said Jodie. "He did that last time he was here."

Stan was playing "Let It Be," and singing along. The house was quiet, listening. He didn't have much of a voice, it was raspy and broke sometimes, but there was great feeling in it that captured all the melancholy and hope Lennon and McCartney had intended.

STEPHEN DEROSA had never been spunkier. His explanation for his great mood was "Prozac, plus, the spirit of God is in me and has filled me up." Maureen assumed his schizophrenia was on an upward crest. Little bothered him. Trouble sleeping? "I don't worry," he said. "I like to lie in bed thinking of bingo and of my brother down at the store, saying happy things."

This man, who on the downward cycle screamed if people closed a door too loudly or ate chicken with their fingers, was now doing imitations. "Have you heard my imitation of Anthony's father? 'Anthony! I've got some new underwear for you. Go over in the corner and try them on.'"

He'd been coming to the community meetings with long lists of things that needed repairing in the house. The others would be ready to end a half hour into the meeting. Maureen caught the hint and would say, "Anything else?" and that was when Stephen pulled out his list, to general moaning.

"I have several things," he said. "Hot water is still dripping in the blue bathroom. I hate seeing that water going down the drain, it's such a waste."

"Anything . . ."

"The toilet in the kitchen bathroom smells," said Stephen, "it needs a new sewer seal . . ."

"Stephen," said Maureen, "If you want to just give me the list after the meeting . . ."

"Item number five," Stephen went on, "pink toilet, you can actually lift up, the bolts are loose . . ."

Teresa, sitting beside Maureen, put her head down on her knees. "Are you all right?" Maureen whispered.

"Item number six. Vacuum cleaner needs new belt. There's so much crap on it I don't know if it can be fixed."

People kept rising out of their chairs, then falling back. Stan Gunter was grinding his teeth loudly.

"Item number seven, grocery list for kitchen . . ."

Stephen seemed to have slowed down. "Is that it?" Maureen asked.

"Yeah," said Stephen. "Oh. I didn't call this an item, but don't forget the bathroom door needs new screws, otherwise it'll come out again . . ."

After a few weeks of this, Maureen did the only sensible thing: she made him the official house handyman, paying him six dollars an hour for odd jobs. When Maureen announced it at a Tuesday meeting, everyone clapped.

"Does a truck come with the job?" someone asked.

Stephen was good at it, too.

This was the period when Stephen cemented his legendary reputation for doing nightly chores. One evening, at 7:15, he went in to clean the bathroom off the kitchen (which is four feet by three feet), closing the door behind him. He did not open the door again until 9:30, when he took a break and had a dish of ice cream. "All I have left is the toilet bowl," he said. "It'll clean up great. All nice and white."

"What are you doing in there?" a friend asked, "building the Panama Canal?"

"That's a good one," Stephen laughed, disappearing behind the closed door again.

He was excited about new things and was more flexible. Usually he'd volunteer as a bingo caller at church only on Saturday nights. Now he'd go to the midweek game, too, if something big was going on. "They have a new microphone," he told Maureen. "I really want to see it. I hear you have to talk into the front, not the side. They might let me try it."

After a ten-year absence, he rejoined the church choir.

He was even enjoying his girlie magazines again, without worrying about hell. "Look at this one," he said up in his room one evening, sliding the magazine from a brown bag. The cover featured a woman in an amateurishly doctored photo with six breasts. "Must be a birth defect," he whispered.

But his major project that fall was wooing Heather. She was nice to him. He hadn't planned on going to the Halloween costume party at the East Hills house, but Heather persuaded him. "I'm too old," said Stephen.

"You're not too old to eat pizza," Heather said.

He went dressed as a handyman.

She explained she just liked him as a friend, but he would not be deterred. He kept inviting her out, to Friendly's, Pastas Cafe, and his mother's for Sunday dinner. Every night he would make a trip down to the deli on School Street and pick up a treat for her—an ice-cream sundae, pastry, cookies. You'd bump into Stephen walking across the living room with a piece of cake and he'd whisper, "It's for Heather. Fattening her up."

Between August and November she gained fifty-six pounds.

Some of that was swelling from an infection which landed Heather in the hospital for a couple of weeks, but either way, she looked more and more beautiful to Stephen.

He was floating around the house, humming like a birdy. "I made up a song," he said. "It goes: 'There's nothing like a woman with a fat can' . . . Wouldn't it be terrible if you were singing it and you were with a woman with a fat can?!" And off he went, humming his merry tune.

ANTHONY'S GOAL for the fall was to get A's or B's in his two psychology courses at Nassau Community College and move out into his own apartment. However, it was not a good omen on the first day of school, when he learned he'd spent the summer reading the wrong five-hundred-page abnormal psychology text.

On a personal level, Anthony's goal was to keep his heart pure, so he could go to Heaven. He was constantly feeling his chest, monitoring the heartbeat. The key to a pure heart was obeying the voices, and they were relentless now. He had to follow their commands; otherwise everything would get out of order and set off a chain reaction that would land him in Hell.

It was quite logical when Anthony laid it all out. Suppose he didn't come downstairs when God told him, or he sat wherever he felt like. Then that would lead someone else in the group home to change where they were sitting. "Then that could lead me to sit in a way—say, putting my knee up like this for example—that would make me think of something terrible that happened a long time ago. Then my heart wouldn't feel full of love, and my heart has to be pure to go to Heaven.

So you see why I don't want to stir up the waters. I just come down-stairs when God tells me."

Anthony was facing forward on the living room couch, when sud-denly he leaned sideways, shifting his position. "The voice just told me to do that," he explained. "I can be up in bed and hear a little sound as loud as a whisper and then, like five seconds later, I know what it meant." He made a loud slap with his hand against the coffee table to illustrate. "That was, 'Get my meaning?' "

The voice was God, or Anthony's father, or sometimes a mix of both. Anthony's psychiatrist kept raising his dosage of Prolixin—it was sixty-five milligrams daily now. He was also taking the tranquil-izer Ativan three times a day.

The voices still got through.

During a staff meeting in the office, Anthony interrupted to get his Ativan and then, in front of all the counselors, launched into a lengthy speech explaining how he knew his father was God. "I have proof. You won't tell Linda Slezak, right?" In a fifteen-minute monologue before the silent counselors, he said he wanted to live in an apartment, go to the hospital, kill himself. He implied he was Jesus Christ, but said he just wanted to be Anthony J. Constantine, a happy-go-lucky guy.

Afterward, Maureen sat with him. "My mother's trying to change my heartbeat," he said. He'd called home that afternoon and heard his mother's voice on the line just a moment, before Dom yelled, "It's OK, I got it."

"Just hearing her voice, she gets inside of me, it's so powerful," Anthony said. "You don't understand my family. My mother's the Devil, my father is God. He never lets up. He's on me all the time. He wants me to be perfect, be a man.

"At Sara Center today counselors were saying sexual things about me, but I handled it beautifully, I didn't let it get to me. But when I have to come home and deal with my father on top of it, I just can't take it."

Anthony had figured out how Dom projected his voice from fifteen miles away in Plainview to the room at the group home. "You won't

MICHAEL WINERIP

tell? He sends it over the telephone wires. My hearing's so good, you don't have any idea. It's like I can hear a pin drop in Alabama.

"I want you to know, Maureen," Anthony said, "I may be smiling at you right now, but I'm going through hell and I need your help. I hope you're not mad at me."

He wanted to talk to his mother and go back to his house for a visit. There were tears in his eyes. "Would you call my mother and ask if I can go home? I want to see my room again."

Maureen said she'd try.

MAUREEN FIGURED it this way: Anthony was angry with his father for not standing up to his mother about visits home. This explained why the dreaded voice in Anthony's head had become his father. Maybe if Maureen could make peace with his mother, Anthony could find a little relief from the voices. If he saw his mother again, it might deflate her importance. A troubled relationship between the two might be better than none at all.

Maureen actually reached her on the phone and was surprised by how much Mrs. Constantine knew of her son's current condition. Clearly, Dom kept her informed. At one point Mrs. Constantine said, "I really, really care about what's going on," and Maureen heard pain in the words. Still, Mrs. Constantine was adamant about never being alone with Anthony again.

That's all right, Maureen said, there are always plenty of counselors around the group home when parents visit.

As a first step Maureen suggested Mrs. Constantine come to the next family forum. These were the monthly meetings held at Melillo clinic for relatives; group home residents did not attend.

Dressed in a plain turquoise pantsuit, Mrs. Constantine arrived at the October family forum with Dom. Every parent in the room understood the significance; no one commented. Mrs. Constantine did not say a word during the hour and a half, though she nodded vigorously several times at others' comments.

Usually Dom lingered afterward. This night he and his wife left as soon as it was over.

She never came to another meeting, nor did she visit the group home or speak with Anthony again or allow him to come home to see his room.

After a few months, when it became clear that Mrs. Constantine would not return to family forum, Fred's father, Mr. Grasso, made a little speech. "I just want to tell you," he said to Dom, "How much I admire what you do."

"Oh it's nothing at all," said Dom. "All of us do for our children."

"None of us sacrifices and works for our kids the way you work for yours," said Mr. Grasso.

THE VOICES intruded more. Anthony missed school a couple of days. "Even in my dreams," said Anthony, "they don't leave me alone. It's like I don't dream, I hear things in my dreams. They keep saying, 'mental torture, mental torture.' That's why I was crying. It takes so much energy to fight them. So much courage. I don't know if I can do it. It's so tiring, they fill up the whole day. Why would my father do this to me? I hate him for it."

OCTOBER 15 was quiet for a Tuesday night at the house. Maureen was away, so the community and staff meetings were short. Heather and a few others played cards at the dining room table. Fred and Teresa watched TV. Stephen DeRosa put on his boots and gloves to clean a bathroom. Anthony was up in his room sleeping or studying.

In the office, Donna Rubin showed Sandra Ford, a new counselor, how to distribute meds. Donna explained that the residents were to swallow their pills in front of her, describing what they were taking and the dosage.

Around nine, Anthony came down. "Prolixin 10, two tabs," he said.

"What?" said Donna. He was on three at night.

"I said three tabs, Prolixin 10."

"Sorry," said Donna. "Thought you said two." She was the easiest-going counselor at the house. During his first year, Anthony had a big crush on her.

Suddenly he yelled, "I'm sick of people in this fucking place telling me what to do. I'm a man and I should be treated like an equal. I'm not some boy. I deserve respect." He coughed, spraying the two counselors.

"We do respect—Anthony, please," said Donna, "cover your mouth when you cough."

"I don't need to be told to cover my mouth," he said, "But next time I won't do it," and he coughed, spitting on them again.

She suggested he go upstairs, cool off, and then they'd talk.

Anthony walked out but wheeled around, returning to the office door, and Donna. He knew what was going on. She felt so superior because she was getting her Ph.D. in psychology and he was just taking introductory freshman courses at a puny community college. Anthony J. Constantine would show them. "I'm not afraid of you," he screamed. "Fuck you. You can't tell me what to do. I'm not going upstairs and calm down. Fuck you!" He stepped toward Donna, who was about half his weight. She held her ground—she didn't want to show fear. Anthony suddenly shoved her hard with both his hands, slamming her into the office door. Sandra was behind her and cushioned the impact, but it hurt.

Anthony rushed up the stairs, then came back. In a high, angry voice, he yelled, "I never did this before in my life. I'm going to get her fired."

Lauryn Schelfo, another 105-pound counselor, came up behind him. "I want you to look at me, Anthony," she said in a firm voice. "No, no —I want you to look at me. Anthony. Look. I want you to go upstairs —upstairs. I just want you to go upstairs and calm down. I need to have a smoke and calm down myself. You know, Anthony, things like this have happened before and we've worked them out. Now we're just going to calm down."

Residents watched from a distance, then quickly returned to what they were doing.

"Another hospital case," said Heather. "They didn't take him away when he hit Joe. Maybe now that he hit a counselor they'll do something."

Sounding like Dan Rather, Fred provided the trailer for the eleven o'clock news: "Violence at the group home," he said, before going silent again.

Stephen DeRosa emerged from the pink bathroom totally oblivious, lugging a bucket and a gallon of Lysol. "It's ready to be checked," he told Sandra cheerfully. "You should've seen all the hairs in the sink,"

LAURYN WAS the overnight counselor, alone from 11 P.M. to 7 A.M. She wanted Anthony out of the house. He'd broken a rule. All the residents had witnessed it. Everyone needed to see there were consequences. She called Debbie Dombrowski on the emergency beeper. Debbie spoke with Anthony. He said he was mad at himself for what he'd done, but he'd felt picked on. He kept apologizing. "Are they going to call my father?" he asked. He promised to go to bed. She knew his history—he'd blow up, then feel enormous guilt. It was the same thing when he'd hit Joe and threatened Stan.

Debbie had been through her share of crises as manager of the Glen Head house. She'd once called the police on a resident who'd put a knife to another resident's throat—albeit a kitchen butter knife. From what she'd heard, she did not believe Anthony was dangerous now.

"I want him out tonight," said Lauryn.

"Where?" said Debbie.

Lauryn suggested the Crisis Residence, a building on the grounds of Pilgrim State Hospital that took people in trouble who needed a few days to collect themselves.

"It's closed," said Debbie. The state had shut it down earlier in the month during budget cuts.

Lauryn was fuming after hanging up. "Why did she ask me about getting him out of the house, if she wasn't going to listen? There's no protection for counselors, no rules, you can do what you want."

Lauryn was a sharp, hardworking twenty-two-year-old who'd graduated the previous spring from the state university at Albany. She was clocking thirty-three hours a week at the group home; two shifts a week as an aide on 3-West at Glen Cove Hospital; plus taking a course toward her master's in social work. She was the type of person who, when she had the Friday overnight, would bring in a couple of half gallons of ice cream and a tape from Blockbuster Video to brighten people's weekend.

Around midnight she sat in the living room of the quiet house, having a smoke. All the residents, including Anthony, were in bed. "I feel a lot safer working at the hospital," she said. "You're working with lots of other staff. If a patient hits an aide, they put him in restraints.

"I could have had a job at the hospital full-time making ten thousand more a year. You work the night shift, it's quiet, you listen to the radio. Here I put in and can't get a day off a month ahead. If you can't find someone to replace you, you can't have it off. I couldn't even get the night before my sister's shower off."

The funny thing was, she preferred the group home. She liked the people, found it more challenging, felt she had more impact.

A little before 1 A.M., Lauryn locked the office door and climbed into bed. She fell right asleep. In the middle of the night she thought she heard furniture moving, but it was just someone in the room above the office, turning over.

Anthony came in early for his meds Wednesday morning—he probably hadn't slept much either. He was taking them so fast, Lauryn asked him to slow down, and he raised his voice.

"Look," said Lauryn, "It is 7 A.M. and I can't deal with you and anyone else yelling at me. If you need to yell at me, please leave."

"All right," Anthony said. Midmorning, he went off to his volunteer job at a local nursing home, and did fine.

When Maureen later suggested he sit with Lauryn and talk about what happened, Anthony said, "I can't. I'm afraid of Lauryn. She scares me."

FOR DAYS the incident dominated the counselors' conversations. Several complained to Maureen; Lauryn went directly to Linda Slezak to voice her distress. At the October 22 staff meeting they argued that there should be a rule about hitting a counselor—or resident—and that Anthony should have been automatically removed.

Maureen answered them with questions. Where should Anthony have been removed to? Most agreed he didn't need the hospital. There was no more Crisis Residence—and suppose there was? Do you ship him in the middle of the night to an unfamiliar place thirty miles away in Suffolk County? What if he resisted? Do you put him in restraints? How do the other residents feel seeing that? The counselors knew Anthony, he knew them, they knew his behavior patterns. When he was most fragile, they wanted to hand him off to someone else? Tragedies in the system often came between workers and patients who were strangers. In New York State in the previous decade, 104 mental patients had died while being restrained, mainly at large state hospitals.

"We don't want to punish him for being sick," Maureen said. "You have to think about what's going on inside someone. Anthony was psychotic at the time, hearing voices constantly. It's hard for him to distinguish what's inside and what's outside. The phone, the TV, it all blends, all this noise, all the confusion trying to hear through all the noise.

"You know how guilty he feels," Maureen continued. When she'd come back on Thursday, he'd told her, "I did something terrible. I hit a girl. My father says a man never hits a girl."

"It's hard," said Paula Marsters, "really hard, the whole thing is a hard situation."

"It is hard," said Maureen, "especially in light of the limited mental-health system. You have to think of it this way: What do you think will help Anthony the most?"

They were quiet. "You did the right thing," said Maureen.

"I did?" said Lauryn.

"You did," said Maureen. Maureen didn't say it, but getting pushed around once in a while was the price they paid for running a show with a little humanity.

THE DOCTOR had Anthony up to seventy milligrams of Prolixin daily now—a tremendous amount of antipsychotic, and twice the dose when he was at his best. Side effects worsened at such a high dosage. Anthony was tired all the time. He was sloppy, his shirt was never tucked in. On Sundays, when Dom took him for the day, Anthony fell asleep in the car and at the movies. His legs shook, he rocked back and forth in his chair and rolled his tongue—the involuntary movements that large doses of antipsychotic medication can cause, known as tardive dyskinesia.

Still the voices broke through.

The main thing Anthony hoped for now was to hang on at school. Maureen told him it was OK to lower his expectations at a time like this. Just passing would be great. She wished to hell he hadn't insisted on taking abnormal psych. She could imagine what the classes were like for him.

He got a C on a test and said he was satisfied. "It's really hard for me to read. I can't understand it, it's so hard." Dom talked about how proud he was of Anthony, how well Anthony was doing, especially with what he was going through. Dom urged him not to put too much pressure on himself, and many times reminded Anthony that if he wanted to drop out, there was no disgrace in it, people did all the time.

His father could not have been more supportive or understanding.

However, the father's voice in Anthony's head was ruthless, pressing him to work harder, taunting him for not being a man.

Anthony told several counselors, "My father's putting so much pressure on me for school, he never lets up."

On his next test he got an F. "I was hearing voices the whole test. My brain's not working. It's going all the time, but it's not always me thinking." He said he might quit after that semester.

The next Sunday he argued with his father at Roosevelt Field mall. Back at the group home, he punched a hole in the wall.

The three-hour abnormal psych lecture the following Tuesday was on mood disorders. The professor contrasted them with other mental illnesses. The professor had a light, jocular speaking style:

"... *Psychotics are very different. They can't deal with reality, they don't understand the world around them ... With the major psychotic disorders there's no triggering event. It's a hard question: Why did this person go nuts?* ...

"... *The problem you're having, you're trying to provide logic to psychotic behavior. These people think, I am the Queen* ...

"... *True maniacs flail about, their arms, their legs* (laughter from the class) ... *There's a case of a man chiming the time for three days.* (Loud laughter. An eighteen-year-old freshman with teased hair shouted, "That's sick!" More laughter.)

"*These people ... these individuals ... these types ... their behavior* ...

"*Even if we're really out of it, there's going to be a few things we enjoy. Not these people, these people are really out of it ... Someone else have a question? No? Sorry. I'm hallucinating!*" (More laughter.)

At the end of the lecture the professor said, "Next time we will talk about schizophrenia."

In the right kind of world Anthony would have been the guest lecturer, but though he tried several times that week, he could not read the two chapters in the text on schizophrenia.

He was scared to death of being unprepared for the schizophrenia lecture.

On Tuesday the phone rang at the Constantines' in Plainview. It was Anthony. Dom was surprised—he was supposed to be in class. "I'm hearing voices," Anthony said. He was sobbing in a phone booth at the student union. "They're really bad, Dom. I can't go to class. No one saw me crying, but I can't go. Dom, I tried."

Mr. Constantine drove to get his son and brought him back to the group home. Anthony never returned to college.

TWICE THAT FALL Jasper was hospitalized. Both were short stays. They changed his antipsychotic, but it didn't make a difference.

He was laughing to himself constantly, seeing more Gambinos, telling his imaginary friends he'd be right back, he had to go take his meds. These last six months, Maureen felt like he'd just given up and slipped away from them. His obesity, his odor—he'd built a fat, smelly wall around himself.

When he returned from the hospital on October 24, she sat him down in the office. "Glad to have you home, Jasper," she said.

"It's good to be here, Maureen," he said. "Don't worry, I'll tell you when I'm getting sick, if I need another hospitalization."

"That's great, Jasper. But is there anything we can do to help? How can we help you? What do you need to stay out of the hospital?"

"I need love," said Jasper.

"Well, you know, we all love you here," said Maureen.

"That's good," said Jasper.

HE DIDN'T need that kind of love. An admitting nurse in the Glen Cove Hospital emergency room told Lauryn Schelfo that she'd known Jasper a decade ago at Glen Cove High and he'd been quite the smoothie with the chickies. "He was *the* man," she said. Jasper himself had said to Jodie Schwartz, "I used to be a clean dude and fared well with the ladies."

Maureen believed that on some level, Jasper still saw himself as that high school dude. At a staff meeting, Paula Marsters described how she'd overheard him asking another resident, "You want to buy some cheeba?" Paula gave him a hard time, saying "Jasper, you can't say that anymore."

Sandra Ford and Charles Winslow, two of the black counselors on the staff, could not stop laughing. "How old is he?" Sandra asked. "That word is so old. Nobody says 'cheeba' anymore."

"His old homeboy talk," Maureen said softly.

Jodie told them how she'd caught him heading out to program one morning wearing a dirty shirt, dirty sweatpants, a tweed jacket with the collar up, and dark glasses. "I said, 'Jasper, you can't go out like that.' He said they're his homeboy clothes."

About the only time he showed initiative now was if there was a social function with women. At a community meeting, Maureen brought up the Halloween party for the three houses.

"What did we do with my costume from last year?" Jasper asked.

"Yeah, you were a ghost," said Maureen. "Maybe it's in your drawer."

"Yeah," said Jasper.

"We had to get a special sheet," said Maureen. "Remember, you didn't want to go as a flower ghost?"

He'd invited most of the female counselors into his room at one time or another and tried to get something going with the new women at the house. Always he was gentlemanly—persistent—but Jasper knew when to stop. After trying to get a kiss from Lauryn, he'd asked her, "Are you scared of me?"

"No," said Lauryn, "should I be?"

"I never hurt anybody," said Jasper.

"I know," said Lauryn.

"I'm a sensitive guy," said Jasper. "I could never kill anybody."

The new resident at the house, Marie, who was attractive and in her twenties, was nice to him in the weeks after she moved in. She was fearful about being in a new place and would take any friend she could find; Jasper had his own ideas. He'd make comments to her about music or offer her a Popsicle. When he'd asked for a kiss, Marie would say, "Jasper!" in a shocked, teasy way that wasn't exactly a no. In late October, Marie was playing cards at the dining room table after dinner. Jasper stood in the doorway watching. He eased closer, then sat down beside her. He didn't talk, just sat close, and finally, Marie said, "Jasper, please, you smell like a skunk."

Jasper returned to the living room couch and soon was laughing loudly to himself.

AT A TUESDAY night meeting, Maureen worked on getting them to put their cups and plates in the dishwasher after snacks. Fred had been doing a lot of extra cleanup work for the others, particularly

Jasper, the grand snacker. "How could the rest of us help Fred out?" Maureen asked, trying to plant a seed.

"I don't think we should put this kind of pressure on Fred," said Jasper.

"Really, Jasper?" said Maureen. "What do you think we should do?"

"Get a maid," said Jasper.

COUNSELORS WERE now wearing rubber gloves when they had to touch his things. During a hospitalization, he needed more underwear, and Jodie told Sandra, "You don't have to touch it; just take his whole drawer and dump it in the washing machine."

They tried to reach his mother when he was hospitalized, but she'd moved without telling Jasper and her new number was unlisted.

At night he'd stand by the microwave, the timer bell going off every few minutes, as he warmed up plate after plate of food.

One dark, chilly morning, at 4:30 A.M. the overnight counselor, Charles, heard someone walking around, got up to check, and found Jasper outside on the lawn, dancing. When he asked Jasper to come in, Jasper said, "That's cool, Charles."

ON NOVEMBER 12, Lauryn, the overnight counselor, was playing cards with a couple of residents when, a little past 10 P.M., Teresa came over and said softly, "I need you."

Lauryn asked if it could wait until the end of the hand and Teresa said, "I don't think so."

Teresa had cut a gash in her arm that would take eighteen stitches to close. She hadn't been trying to kill herself; just cutting.

Lauryn was going to take her to the hospital, but first had to arrange for a backup counselor to watch the house. Teresa waited in the sitting room, puffing a Winston, her arm wrapped in a towel.

Several residents gathered.

"I'm sorry you're not feeling well," said Stephen.

"Where you going, Teresa?" one of the men asked quietly.

"Don't know," she said.

"Long Island Jewish is really good," he said, his voice rising from nervousness. "They give you hamburg and a salad for lunch. You can have chicken. It's really good, you have a choice."

"It is good," said Marie, "I was there."

"The hamburgers are thick," said another.

Teresa wanted to know if you could smoke.

"No. But you can step outside for a smoke. It's no big deal. I was there twice. I got better there. It's a good place."

Lauryn walked in carrying Teresa's suitcase. "Ready?" she asked.

THE GRAPHS tracking Stan's physical and mental health were racing off in opposite directions now. On the same day he put away his cane for good, the voice of God returned, the same deep voice that had tricked him into jumping. It woke him after midnight, chanting, "Kill yourself, kill yourself."

After five months of quiet, Stan was terrified. He told the voice, "I remember what happened, I'm not going to listen to you," and it stopped. He reported this to Donna Rubin the next morning. She asked if there'd been more incidents.

None, he said. "Except I can always conjure up the Jesus voice, but he's never harmed me. All I have to say is, 'Jesus, do you love me?' and he says 'Yes.' When I had my first breakdown, I had a problem eating, I was anorexic. To this day when I'm going to eat, I hear Jesus saying, 'Eat, eat, eat.' I don't know where that's coming from."

Maureen assured him that this time he wasn't alone, he had people to talk to round the clock and a doctor who knew him. Dr. Rieben upped his dose of Navane.

Two weeks later the voice commanded Stan to jump off a balcony and become a saint. The voice warned Stan not to dare tell, but he reported it to Maureen.

His Navane was upped to thirty milligrams, three times his dosage at the time of the jump.

On November 25, the voice dangled sainthood again, if he'd just go to the kitchen, get a knife, and kill himself. He told Maureen he needed the hospital. He went to the Glen Cove emergency room with a counselor, but because of a foul-up by the hospital was kept waiting six hours for a screening. Donna Rubin joked with him, talked to him, did anything to divert him, but he grew quieter and quieter, his color draining. "How you doing?" she asked five hours into the wait.

"Not so good," said Stan.

"Voices?" said Donna. "What are they saying?"

Stan was distracted, listening. "They're telling me they're God."

"Both of them?" asked Donna.

"Yeah," said Stan.

He spent Thanksgiving, Christmas, and New Year's hospitalized.

FRED WAS talking more. He was actually initiating conversation. Someone at the house wore a new sweater and Fred was the first to compliment it. Maureen came back from vacation and Fred asked how her camping trip to New Hampshire went. She did a double take. "Fine, Fred, nice of you to ask." In the late afternoon, he'd take the house ten-speed for a spin around Glen Cove and neighboring Locust Valley. If the gear shift was jammed or the brake pads off center, Fred repaired them.

At night, when he got up to use the bathroom, he was remembering to put on his bathrobe instead of wandering around in his underwear —much to the female residents' relief.

He carried his wet bath mat down to the laundry room.

The improvement appeared to be the result of an additional drug Fred's psychiatrist was trying him on—Eldepryl, a mood elevator. In tandem with clozapine, it was having an effect.

It was another reason Mrs. Grasso so valued the group home. Because of the supervision, it was a safe place to try out new medications. If there was a bad reaction, the staff could be counted on to pick it up. In 1989, after Fred had been at the group home nine months, his doctor reduced his clozapine from three hundred milligrams daily to two hundred. Within a week, counselors noticed he'd stopped interacting with others. He was having trouble getting up in the morning. Jeanne McMorrow at Sara Center reported that he wasn't eating lunch, seemed lethargic and unable to concentrate. If Fred had still been living at the Boerum Hill institution in Brooklyn, Mrs. Grasso said, no one would have noticed until Fred needed to be hospitalized. It had happened several times there (at considerable extra cost to the taxpayers who footed the hospital bills via Medicaid). The group home permitted a psychiatrist to fine-tune the meds without a crisis: three hundred milligrams daily worked for Fred; two hundred milligrams did not.

During the past summer, his psychiatrist had started him on Eldepryl, and by September, when there hadn't been a change, doubled the dosage.

Because staff saw him round the clock—rather than for a forty-five minute weekly or monthly visit to a psychiatrist—small changes registered. Fred hadn't turned into Phil Donahue. He was still pretty much the Sphinx of 9 Highland. An outsider would not have noticed. But as Maureen said at a staff meeting, "Fred just seems to be a little more there lately." He'd been telling her all about his old Triumph Spitfire.

"He's getting better," said Charles.

"A sweetheart," said Paula.

DURING ONE OF the fall holiday weekends, Patty Rogers, a Harvard graduate and professor at Plymouth State College, usually brought her young son and daughter down from New Hampshire to Oyster Bay, Long Island, where she'd grown up, to visit her parents. Sometimes she'd catch a glimpse of Fred Grasso, home for the holidays, too. She was thirty-three and hadn't talked to him in nearly fifteen years, though she still dreamed of him.

Fred had been Patty Rogers' first serious boyfriend. They were next-door neighbors. He is two years older and Patty developed a major crush on him as a teenager in the 1970s. She thought he was terrific looking. She loved Fred's sardonic humor and his unforced, natural intelligence. On summer nights, eight or ten boys and girls from the block would hang out under the streetlight near Fred's house. He was the leader among the boys. Sometimes they'd gather by the beach at the end of the street. When she was fourteen, they started dating. He'd take her for rides in his Triumph convertible. They were a striking couple. He was tall, lean, and dark; she was five feet nine, with long, straight red-brown hair. Pat had ambition, too. She was near the top of her class, on the staffs of the yearbook and newspaper, and student government vice president.

She loved his kindness. He played with the little kids on the street, spinning them on the front lawn, giving them piggyback rides, chasing them. Her parents adored Fred and he spent lots of time hanging out at the Rogers' house. They rarely went to Fred's. The Grasso house was always so fastidiously clean, and Patty was intimidated by Mrs. Grasso. Fred's mother seemed so judgmental and strong-willed to her. Patty had a sense that Mr. and Mrs. Grasso didn't approve of her; she wasn't Italian and perhaps was a little smarter and more independent than they thought a girl should be.

Fred was more mature than most boys she met. She had an infant cousin who suddenly became ill one day. The baby's mother was frantic, and though Fred was just sixteen, he took control, driving them to the hospital. He was so gentle, he calmed them. Another time, Patty's five-year-old brother was riding his bike, flipped over, and blacked out on the street. Fred was there first with a blanket, then carried the boy home.

He was easy to be with—they'd drive around talking about nothing for hours. She used to go to his baseball games. She loved the way he moved. He gave her a chain of beer can tops and when his family went away on trips, he mailed her postcards with funny comments. She wrote him poems and bought him a Saint Christopher's medal for his car. They had a song, "Without You," by Harry Nilsson.

Patty saw a change his eleventh-grade year. He'd always been in the college prep courses, but now seemed to have a lazier attitude, dropping chemistry though his teacher objected. He started hanging out with a kid at school who had a lot of money, did drugs, and was a primo jerk—the kind of person Fred had never mixed with before. Fred smoked a joint with him after school each day, though Patty never really thought of Freddy as a druggie, more as a follower.

Fred had always been gentle, but now he'd push for sex, at times in a mean, heavy-handed way. She felt it wasn't so much Fred as the friend egging Fred on.

Fred and Patty would break up, then get back together in the summers. By the time she was a junior he was at Nassau Community College. If she spotted him in his yard, mowing the lawn, she'd play the piano—not her classical music—but "Yesterday," "Theme from *Love Story*," "Can't Live without You." Fred never commented, though she'd see him stop the mower and linger.

He broke up with her for good toward the end of her junior year— said he was taking someone else to her junior prom. "I remember him telling me he was going to take a sleeping bag and go to the beach with this girl. It was so mean to say that. It wasn't like him. I thought it was cruel and out of character. I ran into him at a party prom night. He was sitting on a couch staring up at the ceiling, really wasted. He looked unhappy with himself."

In 1976 Patty Rogers went off to Harvard. Spring break she brought home a Harvard classmate, her new boyfriend (and future husband), who stayed part of the week. "Fred came over to my house later in the week," she recalled years after. "I was alone. We were in the kitchen. He barely talked, just sat there in the chair, staring around. He made a few weird remarks. He asked if that was my boyfriend, if I had boyfriends and if I was having sex. He wouldn't look me in the eye. I felt scared, threatened by him. He sat for a long time, not saying anything. I was afraid to be alone with him in the house. I finally said I had to go someplace so he'd leave. I didn't have to go anywhere, but I went out, just so he'd go.

"The summer after my freshman year, Mrs. Grasso came over. She said, 'Have you seen Fred? Does he look different to you? Can you talk to him and see what's the matter?' I didn't tell her, but I didn't want anything to do with him. I was amazed she came over to our house. It was one of the first times I can remember Mrs. Grasso in my house. I think I was in their house maybe seven times in my whole life.

"I didn't talk about this to anybody, I felt so terrible. Fairly soon after this, my mother told me he was up in the tree crowing like a rooster and his family took him away.

"When I came home to visit my parents I'd catch a glimpse of him. He had a funny pallor to his skin. A few times he'd say hi. He had glazed eyes, sort of dead eyes, very dulled. I'd see him mowing the lawn, very methodic, just doing his job.

"I didn't see any spark, and I don't think he knew who I was. A couple of times he looked away. I thought then, maybe he knew, and was embarrassed.

"I always imagined he was living in a hospital. I knew his parents went and picked him up somewhere and brought him home and brought him back. My mother told me he had schizophrenia, but I never witnessed his schizophrenic behavior.

"About five or six years ago his sister Rebecca came over trying to figure out what happened. I felt it was the drugs, maybe he'd burned his brains out. I'd never been comfortable discussing it with the family. Rebecca's theory was he'd self-medicated the schizophrenia.

"I never really spoke to him after my freshman year in college. I have such a really terrible feeling about that. That last time I talked with him I felt terrible about being so frightened of him and terrible about how much he frightened me.

"I still always think of him on his birthday even if I'm trying not to. I've had nightmares for years, nightmares of being chased by Fred and he'd hurt me. A couple of times I dreamed Fred was dead."

Professor Pat Rogers and her family live in New Hampshire's White Mountains, not far from the cold, clear rushing waters of the Swift River, one of the more pristine slices of northern New England. It is a world away from suburban Long Island where she grew up. Even so, a few times a year she will jolt awake in the middle of the night sweating and breathing hard, and her husband will say to her "The Fred dream?"

. . .

On the face of it, Heather's fall sounded like an extraordinary disaster. In September she returned to self-mutilation, cutting herself with razor blades. In October her car was repossessed. In November she was hospitalized for two weeks because doctors feared she might have a serious heart condition. By December she was ready to leave the group home and get her own apartment.

Through the worst moments, her therapist, Dr. John Imhof, kept saying she was getting stronger, and he was right. In a way it was one last grand tour of self-destructiveness before moving on. Heather seemed to have a need to sample trouble firsthand to be reminded why it wasn't advisable. She had to spend two final weeks vegetating on a psych ward in August to realize she never wanted to do that again.

In the last several years she'd gone from drug abuse to suicide attempts to self-mutilation to letting her financial responsibilities slide, and finally, by the end of the fall, to excessive smoking and overeating. Slowly she was progressing to more socially acceptable forms of self-destructiveness.

Heather and her best friend at the house, Teresa, fed off each other's problems these months. There was a one-upmanship to it. Maureen would say, "If Heather coughs, Teresa gets pneumonia." They were a little club, the two borderlines, wearing matching socks, trading coats, eating by themselves, going to the emergency room together for their breathing problems. Teresa would stick one of her Winstons in Heather's pack of Marlboros to see if Heather noticed. They'd talk about cutting themselves and how good it would feel.

A few times that September Heather used a razor blade in her room and carved up her arm, but cutting lost some appeal after Teresa's eighteen-stitch gash resulted in a prolonged hospital stay.

Heather's brother had warned her several weeks ahead that her car was in danger of being repossessed for missed payments, and gave her a lawyer's name. But Heather did not contact the man and woke one morning to find the car gone. She'd owned a car all her adult life and was miserable depending on buses. She was sure the group home counselors were picking on her because they did not drive her to more of her appointments.

Heather's health problems were real. Her body swelled, taking on twenty-four pounds of fluid in November, and she needed to be hospitalized and treated with diuretics. (The cause was never found.) However she didn't help matters by smoking heavily, overeating, and getting no exercise.

Through it all, Dr. Imhof always held out hope because he knew she had the power to stop this. She'd abused cocaine eight years and quit. The difficulty was reaching the root of her problem in therapy, getting her to talk about her father's sexual abuse. He believed Heather had much yet to tell, but they made little progress that fall.

B Y D E C E M B E R she was physically healthy and ready to move on. "I can't wait to get my own apartment," she said. "I can't take this place anymore. One person's laughing to himself, one's hearing voices. This place is sick." Heather was noticing, a sure sign it was time to go. Maureen strongly recommended her for a supported apartment.

Unfortunately, the state Office of Mental Health hadn't funded any of the three hundred new subsidized apartments that had been pledged for Long Island that fall. Heather waited months for a place.

It wasn't a waste only for Heather. Just as it was a waste of tax dollars to keep people in a state hospital ($120,000 per bed a year) when they were ready for a group home ($35,000 a year); it was a waste to keep Heather in a group home when she was ready for a subsidized apartment ($9,000 per bed a year).

T H E F I R S T W E E K of December, Jasper went back into the hospital. "This is his fifth or sixth time in a year," Maureen said at the Monday meeting with Linda Slezak.

"I remember the latest hospitalization," Linda said. "He didn't come out significantly better."

"I have the feeling it'll be the same," said Maureen. "I feel so bad for him, so bad for him."

Linda didn't say anything. She was still waiting for Maureen to make the decision.

Later that week Maureen visited Jasper at Central General. At the end of the visit he took her arm and said, "I have to show you something." He dragged her into the shower.

"You see that shower massage head?" Jasper said. "I can hold it in my hand. That's the kind of shower I need. I can get clean!"

WITH ANTHONY'S college career over, Maureen and his father felt it was time to try him on clozapine. The drug, widely considered the most important advance in schizophrenia treatment in twenty years, now cost half what it had a year before and was routinely covered by Medicaid.

Maureen and Linda Slezak—like most mental-health professionals —wanted all the chronic schizophrenics at the house tested on it. Against such a bleak illness, you pursued any hope. At the end of 1991 and the start of 1992, Anthony, Stan, and Jasper were all put on clozapine.

During this period the mainstream press was discovering the drug and extolling its powers. In January 1992, a *Los Angeles Times* series was headlined MENTAL PATIENTS AWAKEN. The story featured a photo of Robert DeNiro coming back to life in the popular film *Awakenings*. In June, *Time* magazine ran a cover story called "Awakenings: A New Drug Brings Patients Back to Life." The lead photo featured a schizophrenic man in a dark pinstriped suit dancing with a lovely blond counselor. Schizophrenics profiled were now working as a teacher, drill press operator, and maintenance man. In October, a front-page *Wall Street Journal* story headlined A NEW DRUG SEEMS TO HOLD PROMISE OF A NORMAL LIFE AFTER BOUTS IN HOSPITALS described the remarkable recovery of a thirty-three-year-old woman on clozapine.

But the press—even when well-meaning—zeroes in on the most sensational and dramatic, the small group of "miracles." There was a humanitarian motive for this. Many states, like New York, facing fiscal crises, were tightly rationing the distribution of clozapine to schizophrenics in state hospitals. There were long waiting lists. At places like Bronx State Hospital, only twenty-five of three hundred schizophrenics were being tried on it at a time. News accounts that described miracle successes put pressure on state legislators to allocate more money.

A couple dozen people had been tried on clozapine at Melillo's group homes, and while many were helped, Linda Slezak was still waiting for her first awakening.

Fred Grasso's experience is probably much more typical. Those involved with Fred all agree clozapine has helped. Fred was hospitalized several times from 1979–85, but not since he started clozapine in May 1985. Linda Slezak believes that Fred would be on the back ward of a state hospital by now if not for clozapine.

If you didn't know Fred and just spoke to his parents, you might think Fred was a clozapine awakening, too. When they talked of the drug, they compared the schizophrenic Fred on clozapine with the schizophrenic Fred previously on other antipsychotics.

"Before clozapine, he was really unresponsive," said Mr. Grasso.

"Like a zombie," says Mrs. Grasso. "As soon as he went on clozapine he perked up."

"Became social," said Mr. Grasso. ". . . More bushy tailed, more personality."

This was also how psychiatrists would be likely to describe Fred's improvement. They would not have observed someone like Fred until he was already very ill with schizophrenia, and they would be heartened by this progress.

However, if, like Fred's sister Rebecca, you compared Fred on clozapine to the Fred she once knew, before schizophrenia, Fred with the Triumph Spitfire, Fred with the Harvard-bound girlfriend, there was no awakening.

"I go home and see Fred and it's painful," she said. "What do you talk about? Occasionally since clozapine he may volunteer a thought. Occasionally I see the old Fred, a look in the eye for a split second, an animation, a gleam. And as quickly as it comes, it's gone. He might say, 'Oh right Beck,' the way he used to, and then it's gone.

"I describe to people, my brother Fred is dead. It's like *Invasion of the Body Snatchers*. It's his shell walking around and he'll sneak out for a split second, but then he's gone."

FRED'S OPINION was, "It's a good one, that clozapine, takes the tension out of your muscles." He preferred it to Prolixin, which he said gave him muscle spasms. When asked if he saw other effects, he answered, "I'm not sure. I'm not too in touch with my body parts."

The residents of the group home didn't need *Time* or *The Wall Street Journal* to formulate their opinions on clozapine. They were quite realistic about what to expect. At one point, when Maureen talked to Anthony about the possibility of going on clozapine, he said to her, "It doesn't mean I'm going to be like Fred, does it?"

DECEMBER 17, Maureen bought the house Christmas tree and that afternoon, several decorated it. In the living room now, instead of the usual smoke, there was a whiff of pine forest. Stephen DeRosa made everyone cards, which he hung on the tree. (He'd explained to Maureen, "I put stamps on all the envelopes. I didn't want to seem cheap.")

On top of the piano were cards to the group home from JoAnn up in Vermont, the electrician, and the plumber.

Before opening presents, Stephen walked down to the deli and brought back Heather ice cream. "You're in a good mood," said Maureen. He was humming something.

They all got a gift from the house. Jodie and Lauryn did the shopping: a hat, scarf and gloves for Heather; denim work shirt for Fred; a blue button-down dress shirt for Stephen; a Tom Petty tape for Anthony; cologne sets for Stan and Jasper.

The party was at the East Hills house that year. They drove over in

MICHAEL WINERIP

several cars. Stephen was fussing over his clothes, so he was the last one ready. He looked handsome in his dark gray suit.

The East Hills house was mobbed with residents, parents, counselors, alums, and Melillo board members. You could barely move. Everyone was dressed for the holiday. Julie Callahan was there, looking gorgeous in a navy blue business suit she'd bought on sale at a thrift shop for six dollars. The Grassos had come, and so had Dom Constantine, of course. There were trays of hors d'oeuvres, fancy deli sandwiches, cakes, cookies, juices, and plenty of soda in two-liter bottles.

A woman from the Glen Head house was showing people a poem of thanks she'd written entitled "The Melillo Pillow." Stephen DeRosa kept wondering whether he should ask this beautiful fat girl from the East Hills house for a date. "She says she likes my suit," he whispered, "but I don't think she likes me."

Christmas Eve, Jodie Schwartz drove Heather an hour to her brother's house, where she spent the holiday. For the first time in months, Heather dressed up—in a red sweater, black tights, and two small green earrings in each ear. Everyone remarked on how pretty she was.

Jodie, who is Jewish, volunteered to work a long shift Christmas Day so the rest of the staff could have off. They baked a ham and made corn and mashed potatoes. Four residents were there for dinner, including Jasper and Stan, who'd come over in a taxi from Glen Cove Hospital. (His parents had gone to Florida for the holiday.)

After celebrating at home with his wife and daughter, Dom Constantine arrived in the early afternoon to pick up Anthony. The father and son went to a matinee at the Glen Cove Cineplex Odeon, then out for Christmas dinner at Uncle Dai's Chinese restaurant.

chapter 16

DEFUNDING THE EMPOWERED

THE YEARS 1991 and 1992 were a watershed for group homes for the mentally ill in New York State. If ever there was a time when the group home system was going to be dismantled, this was it. The country was heading into a prolonged recession. Social services were not a priority for the Bush administration. State government, feeling the cumulative pinch, undertook extensive budget cutting, with Governor Cuomo ordering a 10 percent reduction in the state workforce.

In these years there was virtually no new funding of homes. In 1993, only 166 beds were opened statewide—about a dozen homes, the lowest since serious building began in the early 1980s. The numbers were particularly distressing when you considered the need: in 1991 there were an estimated ten thousand homeless mentally ill people living on the streets of New York City alone.

Pressure on group home program directors like Linda Slezak kept building. In the four budget years between 1989 and 1992, publicly funded nonprofit agencies like Melillo running group homes received state funds for only one cost-of-living raise for their workers. During the same period, unionized workers at state mental hospitals—who already made 50 percent more than the group home workers with comparable jobs—received more raises, and those raises were larger. Salaries for senior counselors at group homes (which rarely were unionized) started at eighteen thousand dollars; at unionized state hospitals, twenty-seven thousand.

In these months Linda Slezak found a large part of her time devoted to fighting for the homes' survival. There were constant meetings and phone conversations with officials from the group home association, the county and state. The group home association was trying to put pressure on the politicians to fund more homes, and so Linda made the rounds.

She visited her local assemblyman's office in Great Neck.

December 20, 1991, she was one of the eighty protesters demonstrating in the cold in front of the Oyster Bay, Long Island, office of state senator Ralph Marino, the powerful Republican majority leader who'd called for a freeze on group home development. "What do we want? Housing!" Linda chanted as she marched along the main street of one of Long Island's richest towns. "What don't we want? The streets." For Linda it was humiliating to resort to this; she was supposed to be a professional delivering a service, not a community activist.

A few months later she was in Albany for the group home association's annual lobbying effort. Most years she stayed at a Ramada Inn for the two-day campaign, but this year, because of budget constraints, she did not remain overnight, driving the three and a half hours back to Glen Cove at the end of the long day.

The media was not much help. It was so hard to make even the newspaper reporters understand the key issues, let alone the general public. If you said "state mental hospital," people got an immediate image. But group homes? By their very nature they were inconspicuous and scattered about. Few reporters had ever seen one, let alone been inside one. The group home was regarded by most as a novelty program, even though there were now as many New Yorkers living in state-financed group homes and apartment programs as in state mental hospitals.

For newspapers, and even more so for TV, it's always easier to report matters in black-and-white. The group home was a hybrid—not a state program, not a private program, but a state-financed program run by private nonprofit agencies. When Linda's association held a press conference at the courthouse in Mineola, Long Island, to dramatize the need for the state to give group home workers a cost-of-living raise, reporters had a hard time understanding the most basic issues.

AROUND 9 HIGHLAND and the Melillo clinic, the cuts were felt in big ways and small. If residents lost their therapist, it could take months to get another one, and she (few were men) would likely be an unpaid intern. A county-funded drop-in breakfast program at the clinic that was popular among the sickest residents limped along several months before dying. (In hopes of keeping it alive until new funds arrived, clinic director Dan Vogrin and therapist Heidi Kominsky paid for food out of their pockets for six months, then gave up.) In March of 1992, Maureen was informed that the supported apartment program wasn't taking any more applications because of the cuts.

The low salaries had long contributed to a rapid turnover rate—for some group-home agencies it is 60 percent a year—and now it was worse. Jodie Schwartz, the last of the original counselors at 9 Highland, left in June 1992 to take a job selling mattresses. Paula Marsters, who'd been at the house two and a half years and was making eighteen thousand dollars, left to be a case manager for twenty-three thousand dollars. A group home manager like Maureen, with a master's degree, was making between twenty-five and thirty thousand dollars, less than half of what a Nassau County patrol cop made (for what had to be one of the safer policing jobs in America).

At the weekly Monday staff meetings with her three group home managers, Linda Slezak used to order in lunch for the four of them from a local deli. It was a rare perk of the job. The bill came to about fifteen dollars for all of them. In January 1992, worried about the budget, Linda stopped the expense account sandwiches.

Some of the belt tightening wasn't so terrible; it was just the cumulative effect that wore you down. When a few residents requested locks on their room for privacy, to save money Maureen put them on herself. When the interior of the house needed painting, she hired residents to do it for six dollars an hour. She cut the number of videos the house general fund would pay for from two a week to one. She replaced the battered living room furniture with two couches and a chair for $750, from Seaman's overstock rooms of damaged items.

THE BUDGET cutting would have been easier to take if the pain had been distributed evenly throughout the mental health system. But it was not. Incredibly, the Office of Mental Health continued to pour most of its funds into the antiquated state mental hospitals. Despite the enormous amount of dumping of patients from state hospitals in the 1960s and '70s, New York went on merrily adding new mental hospitals, without closing old ones.

In 1953 there were eighteen state hospitals in New York housing 93,000 psychiatric patients.

In 1992 the state hospital population was down to 11,000, but there were now twenty-two hospitals.

By the early 1990s there were 170,000 mentally ill New Yorkers living outside hospitals in the community. And yet the state Office of Mental Health was still spending two-thirds of its budget on hospital care.

The blame did not rest with state mental-health officials alone. Before they could close a hospital, they had to have legislative approval, and many of the more conservative upstate legislators regarded their local mental hospital as a public works project. A place like Willard Psychiatric Center in Romulus, New York, was the third largest employer in rural Seneca County. The most blatant example of this featherbedding was Gowanda state hospital, near Buffalo. Legislators in that area refused to let it close until they were promised a public works project of equal magnitude. For the last few years Gowanda state hospital has continued to operate with just twelve patients and an annual budget of two million dollars. Advocates joked bitterly that it was the most expensive group home in America.

Closing the hospitals was made harder by the public employees' unions, which fought fiercely to hold on to jobs, regardless of need. When the legislature finally agreed to close Harlem Valley State Hospital in upstate Duchess County in July of 1993, the civil service employees' union went to court and obtained an injunction delaying the closing. Stories on state hospital workers protesting layoffs got large, sympathetic play on TV and in the paper. For the six o'clock news the visuals were good: state workers facing layoffs marching in front of a mental hospital. The message seemed obvious—more cold-hearted budget cutting by government. Rarely was the true context given: that shutting these hospitals was an enlightened way to save tax dollars that could be used to treat people more humanely in the community.

Somewhere along the line, you would have thought that it might dawn on union leaders to get out and organize the jobs of the future— the underpaid group-home workers—rather than protect the dinosaurs. But few group-home agencies were targeted for organizing drives.

In the early 1990s politicians from President Bush on down to village mayors were preaching about the need to make the hard choices if taxes were to be reduced. Here was a perfect example of that kind of choice sitting under their noses—and no one wanted to make it. Group homes could be operated for a quarter of what a state hospital cost. What made the choice hard was that few people wanted one in their neighborhood and even fewer politicians wanted to be associated with one. Failure to close most of the hospitals and move the capable patients into community care was a classic failure of political will.

Advocates for the mentally ill understood this and knew exactly what they needed: a court to order government to do the right thing. In a strikingly similar situation, courts nationwide had done this for retarded adults in the 1970s. In 1975 a federal judge ordered that Willowbrook state institution for the retarded in New York City—a real snake pit—be emptied and residents placed in group homes and apartments. In the next few years, forty states were put under similar court orders. The court order took the decision out of the political arena. The debate was over; you had to build group homes for the retarded. There was no hand wringing over budget shortfalls.

Beginning in 1984, Bob Hayes, attorney for the Coalition for the Homeless in New York City, labored at establishing a similar landmark case on behalf of the homeless mentally ill. His efforts have dragged on in court for years. In February 1993, a New York State Supreme Court judge finally ordered the city to provide housing to all homeless mental patients discharged from public hospitals. But exactly what the quality of that housing will be could take several more years to litigate. The Coalition for the Homeless argued that the city's huge barracks-style shelters were loosely supervised havens for crack dealing and violence and should have been replaced by supervised group homes, apartments, and single-room-occupancy hotels. The City contended its shelters were adequate.

Absent a judge's gun to the head, even liberal politicians like Governor Cuomo or former New York City mayor David Dinkins felt little pressure to do for the mentally ill what the courts ordered for the retarded. Absent a judge's gun, this neglected, mistreated group of people will continue to devalue the quality of life for everyone in America's big cities.

The impact of court intervention is made plain by comparing public spending figures for the retarded versus the mentally ill. During the 1980s, states spent one-fourth as much on community programs for the mentally ill as they did for the retarded, according to a 1992 study by Dr. David Braddock of the University of Illinois published in the *American Journal of Psychiatry*.

New York spends 3.5 times more money building group homes for the retarded than for the mentally ill.

Many sociologists and politicians seek to blame the civil liberties movement for all the mentally ill living on the streets. The argument goes that if we had stronger laws allowing us to lock up the dangerous crazy people, we could clean up the streets fast. Yet if civil liberties issues were truly at the heart of the problem in dealing with the severely mentally ill, you'd think group home administrators like Linda Slezak and Maureen Coley would constantly be requesting commitment hearings for recalcitrant residents. That is not the case. Linda and Maureen had seen firsthand that if you knew the residents well and provided a humane place for them to live and guaranteed that their group home bed would be held while they were in the hospital, they'd virtually always agree to be hospitalized voluntarily. (And this wasn't because 9 Highland was in an upscale suburb. It was the same for Bruce Stewart, who managed a home for male schizophrenic crack users in Bedford-Stuyvesant, Brooklyn. If you asked Bruce Stewart where he stood on the question of committing people against their will versus protecting their civil liberties, he'd answer, "A totally bogus issue. In my two years I have not had one instance—not one— when a person was angry and decompensating and the staff has not been able to get him to go to the hospital on his own by talking to him.")

To the Lindas and Maureens, the core societal problem wasn't forcing sick people on the streets to go into the hospital; it was having a humane place for them to live when they got out. There was no turning back to the large-scale warehousing of the mentally ill. The introduction of psychotropic medications—beginning with the antipsychotic Thorazine in the 1950s—had forever closed off that way of life. Few needed to live that way now for a long period. Maybe for a short hospitalization—maybe for several short hospitalizations a year. But to attempt to lock up most of this population long-term now would be a violation of basic human rights.

And yet, even with medication, large numbers were not well enough to live on their own, either. To Maureen and Linda it was obvious: If you built enough of these supervised programs to replace the state hospital wards that had been closed down in the last forty years—enough group homes, apartment programs, supervised single-room-occupancy hotels—your mentally ill homeless problem would disappear. The state hospital population had been reduced by 80,000 in New York in the last forty years, yet only 11,000 beds were funded in the community in that same period.

SADLY, the most serious threat to the group homes for the mentally ill in these years came from the people who should have been the houses' biggest friend, the state Office of Mental Health. When the fiscal crisis hit, the state commissioner and his bureaucrats didn't blast the unions; the unions were part of the Democratic party's constituency (and gave generously to the Republicans, too). They didn't make speeches about cowardly, knuckleheaded legislators; the Democratic governor needed many of those legislators to get his high-priority programs passed. Instead, they tried to beat up on the newest, least entrenched player—the group home association.

In the fall of 1991, at the height of the crunch, state officials proposed new group home regulations. Staff would be cut and the group homes would be turned into glorified boardinghouses. Under the proposal, counselors would no longer help residents manage their lives. The best thing about the group home—the case management function that helped keep people from falling through the cracks in the system —would be removed. It would be turned into a housing program with a manager who was more like a building superintendent than a social worker.

A boardinghouse/group home would not have a Maureen Coley or Tim Cook running it; would not have staff to catch Julie Callahan's multiple personalities; would not have the time to diffuse Anthony Constantine's voices; would not care if Jasper stayed or went; would not be able to monitor the change in Fred's medication dosage.

The state's proposal was to assign everyone a case manager who would visit the house. But again, if you knew the system, you knew how unreliable the case managers tended to be. Typically they were overloaded with cases; the turnover among the case managers was great; they weren't around at night or at the moment a crisis hit; and they didn't know the person the way a counselor sleeping under the same roof did. People like Julie, Heather, Jasper, who had case managers at the group home or in apartment programs, rarely if ever saw them.

Linda Slezak looked at the proposed guidelines as a cynical, underhanded way to cut the cost of running a group home. But it was worse than that. There was also a subtle power struggle going on. The growth of group homes over the previous decade had created a brand-new class of leaders in the mental health system—the Linda Slezaks—who were threatening to both the traditional state and county bureaucrats. Across New York State, there were now one thousand directors, assistant directors, and managers of nonprofit group home programs for the mentally ill. These people were professionals with master's and doctorates. Their sponsoring nonprofit organizations often carried considerable weight locally. Some, like Catholic Charities, were national powers.

One thousand Linda Slezaks were an important check on the power of the state and county mental-health directors. In New York, the people who ran the state Office of Mental Health answered to the Democratic governor. In Nassau County, Long Island, the people who ran the county mental-health programs answered to the Republican machine. The heads of nonprofits were an independent mix. As a result, they lacked a political godfather to protect them at a bad moment. But they did have an ace in the hole: they ran a cost-effective operation that worked and was needed.

The state bureaucrats tried to bully the Linda Slezaks on the change in group home regulations, but did not succeed. On September 16, 1991, state officials on Long Island held a discouraging meeting with group home directors. John Iafrate, the state's top regional bureaucrat, droned on in highly civilized fashion about removing the case management function from the group home. "We feel the consumers are not very happy with limited options of consumers living in the same place [where] they get their case management services," he said. "And the philosophy on Long Island has always been consumer oriented."

Fortunately, the real consumers and advocates knew the truth. When public hearings were held to collect comments on the gutting of group homes, people from all over the state spoke in their defense. A

1988 survey by the New York State Alliance for the Mentally Ill—the principal mental-health advocacy group—rated the group home the single most helpful program in the mental health system. (The state Office of Mental Health officials knew this; they were cosponsors of the survey.) In that survey, fifteen hundred family members of mentally ill people were asked what programs (or people) they'd found "moderately to very helpful" for their relatives. Sixty-seven percent rated group homes helpful. This compared to 50 percent for private psychiatric hospitals; 46 percent for state hospitals; 40 percent for community hospitals with a psychiatric unit; 38 percent for adult homes; 30 percent for the clergy; 25 percent for nursing homes.

These people wrote passionate letters to state officials. They wanted to know why on God's earth the state was tampering with the thing that seemed to work best.

Among the letter writers was Anthony's dad, Dom Constantine. "I find it difficult to explain what this group home has meant not only to our son, but also to our family," Mr. Constantine wrote. "It has offered my son a quality of life that is as normal as possible for him . . . When you visit the group home as often as I have you come away with a sense of family. There is warmth, concern and dedication that we have never experienced in any other government institution.

"In the 15 years that Anthony has been ill, the group home has been the ONLY bright light our family has experienced in a sea of darkness and despair."

In the spring of 1992, the state Office of Mental Health backed down.

SIZING UP this bleak economic and political scene, the Not in My Back Yard crowd spied opportunity. They used budget problems as a smokescreen to kill group homes. In 1988, a team of state and county officials approved a group home for New Hyde Park, Long Island, that was on the same block as a local high school. It brought huge, vicious, prolonged neighborhood protests—bigger than Glen Cove's. The Parks Civic Association asked in its mailings, "How can parents rationalize that the welfare of 10 to 14 potentially dangerous medicated psychiatric adult patients including those with violent histories and previous criminal records including sexual and substance abuse—take precedence over the safety of the 1200 [high school] children?" The school superintendent, George Goldstein, knew a popular issue when he saw it, equating the proposed house's location to "placing a nursery school on the Long Island Expressway."

The house was approved in an administrative hearing, but the local politicians kept pushing for new hearings and the Office of Mental Health—under pressure from the governor's office—kept caving in.

Repeatedly, the courts ruled in favor of the house and by the spring of 1991, it seemed close to opening. This was one of the rare group homes that the state had intended to run itself, but when the political heat got to be too much, state officials went looking for a nonprofit to step in. The first four agencies approached felt it was too controversial and said no. Then the state asked Melillo.

By then, the Melillo board of directors that had nearly collapsed during the 9 Highland battle was rebuilt. These were people who cared. Several had gone on their own to see the New Hyde Park house. They asked clinic director Dan Vogrin if he thought Melillo could handle a fourth group home. He said he'd hoped by this time that the agency would have had five, and that Linda Slezak was eager. Jack Williams, a social worker new to the board, said, "If we don't do it, who will? Ten people might not have treatment if we back down."

"The downside," said Dan, "is we have to muddle through the political mess that's been created. However, we did work through the Glen Cove scenario."

"It couldn't be worse than that," said another.

Board president Gil McGill wanted to take on the controversial New Hyde Park house. But he also knew unity was crucial. "We learned through the Glen Cove experience," he said. "This board was torn apart by the Glen Cove house. We have to stick together. We have to make a decision together, one way or other."

"I'll make a motion to accept," said Carolyn Wilson. There was a quick second, by Henry Holman. The vote was unanimous.

BUT IT WAS not to be. As strong as the state law was in support of group homes, it was no match for a bipartisan coalition of the state's top politicians determined to circumvent it. The neighborhood people were fortunate that the New Hyde Park house fell in the districts of powerful Republican senator Michael Tully and Democratic town supervisor Ben Zwirn, two leading NIMBY politicians in the county. Senator Tully worked through Republican state majority leader Marino; Zwirn through Frank Jones in the governor's office. It was a rainbow coalition forged in NIMBY heaven.

A deal was cut and the state Office of Mental Health was called on by Governor Cuomo's office to do the cheesy act. The scheme was transparent: a temporary group home moratorium was declared by the office because of "budget cuts." (The only place in the state this moratorium applied happened to be Long Island.) Suddenly state mental-health officials were concerned they'd overbuilt Long Island with group homes. Three months later the state quietly announced that the New Hyde Park house was officially dead. So was an unpopular group home planned for wealthy, Republican Garden City.

The money could be better used for small, scattered apartment-living programs, state officials said.

After a respectable amount of time had passed, new group homes were again planned on Long Island.

AS SHE DROVE to work on the morning of July 14, 1992, Maureen listened to National Public Radio. The announcer was describing several key demonstrations planned for later in the day at the Democratic National Convention in New York City. Police were worried about violence at an AIDS march, as well as antiabortion and prochoice rallies. The newscast did not mention the demonstration sponsored by the National Alliance for the Mentally Ill that several house residents and counselors would be attending, and Maureen remembered thinking, the problem with the mentally ill is they're not violent enough.

They'd made signs ("We deserve housing, too"; "More housing for us") which they carried on the 11:03 train into the city. A little past noon they joined a few dozen others at the protest site, on 8th Avenue across the street from Madison Square Garden, where the Democrats were about to nominate Bill Clinton for President. This was the officially sanctioned block for convention demonstrations. The sidewalk was sectioned off by blue police barricades so that several protests could be held at once. Leaders of the National Alliance for the Mentally Ill took turns speaking from an elevated podium. About 100 people marched in an orderly circle, chanting, with another 50 supporters standing nearby.

The heat was awful and several house residents, including Anthony Constantine, were quickly drained, retreating to nearby Penn Station to rest. For most, the highpoint came in midafternoon, when Bob Boorstin, an assistant communications director for Bill Clinton, addressed their rally. Boorstin mentioned that he's manic depressive and said Mr. Clinton was sympathetic to their cause.

Maureen bought them all ice cream cones for the train ride home.

At the house they turned on the TV, switching channels to see if they'd made the six o'clock news. There was footage of 10,000 pro-choice marchers in Times Square and an AIDS demonstration. There was a piece questioning whether police had forced the homeless from their usual haunts around Madison Square Garden to give the city a better image for the convention. But there was nothing on the successfully housed homeless mentally ill asking for more of these exemplary housing programs. A few residents made cynical remarks, although counselor Paula Marsters said, "When the Clinton guy came out I felt we made a little difference."

That night at the community meeting the main topic was a complaint from the neighbors on Douglas Drive, the side street that borders the house. They were upset that group home residents had been seen walking up the cul de sac at night, smoking and sipping coffee.

These neighbors felt this was intimidating. The neighbors were also concerned that on summer evenings, two or three residents were seen sitting in chairs on the patio in front of the house. The neighbors told Dan Vogrin at the Melillo clinic, "In our neighborhood, we don't sit in front of our houses; we sit out back." Dan asked the residents to discuss it, and let him know how they wanted to handle it.

After seeing what a day of orderly, well-behaved protesting got you, Maureen had some ideas about what the neighbors should do with their latest gripes, but she controlled herself. There was lengthy discussion, and as usual, she found the group home residents too forgiving. Stephen DeRosa said, "I know a lot of people are against this group home, but I look at it—maybe I would've done the same thing if I wasn't a mental patient."

Finally, Maureen said, "You can do what you want, but I personally don't think you should change your behavior in any way that is uncomfortable for you. This is your house." She asked for some consensus on what to tell the neighbors.

"Mind your own business," said Marie, and it carried unanimously.

AMAZINGLY, the recession, the budget cuts, the NIMBY politicians and neighbors, the Highland Road civic association, the state and county bureaucrats, could not undermine the group home for the most basic of reasons: it was an exemplary neighbor. The damn thing worked. In time, even several of the original opponents of the Glen Cove house admitted as much.

Anna and Jim Iversen—the private investigator who had worked closely with the mayor to defeat the house—had moved into the neighborhood in 1987. The couple had no children and came from Queens in search of the suburban life, paying $365,000 for a handsome five-bedroom house on a half acre, with three and a half bathrooms and a pool. "We didn't know anything about group homes," said Mrs. Iversen. "When we heard one was planned three blocks away, we went to the meetings and we didn't like what we heard."

By the summer of 1992, with the group home opened three and a half years, she'd changed. "A lot of it now I see was fear of the unknown. We felt this was being shoved down our throats. Now I can see maybe we overreacted, maybe we said and did things we shouldn't have. My husband liked controversy. He dwelled on it. The more controversial, the better." (Mr. Iversen died in the fall of 1989).

"At this point, to be honest," said Mrs. Iversen, "I don't know it's there."

If anyone in Glen Cove should have been aware of the group home's shortcomings, it was Anna Iversen. She'd come to know Mayor De-Riggi well, and in June 1988 he made her deputy mayor of Glen Cove, a post she held for the next four years. A key part of her job was fielding citizens' complaints regarding municipal services. Anyone unhappy about the group home who called city hall from 1988 to 1992 would have spoken with Anna Iversen.

In that time, she says, there were "a few minor complaints" about 9 Highland. A few times neighbors called about too many of the counselors parking their cars on the bordering side street, Douglas Drive. Even though the cars were legally parked, Linda Slezak told the staff, as a courtesy, not to use the side street.

"Once the parking was straightened out there was never a problem," said Mrs. Iversen. A few complaints were so petty the deputy mayor wouldn't pass them on. "Someone actually called complaining about the way a tree was pruned," she said. At first, people watched the house like hawks. Every day on the way to work Mrs. Iversen drove past, looking for problems.

She toured the house with several opposition leaders the summer after it opened. "I was surprised," she said. "I didn't think with the square footage they had they could have made it so livable. When we went in, it was actually quite pleasant. The rooms were very bright. I didn't expect it to look that nice. They made coffee and cakes and we were able to talk with the residents. People were more social than I thought. They talked about biking and going to crafts fairs all over the county.

"Some stared, making me uncomfortable. A few sat and didn't say anything. There was a big heavy guy, really weird, I remember, very,

very heavy." She was surprised to learn the huge fellow was from Glen Cove. "Really? I wouldn't have guessed," she said.

"I don't think about the house anymore," she said one afternoon, sitting in the den of her immaculate home. "I don't think it would make a difference if I was to sell my house. I myself haven't heard anything about the house in years, negative or positive."

MANY PERFORMED small, subtle kindnesses toward the house and its residents. The Reverend Richard McCall from Saint Paul's Episcopal Church on Highland preached sermons that in a gentle way made it clear where he stood. About a half dozen leaders of the parish came to him privately, looking for guidance on the issue, and he said he knew group homes to be good places.

What struck Dr. Ed Woodman, the Porsche-driving dentist who lives across the street at 11 Highland, is how much better the property is kept as a group home than it was by the family who lived there previously. "Before the group home, the house was awful," Dr. Woodman said. "The grass was never cut. The kids were noisy and abusive to each other. They had cars up on cinder blocks. One July 4, one of the kids set my shrubs on fire."

Dr. Woodman had been part of the opposition, but he changed after the house opened. "Once you see it's a fait accompli, you can stand aside and bitch and piss and moan," he said, "or you can join it and try to guide it." He joined—the Melillo board of directors—becoming a respected and active member. He went to consumer subcommittee meetings with residents. At one point the busy dentist drew up posters for Melillo's three group homes, explaining how residents could qualify for a half-price transit pass for the disabled.

A patient of his from East Williston, Long Island, mentioned that she has a retarded son and they were trying to get a group home opened. She wondered if Dr. Woodman would be willing to speak at the public hearing.

He did. The onetime group home opponent began his speech by

telling them about his $350,000 house, his Porsche and Mercedes. "I have a two-week-old daughter," he said. "And I'm very concerned about her safety and well-being." When he finished he was surprised at the clapping and would later say, "I practically got a standing ovation."

"It's easy enough to say I don't want those mentally incompetent assholes living next door," Dr. Woodman would say one morning over breakfast. "But when you get an idea of who they are, they're not incompetents. They're people living destroyed, painful lives. If you're a compassionate person, you have to say, 'What can be done for these people?' rather than throw them out to the Bowery in New York City. It's like wearing a seal coat and then you see the little seal clubbed to death and afterwards you don't look at the coat the same way. When you see the seal's eyes it becomes a national emergency not to harm seals. It's a difference of perception. Instead of seeing them as demented, deranged and dangerous, they need to be viewed as sick and more dangerous to themselves than the community. It's not cut-and-dry, but it's not threatening either."

THE NEXT-DOOR neighbors on Douglas continued to be bitter. They never accepted invitations to visit and spoke to residents or staff only if they were upset about something. When a new female resident of the group home made the mistake of parking too near their property, the wife called out, "Are you with that house?" She threatened to call the police when another female resident, dressed in T-shirt and shorts, sunbathed in the group home's front yard.

During the first five years the house was opened, this neighbor made several dozen complaints of this order and Maureen felt all but one were small and mean-spirited. One afternoon in November of 1992, a male resident, Richard, was out front of the house, saw a car turn the corner from Highland to Douglas, recognized it as Donna Rubin, a group home counselor, and jokingly ran in front of the car, pretending to block its path. To his horror, he realized it was not Donna but the adult daughter of the couple next door. If there'd been some kind of a relationship with the neighbor, this all would have passed in an instant with a quick apology, but instead the woman pulled into her driveway and called the police about a crazy man running in front of cars. When the police arrived, counselor Charles Winslow explained and apologized.

That was as bad as it got in five years.

The next-door neighbor viewed the incident as proof that there was no supervision at 9 Highland. "These people wander the streets," she said. "They don't belong out on the street, they just don't."

She blamed Mayor DeRiggi for not opposing the group home aggressively enough. "DeRiggi just let it go in," she said. "He didn't do anything to stop it."

As much as she despised having the home next door, she acknowledged that group home residents were never noisy. "Look, I think the idea of these houses is very good, great," she said. "If I had a problem or one of my children needed it, it's great. But how am I expected to react? If we were just three or four houses away, I wouldn't feel so angry. If I lived down the street, I could look left and right and see people. Not that these aren't people. But the mere fact I see them when I look out my window is unpleasant."

ROY SPEISER, the chiropractor who led the opposition, lost interest in the house within months after it opened. He lived around the corner a couple of blocks away in a location untouched by the group home. Soon after it opened, when a neighbor complained about parking on Douglas to Speiser, the chiropractor suggested she call Dr. Woodman.

Speiser probably benefited from his high-profile opposition and his NIMBY alliance with Mayor DeRiggi. The Mayor had the chiropractor come to City Hall a few times to speak to city employees about how they could avoid back problems in the workplace. And the City hired Speiser to examine city employees who'd filed workman's compensation claims involving back problems.

. . .

MUCH OF THE immediate neighbors' concern revolved around what would happen to their property values. For several years in the Northeast, real estate values had been stagnant or dropping. Even in the priciest neighborhoods on Long Island, few houses were selling. Logic would indicate that, given general prejudices, if your house is right beside a group home, fewer people will be interested. A couple of doors away it probably will have little effect, and a block away or more —people like Roy Speiser or Anna Iversen—the impact is nil.

After 9 Highland opened, there was no panic. Basically, what happened is nothing. Of the two dozen closest homes, three were sold between the winter of 1989 and the summer of 1993. In 1991, with the real estate crisis at its worst, the next-door neighbors to 9 Highland put their home on the market for two years without selling. They'd bought in June of 1983 for $122,500 and were asking $289,000.

On March 19, 1990, fifteen months after the group home opened, John and Karen Picciano sold their house, a few doors away, at 8 Douglas Drive. The Piccianos had purchased their house back in 1977 for $45,000; they sold it for $350,000 to Thomas Devine, a sales manager for a pharmaceutical company, and his wife Stephanie, a manager for AT&T. The Devines have two young children and liked the safety of living on a cul-de-sac.

The Devines did not know there was a group home until they'd lived on the street for six months. They've had no problems with it. "None at all," said Mr. Devine.

The Devines still might not know, except that six months after moving in, they invited over their cousins from the next block, the Speisers. "That's when we found out," said Mr. Devine. If Mr. Devine is walking past with one of his children and sees someone sitting in front of the group home, he waves. "We try to be sociable neighbors," he says.

. . .

SIX YEARS after leading the city's effort to kill the group home, Mayor DeRiggi said, "I was a new Mayor then, and this has been a good education for me. The fact of the matter is, it hasn't been a problem."

However, he still believed the location was wrong. He questioned why, since there is little interaction between group home residents and neighbors, the place had to be in a residential neighborhood. "I think the fundamental cause of our mental health problems is the Governor went around saying close places like Willowbrook and Pilgrim State. Many of our homeless problems have been caused by closing these institutions. They should have been upgraded instead.

"I don't think it's fair to have questionable people living next door to a family that has children. I don't know who can make the decision to thrust them upon regular people. To put that beside people who've saved to put their children and family in the best possible environment —it's not right. People don't bargain for that when they move to a suburban community. They make a lot of sacrifices, pay a lot of taxes to get away from that element."

Donald DeRiggi was twice reelected mayor of Glen Cove and in 1993 won a race for county judge.

THAT SPRING OF 1993, Dr. Woodman's wife, Francesca, got a call from another neighbor. They were planning a block party for the Douglas Drive section of Highland Road and didn't want to invite the group home. They were looking for guidance on how to handle this delicate matter. How to tactfully not invite someone? Mrs. Woodman called Dan Vogrin at Melillo. There was a time when Dan would have agonized over the question, in hopes of being the perfect neighbor. Once Dan and Linda had asked group home residents to go door-to-door to invite neighbors to an open house at a new group home—the very same neighbors who'd spewed all kinds of prejudice at public meetings. No more. Dan and Linda had learned. They were done asking group home residents to live up to a higher standard than their normal neighbors.

"I don't know what to say," Dan said to Mrs. Woodman. "Just tell them to follow their consciences."

Mrs. Woodman relayed Dan's message to the neighbor. An hour later Mrs. Woodman's phone rang again and the caller said, "I guess they'll be invited."

chapter 17

THE BEST CHRISTMAS EVER

CLOZAPINE BROUGHT no awakenings at 9 Highland. In Stan's case it had little noticeable effect. With Anthony it lowered the volume of the voices, reducing their powers, although, over all, Anthony wasn't much changed.

Jasper was still Jasper, but more alert and chatty. He began talking about wanting to see his mother. He'd heard she'd moved into a nearby apartment house and much to everyone's surprise went to check on it himself. "I was looking at the names on the buttons to see which one to push," he told Maureen. "There were forty or fifty names, but I didn't see hers." Donna Rubin drove him to his uncle's, in hopes of tracking her down. They sent Mrs. Santiago invitations to Melillo's monthly family forums; the notices came back "address unknown." "She just skipped on him," Maureen said. At a Tuesday night meeting March 17, 1992, Maureen mentioned to house members that a new woman was moving in.

"Has she got parents?" Jasper asked. "I'm glad I don't have anybody. It messes you up."

Clozapine did not make Jasper's hallucinatory world go away. In

426

March they were discussing how to spend the fifty dollars they had collected by saving refundable bottles and cans. Most wanted to have a weekend party and invite friends.

"Yo," said Jasper, "S5K994721."

"Jasper, what are you talking about?" asked Maureen.

"Nothing," laughed Jasper. "Let's go to the Holiday Inn, order ten Whoppers and ten french fries."

"Hold on, Jasper," said Maureen. "We're discussing whether you want the party on Friday or Saturday."

"That's what I'd do," said Jasper, "go to the Holiday Inn, order ten and ten."

Residents were excited about a chance to dance and cut loose, and used the bottle money to order a six-foot-long hero from the local deli as the main refreshment. After the party, a counselor cut the leftover hero into sections and stored it in the refrigerator. Over the weekend people had to fend for themselves at meals, and were looking forward to a piece of that leftover hero.

Jasper ate it all in one night.

It almost caused a riot. "They're upset about that hero, really upset," said counselor Sandra Ford at the next staff meeting.

"He ate it all?" said Donna Rubin. "There was four feet left!"

"All four feet," said Sandra.

"We're going to have to lock up the kitchen," said Maureen. "The residents keep saying, 'What are you doing for him? Fix him!' "

They discussed getting him his own small refrigerator and restricting him to what was in there, then settled on labeling his food and limiting him to that. From now on he was supposed to check with a counselor if he wanted to eat between meals. "The guy is growing by leaps and bounds," said Maureen. "He's going to have a heart attack."

"He hardly fits in my car," said Lauryn Schelfo.

A new living room chair that Maureen had bought just a month before had a broken leg, and Jasper was the prime suspect. He'd broken three others downstairs just by sitting on them. "I'm thinking of giving Jasper his own chair and that would be the only place he could sit," said Maureen.

His primary counselor, Charles, often caught him eating at night, but it was hard to get angry. "I know," said Jasper, "I just can't help it, Charles." Lauryn would sit with him while he ate. The idea was to make him aware of how much he was consuming. "I try to talk to him," she said, "but when he's eating, it's like he's in a daze, zoned out, he's not there."

In January, Maureen got him out of the state day program into Sara Center, where staff tried to help, too, but the problems were the same. Jeanne McMorrow caught him finishing a cheesecake meant for six people.

At least Jeanne reported his lapses. One day at program she noticed what appeared to be feces stains on his pants, and called Maureen. When Jasper got off the bus, he was told to shower immediately.

Jasper refused. He said he wasn't dirty. For sanitary reasons, the counselors made him eat in a separate room, alone. He was told not to touch anything. A counselor dished him out a plate of food. In the midst of dinner, while they were all in the dining room talking and eating, Jasper poked his head in. "Can I have some more please," he said in a small voice.

HE COMPLAINED about his ankles swelling and they took him to the doctor. "Do you eat a lot of junk food?" the doctor asked.

"Oh no, no," said Jasper.

Maureen searched for a program that would treat a schizophrenic with an eating disorder who was on Medicaid, but not even the National Institute of Mental Health had any ideas.

Jasper rarely went out in public anymore. There was a time he liked being seen around Glen Cove with the good-looking female counselors, but now not even his favorite, Donna, could get him out for a walk. He wouldn't go down the hill for cigarettes, or to the Y. Julie Callahan visited the house that spring and for the first time, Jasper would not join her out front for a game of catch.

And people didn't want anything to do with him. When he was hospitalized so he could be put on clozapine, several 3-West patients walked out of a group therapy session, upset about his behavior. Jasper was their worst nightmare—ugly, smelly, laughing at the wrong time, constantly acting loopy. Maureen and Donna tried to get him to talk about his feelings, and though he never would, on some level Jasper plainly understood his metamorphosis into a monster. One evening several residents were discussing seeing a movie, and someone suggested *Beauty and the Beast*.

"I saw that," said Jasper, who'd gone on a field trip from Sara Center. "It was a good movie. I cried."

APRIL 28, four days shy of Jasper's third anniversary at 9 Highland, was a perfect spring day. After dinner the house was filled with a wonderful, golden light. Jasper went into the bathroom near the office. It's a half bathroom—just a toilet and sink—and must have been a terrible place for him to maneuver. He'd been in there awhile, when water began streaming under the door. Jasper opened it and a horrible stench quickly filled the house. The toilet was overflowing. Jasper was naked from the waist up. He'd stripped off his shirt and was trying to clean up the mess with it. Feces was smeared all over his pants. Several residents gathered around in the hallway and stared while the shirtless Jasper, barely able to bend over his stomach, tried to clean himself up. They looked shocked. Was this the kind of place they lived in? Marie began laughing hysterically. Heather whispered quite loudly, "People will never forget this."

The counselors were in a staff meeting. When they realized what had happened, they shooed everyone away. Donna put on gloves, got a mop and bucket, and cleaned up the mess. It took half an hour.

"What happened, Jasper?" she asked.

"I shit all over myself," he said.

THE NEXT WEEK Maureen went to Linda Slezak and said, "I've reached the end." Jasper, Maureen said, was actually deteriorating at the house (precisely what Linda had told her a year ago). They did some searching and decided about the only option for him would be an adult home in a suburb ten miles away. It wasn't a great choice —most residents would be older, he'd no longer be in his hometown, and there were no rules to stop him from sitting around all day. But meals were prepared for you and there was no access to food between meals. Jasper might be forced to control his eating.

They'd recently found a scale to weigh him on at Glen Cove Hospital. He was up to 378 pounds; he'd come into the house at 320.

Maureen discussed it with Jasper, but he was no help. "If you think it's time for me to move," he said.

She asked if he could think of a good place.

"Pilgrim?"

"That's a hospital," said Maureen. "You think you need a hospital?"

"I don't know, maybe," said Jasper. "I'm going to have to think of a speech."

"What do you mean?" said Maureen.

"Everyone who leaves here makes a speech," he said.

Jasper went for an interview at the adult home in mid-May and was accepted. When the social worker asked if he wanted a tour, he said no.

He stayed at 9 Highland long enough to get his June birthday lobster. For a going-away gift Maureen presented him with a Walkman and extra batteries. He played it at such high volume, you could hear the music through the earphones on the other side of the room. "It works," Jasper said. "All right. Thank you." That was his speech, and then they all went into the dining room for the usual Carvel ice cream going-away cake.

A few weeks after he left, his mother showed up at the group home. Maureen told her where her son was. "It would have been nice if you'd visited him here," Maureen said.

Mrs. Santiago began crying. She said she couldn't stand seeing Jasper like he was now.

"It is sad," Maureen said. "But he's a person."

Maureen didn't have it in her to console this woman.

· · ·

JASPER LIVED in the adult home for over a year, then was hospitalized at Pilgrim State, building 30, ward 8, a long-term, locked ward. At 2 o'clock one sunny fall afternoon, the ward lounge was full, holding two to three dozen men, many staring blankly, some dozing, a few holding their heads in their hands and mumbling to themselves. Several, including Jasper, watched TV. A single aide with a key attached to her belt sat in a corner at a card table, talking to a workman.

Jasper looked great. He told a visitor he'd lost 100 pounds, but it appeared to be even more than that. "At the adult home there was only one snack at night," he said. His face no longer looked swollen; you could see his eyes and what a handsome man he was. "I'm waiting for my dismissal," he said. His hope was to get a bed at the group home that was on the grounds of Pilgrim State. Every day he was going to La Casita, a program at the hospital for Hispanic patients. "It's good," Jasper said, "They're going to help me see my mother."

Jasper took the carton of Marlboro 100s his visitor had brought and pulled out one pack. "Thanks," he said. Then he walked over to the ward attendant and gave her the rest of the carton for safekeeping.

"I'll put them away," the attendant said, "Otherwise they'll steal them next shift." On the top of the carton she wrote, "David."

"No, Jasper," said Jasper.

"I'm sorry," said the attendant, "I thought you was David."

THINGS CONTINUED to happen at 9 Highland that were amazing, but had no explanation. Paula Marsters had the overnight on Sunday, August 9, 1992. Usually Fred was in bed at 9:30. That night he was up until 2:30, smoking cigarettes and pacing. When she asked if everything was okay, Fred said he just couldn't sleep.

Next day when Paula came in for an evening shift, she noticed Fred was glazy eyed and withdrawn. She checked his meds, which seemed to be in order; the correct number of clozapine tabs were left in his weekly dispenser.

Fred told her that sometimes coffee and nicotine got to him, it wasn't a big deal. But Paula wouldn't let it go. After dinner she took him into the office. Fred began talking in long, detailed sentences, one after another. He said he'd been having violent thoughts about himself and hurting others lately. He said he didn't know what would happen to him, he had no future, his life was so grim, what was the point of living? He felt despair at all it took just to survive. He talked of his battle not to let despair take over.

Paula felt like a shroud had mysteriously lifted and she was getting a peek at a human being buried alive for a decade. She tried to think what could be going on. Was Fred having an awakening seven years after going on clozapine? Had he somehow been dumping his meds? Did something set off an electrical or chemical storm in his brain that was suddenly connecting circuits? Later she told Maureen, "I could not believe what I was hearing. It was like a different person." Fred said more in fifteen minutes than he had in the entire time he'd lived at the house.

She encouraged him to come talk anytime.

They called his psychiatrist and made a special appointment for Thursday morning. But Fred missed the session and they couldn't find him for several hours. When he showed up at the house in the afternoon, he reeked of alcohol—this wasn't just a beer or two—and could barely make it upstairs to his room. The senior counselor, Michael Perry, went up to see him. Fred was making no sense. He told Michael the sun had invaded his body and next thing he knew he was on a beach and was riding his bike and wiped out and killed a kid and then he wound up at a bar. He talked about how peaceful he felt.

The senior counselor suggested it might be best to go to the hospital. The staff had already checked; there was a bed available on 3-West.

"Good idea," said Fred. "I don't feel so good. My stomach's really nauseous."

This was Fred's first hospitalization in seven years. Maureen didn't know what to make of it. Nobody did. But her guess was that for God knows what reasons, Fred had momentarily seen himself clearly and it so frightened him, he drank until he couldn't see anymore.

Paula Marsters visited him on 3-West the next week. He seemed more like his normal self: friendly, quiet, evasive. As part of the therapy that day at the hospital, they were playing Pictionary, a drawing game. During one round, the word was "despair." Fred was supposed to make a picture that would enable the others to guess the word. He drew a stick figure of a man and when Paula asked him about it, he laughed it off. But she had a feeling Fred had drawn himself.

AT THE END of 1992 a state inspection team visited the house to review the cases of residents who'd been there more than two years—Fred, Anthony, and Stephen DeRosa. With the tight state budget there was financial pressure to move people to less restrictive environments. Such places had less staff than 9 Highland and therefore were cheaper to run. Maureen had mixed feelings about this. It was right to move people toward more independence and to make the best use of tax dollars. On the other hand Fred, Anthony, and Stephen would all need places with regular supervision, either an apartment program with daily visits from a counselor or a group home with less staff. The savings in these cases wouldn't be that great, and Maureen felt that if they wanted to stay at 9 Highland—if it felt like home to them now—they should be able to.

Stephen DeRosa hated change and didn't want to go. Fred didn't say much either way, and Maureen knew in his case it would be a matter of convincing his mother. Every time Mrs. Grasso saw Maureen, she'd say, "With Fred in the group home, for the first time in years, I've been able to sleep through the night. I really don't think he's capable of living anywhere else."

Anthony, with his constant striving to better himself, wanted to move into an apartment. He was at the pre-voc program now, learning how to use a computer. Although done with college, Anthony would still go up to his room and try to read most nights. "I'm reading the best ever," he said one night. "I just did seventy-two pages of *War and Peace*."

After three years in the group home, he still didn't have much of a sense of how to casually socialize with people and spent a lot of time alone in his room. He suddenly began discussing this at one of the Tuesday night meetings, much to Maureen's surprise.

"Sometimes I feel like people ignore me, leave me alone," he said. "Maybe because I'm always in my room."

"You have to try and say hello," said Stephen DeRosa.

"Ever since I got to know you," said Heather, "I think you're a nice person."

"Every Sunday for the last three years I've seen a movie with my father," said Anthony. "I don't want to see movies. But I don't know the rules. I don't know what I'm supposed to do. I'm tired of talking about myself. I've been here three years. I've talked about my life so much."

"You don't always have to talk about big things, Anthony," said Maureen. "You can talk about small things."

Anthony said, "I find the small things boring, very boring. I got a call from my father. He said I should watch *A Star Is Born* at 8 P.M."

"It's sort of up to you," said Stephen. "If you want to watch you should watch."

"Did you hear Stephen?" Maureen asked.

"Yeah," said Anthony. "I want to watch it. Thanks for making me feel better."

In the staff meeting later, Maureen said, "I love these people."

On December 1, 1993, Anthony moved into a supervised apartment.

STEPHEN DEROSA's fantastic, jovial, high-energy fall deteriorated into an angry, paranoid, crabby winter and spring, for no apparent reason except the vagaries of schizophrenia. After rejoining the church choir for the first time in ten years during the fall, he was kicked out in the winter. "I had to blow up," he said. "They just don't do things the right way. I told them I was going to kill myself. I guess that upset them."

He also felt a woman was sitting too close to him at church bingo and warned her he was going to call the state bingo inspector.

At a house meeting Stephen asked Maureen to get new blinds for the dining room. "I don't want people to know I'm in here," he said. He got in an argument with a female resident and kept yelling at her, "cuckoo, cuckoo, cuckoo."

He was suspended from his sheltered workshop job three days for shouting obscenities and racial slurs at a counselor.

Stephen continued to labor conscientiously at fattening up Heather, but in the early part of 1992 they had a falling-out. Out of the clear blue one Sunday afternoon, he told her, "I hope I don't kill you. I had the thought in my head." Maureen didn't think Stephen was really violent; she did feel he needed to go into Glen Cove Hospital for a med adjustment, and he agreed. He deeply regretted what he'd said to Heather and called her many times from the hospital to ask her forgiveness, but it wasn't the same after that. "You're my best friend at the house," he told her.

"You scared me, Stephen," Heather said.

"I ruined everything again, didn't I?" he said. It was like that fat girl at Pilgrim State he'd loved and then yelled at. He really was going to wind up in Hell.

At the hospital he bit an aide's finger because she hadn't told him the priest was there to give communion.

When the group home counselors heard, the first thing they asked was, "Is she black?" She was.

By summer Stephen was jovial and energetic again. He took to wearing suspenders, which looked quite handsome. He wasn't even that upset about Heather. Since she'd left the house, she'd been on a diet and lost quite a bit of weight. So it was hard to have the same feelings about her anyway.

HEATHER MOVED into an apartment at the end of March 1992, on the first floor of an attractive two-family house a mile from the group home, near Morgan Park. The rent was subsidized by the state Office of Mental Health, and she was assigned a caseworker, who was supposed to visit once a month, but never did. That was how Heather preferred it anyway.

Her new roommate was difficult, but this was paradise compared to eleven housemates at the group home. Heather had her own bedroom. The kitchen was large and she loved sitting at the table in the empty house, drinking a sweetened ice tea, smoking a cigarette and listening to WNJP, the soft rock voice of Smithtown, Long Island.

She spent most of her time alone the first year. The quiet was soothing. Now that she was out of the group home and didn't have to attend a program, she stopped, but she had no desire to work yet either. Mainly she read, dozens of books. She read Richard Ben Cramer's 1,325-page treatise on the 1988 presidential campaign, *What It Takes; At the Highest Levels*, by Michael Beschloss and Strobe Talbott; *The Homecoming* by John Bradshaw; a ton of mystery novels. She read *Newsday* cover to cover daily, and some days the *Times*, too.

Her inseparable borderline buddy from the group home now snubbed her. Teresa had moved into an apartment, too, found a job at a pharmacy, was taking nursing courses, and dating a guy she'd met while volunteering for the Glen Cove rescue squad. Heather assumed Teresa didn't want this new normal life interrupted by a friend from the crazy past. The last time they'd run into each other, Teresa was wearing a luscious engagement ring.

Heather's main companion was Ruffian, a puppy she'd picked out at North Shore Animal Shelter shortly after moving in.

Outwardly the days seemed uneventful, yet she made good progress in therapy.

For the first time in nine years with Dr. Imhof, she described the sexual abuse by her father in detail. Until this, Heather hadn't said much more than that it had started at age four and continued until she was fifteen. Now she recalled waiting in bed in the dark, praying this would not be a night the doorknob clicked. Sometimes he'd come to her gently, sometimes brutally. In the morning she stayed in the shower for as long as she could, but never did feel clean. Teachers complained because she dozed in school.

Her father photographed her nude, showing the pictures around to men and women interested in child pornography. He drove her to hotels and left her with people who paid to have sex with her. At fourteen she became pregnant. Her father was a good Catholic who did not believe in abortion, but that did not stop him from taking her to a New York City tenement to have one. The doctor (if that's what he was) must have screwed up because she developed an infection, which forced her father to take her to a legitimate doctor who insisted on hospitalization. The father said, 'Do what you can in the office,' and that was when Heather realized he didn't care about anything but himself. Soon after, she began carrying a butcher's knife to bed. One night when the doorknob clicked, she pulled it on him and warned that if he tried again, she'd cut his fucking throat.

And that was the end of it. She now realized he was a terrible coward. This added to her guilt for not standing up to him sooner.

In the spring of 1992 she visited her mother's grave and it brought back memories of a violent argument her parents had had when she was four. The father, who was superintendent of their apartment building, beat the mother so brutally she had to see a doctor they knew in the building. Her parents often fought, but this one stuck out. Years later she discussed it with her two older brothers, who'd remembered it too. They'd been terrified by the viciousness and knew the fight was about Heather, but not why.

Heather told Dr. Imhof that she now believed this beating was the last time her mother had tried to stop the father from his nocturnal rape routine.

That September Heather described a recurring nightmare where she's in the closet and her father keeps reaching in for her. She retreats frantically to the back, behind the clothes, but he grabs her, yanks her out, and takes her to his room. On the way to the bedroom Heather hears her mother laughing hysterically. After Heather and the father have sex, he's mad and drags her to the bathroom, fills the tub, and pushes her head underwater. He pulls her up and pushes her under and she gasps frantically for air until she finally wakes, shaking and sweating and terrorized.

In real life it had been her mother who punished Heather by locking her in the closet and holding her underwater in the tub.

AS SHE RELIVED past violences, her self-destructive habits from those days reappeared. She went through a period of scratching her arms and legs nervously, to the point of giving herself sores that grew infected. A few times, she cut herself with a razor. Her insomnia, from the days of the clicking bedroom door, returned.

But these reactions passed, and what impressed Dr. Imhof was that she no longer talked of suicide and never was close to a hospitalization again. Just a year before, it had seemed like a great accomplishment to avoid a commitment to Pilgrim State.

Slowly, beginning in the spring of 1993, a few close friends noticed a change. Her voice and eyes had more life. She no longer was on medication. Instead of bringing Ruffian outside for as long as it took the mutt to go to the bathroom, she'd play with him in the backyard. She kept the apartment cleaner and began a serious job hunt.

She was more honest about herself. She told the therapist that she'd gone through her childhood without ever being taken care of, and as a result spent much of her adult life acting out to get that care she felt entitled to now—from counselors at the group home, doctors at the mental hospitals, and her therapist. "I finally realized I can't get my childhood back and there's no point in trying," she said. "I just have to accept it." She wanted to be with people. She and Teresa began seeing each other again, but not in that obsessive, crazy way it had been at the house; maybe once every week or two now. On Heather's first anniversary of living in the apartment, they celebrated with a dinner out.

June 7, 1993, Heather started a fulltime bookkeeping job at a Long Island hospital at $11.49 an hour.

IT WAS HARD for Maureen to get used to having Stan at the house this second time around. Except for a slight limp, he looked like the same Stan, but he was not. After an initial burst of activity, he lapsed into a funk. Maureen couldn't tell if it was depression or his schizophrenia worsening. From January of 1992 until the fall, he did not play the piano once or use his ham radio. He'd been the best cook at the house, but now ducked it as often as possible. In the course of making even the most routine dinner, he had to sit down three or four times to rest. One night he promised an original vegetarian dish— something with black beans, rice, and carrots. It was bland and barely edible. Everyone was too polite to comment, swallowing in silence, until at the end of dinner, in his matter-of-fact style, Jasper had said, "That was terrible, Stan. What was it?"

On the first anniversary of the jump, in late May, he complained of voices and was hospitalized a few days as a precaution. Maureen felt quite sure he thought about it constantly. Stan said he didn't.

He would not stick with any day program for more than a few weeks. Maureen alternated between pushing him ("We can't accept his excuses") and worrying that this was what Stan had become. They were considering Sara Center for him, one of the lowest-functioning settings, the program Jasper attended. "I never thought I'd see this," Maureen told her staff.

Stan's father continued to push. He wanted Stan to try Micrographics and learn the microfilm trade. The father felt a new sense of urgency to find Stan an occupation; Mr. Gunter had just been released from the hospital himself, diagnosed with lymphoma.

IN A FEW months Mr. Gunter had aged fifteen years. The big robust man-God who'd so intimidated his grown son now was gray, thin, bent, and tired looking. Doctors installed a tube in his chest to inject cancer medications. Always the engineer, Mr. Gunter offered to open his shirt to show a visitor. "Amazing what they can do," he said.

The parents sat on a couch in their den one fine sunny afternoon in the summer of 1992 and talked of how worried they were about their son's future. "If I was a betting man I would say the odds are against him in this new program, which has me worried," said the father.

"There's no point in being pessimistic," said Mrs. Gunter.

"I'm worried because I see the odds," said Mr. Gunter.

"Of course they're against him," said Mrs. Gunter. "But I've seen him do great things against tremendous odds." She mentioned the time Stan had helped get the family sailboat to a safe harbor during a terrifying storm.

"After he became ill?" said Mr. Gunter.

"No," Mrs. Gunter said softly.

"We're talking fifteen, sixteen years ago," said Mr. Gunter.

Mr. Gunter read extensively on schizophrenia and felt that the most significant studies involved identical twins. If one twin has schizophrenia, the other has a 35 to 50 percent chance of having it, too —or, to look at it the other way, a 50 to 65 percent chance of not having it. Mr. Gunter believed that this showed two people with identical genetic makeups could have the same predisposition for schizophrenia, but that one could remain healthy by avoiding the serious stress that many psychiatrists believe is crucial for triggering the illness.

Mr. Gunter was sure that if Stan had avoided major stress, he would have avoided schizophrenia. And he was convinced he'd isolated the fatal pattern in Stan's life. The father believed that if only Stan had settled for a modest career, like being a high school music teacher, instead of trying to be a composer, he might be fine now.

In his relentlessly logical fashion, the father traced the "stress trigger" to a conversation they'd had seventeen years earlier, when his son was twenty-three and about to head off to a graduate music program. Their talk still haunts Mr. Gunter. They were on the way to the airport. Stan was beginning at the Royal Academy of Music in Manchester, England, with plans to become a composer. Mr. Gunter had made some inquiries about careers in composing, discussing it with a friend whose son was thirty-seven at the time, and much farther along in the field than Stan. This young man had been fortunate enough to have one of his original pieces performed by Pierre Boulez. And yet at thirty-seven, the man was still dependent on his father for financial support.

"On the way to the airport, Stan asked me if I'd be his patron while he established himself as a composer," Mr. Gunter recalled. "I said, 'Stan, I'm an engineer, not a musical connoisseur. I'd do it if I thought you had potential, but I can't really evaluate that. It's up to the Royal Academy to evaluate and ultimately decide if your capabilities justify my being your patron.

"In that conversation, I put him in a corner. He had to succeed. He went up there and failed, and when he failed he had no way out. It pushed him over the fence. I thought it was reasonable. I didn't know I was dealing with a potential schizophrenic." Within a few months at the academy, Stan stopped eating and sleeping, was delusional, and had to be removed from school. He was never wholly healthy after that.

Listening to her husband tell the story, Mrs. Gunter looked pained. This was something they'd been over many times. "What were you supposed to do, just go along?" Mrs. Gunter asked. "Did you want him to be like [that friend], thirty-seven and still not making a living?"

"At least *he* is not schizophrenic now," said Mr. Gunter.

When Mr. Gunter left the room, his wife said, "He blames himself for everything."

Many decent parents of schizophrenics do. In Mr. Gunter's case, he used his engineering training and took the best scientific theory of our time—that certain people have a genetic predisposition to schizophrenia which is set off by stress—then applied it to the problem at hand, his son. Unfortunately, the science Mr. Gunter was used to, the science of bridge building, road and machinery construction—is a lot farther along than the science of the brain. The best theory in psychiatry need not be very well grounded. Though most textbooks mention stress as a key contributor to the disorder, there has never been a convincing study showing that stress triggers schizophrenia, as Dr. E. Fuller Torrey, one of the country's leading researchers, points out. No one knows what sets it off, but Dr. Torrey believes there are a lot of possibilities more plausible than stress, including a viral infection to the brain shortly before or after the birth that lies dormant, taking years to do its damage.

As smart as Mr. Gunter is, he had never asked himself many of the obvious questions. What if Stan had settled for being a high school music teacher as the Gunters thought best? Teachers don't face stress? What kind of stress would Stan have felt if he believed that he had the potential to be a famous composer, yet settled for less, an ordinary schoolteacher's life? Would Mr. Gunter now be sitting in his million-dollar home, blaming himself for pressuring his son into an ordinary career when Stan had bigger dreams?

Is the twin without schizophrenia spared because he lives the less stressful life? Is there such a thing?

Does extreme stress trigger schizophrenia, or is something already at work in the brain, disabling it so the person can't cope with life's daily stresses and complexities?

"Interesting questions," Mr. Gunter said softly that sunny afternoon, before leaving for the hospital and more cancer treatment.

DR. JO RIEBEN, who started treating Stan again after the jump, found it hard to see him so depressed now. One afternoon they were having coffee at a restaurant. As they talked she thought about how much less animated he seemed.

"Don't be sad," Stan told her. "It'll be all right."

She still resents the way officials from Long Island Jewish Hospital's apartment program forced Stan to stop seeing her, steering him to an inexperienced therapist-intern to satisfy some ridiculous policy.

When interviewed about the policy nearly three years after the jump, Dr. Jorge R. Ramos-Lorenzi, director of Long Island Jewish Hospital's mental health programs, said Stan should have been allowed to continue seeing Dr. Rieben; apparently a mistake had been made at the time, he said.

Dr. Ramos explained that when the apartment program began in the 1970s, there was neighborhood opposition, and to ensure maximum control, Long Island Jewish officials insisted that only their clinic's therapists could treat their apartment residents. But after complaints from residents and advocates, he said this policy was changed in the late 1980s and should no longer have been enforced at the time of Stan's jump.

Steve Ronik, who made Stan give up Dr. Rieben, has left the apartment program and moved to Florida, where he directs another mental health program. When he was asked about Dr. Ramos's comments—that Stan should have been permitted to continue with Dr. Rieben—Ronik replied softly, "Maybe I misunderstood."

BEGINNING IN THE fall of 1992, Maureen saw glimpses of the old Stan. He played the piano occasionally again. At the Halloween party he and Jenny dressed as bride and groom. Stan wore one of his father's old tuxedos, a fake mustache, and took the prize for best costume.

One December afternoon he talked to Maureen about the winter sun. "The weak light this time of year always reminds me of when I lived in Denmark," he said. "The sun didn't rise until ten-thirty on these cold mornings and set by three. It's a light that sticks in your mind."

Such moments gave Maureen hope that the Stan she remembered was still there.

MULTIPLE PERSONALITY disorder was first written about over a century ago, but until recent times it was assumed to be exceedingly rare, an exotic freak of nature. As late as the 1960s, child abuse was hardly ever discussed publicly. And if child abuse was not to be taken seriously, neither was a disorder rooted in child abuse.

It wasn't until 1980 that the *Diagnostic and Statistical Manual of the American Psychiatric Association* recognized multiple personality disorder. Today it's evident that the problem is much more prevalent than was believed even fifteen years ago.

How prevalent? No one has an answer. A 1992 article in *Professional Psychology* reviews studies with estimates ranging from as few as 1 in 10,000 up to 1 in 100. Dr. Robert Mayer, in *Through Divided Minds*, describes assembling a conference on the subject in New York City in 1986. Despite a shoestring budget, he was able to locate two hundred therapists, all treating at least one multiple-personality patient.

Further complicating matters is that underreporting of the disorder is common. The typical multiple has gone through three therapists and is in the mental health system seven years before being properly diagnosed. (Thanks to Tim Cook at the group home, Julie's case took half the average time to spot.)

In November 1992, two and a half years after Julie left the group home, another young woman arrived at 9 Highland from the same renowned borderline unit that had once treated Julie. This young woman had been violently abused as a child, her face cut up with a knife by her father. Her behavior was extremely erratic; she'd be sitting quietly at a Tuesday community meeting one minute, then suddenly leap up and run out of the room screaming. The young woman told Maureen Coley that sometimes she felt like she had thirteen people inside her.

Maureen had a hunch and discussed it with the woman's therapist, who said, "No way." When the woman was sent for treatment at North Shore University Hospital, Maureen spoke to the ward social worker, who said, "It can't be, because she wouldn't be aware of the other personalities."

But it was. Twice in three years, a $25,000-a-year manager of an inconspicuous colonial house on a quiet suburban street in Glen Cove had recognized a disorder that was missed at some of the most prestigious hospitals in New York.

FROM 1986 TO 1990, Julie was hospitalized seven times; in the last three years not once. She continued to excel at work and volunteer for a local charity. When she heard about the new multiple at the group home, Julie visited her, giving her pep talks, practical advice, and inviting her over for pizza.

At college, Julie was getting straight A's in her evening courses, and often was the top student in class. Technically, credit for this had to be shared with twelve-year-old Megan, the most studious of the personalities, who popped out to take the multiple-choice tests, scoring 100's with impressive regularity.

However, you couldn't give Julie or Megan too much credit, without Didi popping out and demanding, "What about me? D-i, d-i." And it was true, even four-year-old Di had helped on the academic front, coming up with a way to work her "very, very favorite TV show," *Sesame Street*, into a writing assignment on bias in society. "And we got an A! So what do you think of them apples?" Di said. Forever after, Di would refer to this as "my paper," and cite it as further evidence that she was the world's most amazing person who wasn't even five years old.

Di being Di, she made a number of surprise appearances during Christmas shopping season and Julie would later say, "I can't figure why I bought this silly thing, I didn't plan to." Fortunately, Di had excellent taste for such a young personality. For a pregnant friend of Julie's, expecting her fourth child, Di interceded to pick a five-inch-high statue of a young maiden, cradling a family of baby birds in a fold of her dress. "It's weally bootiful," Di said later, and it was.

Nights were still awful. The Scared One, Betty, and Tess continued to relive horrors regularly. Rare was the night when their boyfriend Jim didn't have to sit on the Scared One to keep her from fleeing the apartment in terror.

Still, people who saw only Julie—her fellow workers and bosses, classmates and professors, and most friends—were struck by what an unusually well balanced and *normal* young woman she was. As insane as it sounds, when you knew the personalities, you also were struck by the balance in the system. Sixteen-year-old Marlena's rage and rebelliousness over what had happened to them was balanced by twelve-year-old Megan's prudence. The Scared One's terror and gloom were countered by Didi, as chirpy a testament to hope as there ever was.

For Christmas, Jim bought each personality a gift. Megan refused to accept hers. She wouldn't speak to Jim. Megan was opposed to getting too involved. "If I accept it, then I have to be nice to him and talk to him and I don't want to have to do that," she said. Though Megan had excellent manners, she refused to say no to him in person. She asked one of the adult personalities, Abigail, to explain that if this relationship was going to last—for example, if they married someday—there'd be plenty of time for gifts. "He doesn't even know me," the Megan personality told the Abigail personality.

In a way Julie's system was holding back a piece of itself from Jim, and the piece was named Megan. "You don't know what it was like, before Jim, when we lived alone in the apartment," Megan explained. "One time the Scared One ran out of the apartment with nothing on except a top. It was a bad neighborhood and lots of people were on the street and it was terrible."

Megan's voice was barely audible as she said, "I just don't want to be raped again.

"Right now the Scared One comes out every night and Jim sits on her. But if it's over with Jim, we'll be alone again and it will be worse, because we won't be used to being alone. Having Jim, and with the big ones being strong, it's still hard every night. If Jim's gone, the big ones will be so upset, they'll be weak.

"I'm scared what will happen if there's no one to sit on us."

For all these reasons, Megan took a pass on Christmas. And then, like a shot from the sky, Didi popped out to say she had never seen a Christmas like it. She was staying busy, searching for superlatives to do it justice, such as, "the greatest best Christmas of ever and ever." Not only did Di want to open her gifts, she wanted to open everyone else's, too.

"I never got presents before," said Di. "And this time I got the most Christmas presents in the whole world. Santa Claus is the bestest Santa Claus.

"I was waiting all day for Santa Claus and waiting and waiting and I was getting sad he didn't come," Di said. "He didn't come last year or the year before. And then we had to go out to deliver some things and when we got home and all the presents were there.

"And you know what? There were so many presents I couldn't open them fast enough. I got a Sesame Street viewfinder, I got *The Little Engine that Could* . . .''

She got the best Ernie doll in the "wold."

"We got a lot of gifts. We really cleaned it up. Some were for the other girls and I couldn't open them. And I said, 'Jim, do you think it would be OK if I opened one by mistake?' "

Every time Jim tried to get Tess to open hers, she started to run out the door. He'd bought Christmas candy for Tammy, a personality who was always starving and ate like a wild animal, but Tammy kept saying God didn't want her to have anything for Christmas. Finally Jim prevailed, but Tammy swallowed it so fast, the hard candy stuck in her throat, gagging her. "We was turning blue," Di said later. "If Jim hadn't pounded us on the back we'd be history.

"Did I happen to say I got a Big Bird piano too? You know what? Sometimes I'll pretend I'm playing, and Megan will come out and do a song and Jim gets faked out thinking it's me, Di."

Then, Jim would say, "That's really good, Di." And Didi answers; "Jim, I don't know how I do it myself.

"And you know what? Santa has the same exact wrapping paper as Jim. Isn't that amazing? I thought so, too.

"This is what I think. I think Santa gave us so many presents because he forgot us last year. And he forgot us when we lived in the mommy person's house. And he forgot us when we were in the hospital. He forgot us a long time. I think he was making up for it, that's what I think."

Thursday morning, December 26, after Didi had played with her new Sesame Street viewfinder, her Big Bird piano, and the best Ernie doll in the entire world, Julie popped out, showered, did her hair and makeup, changed into grown-up clothes, and at her usual time, 8:30, climbed into her car and drove to work along expressways and parkways that were nearly deserted.

AFTERWORD

IN 1991 AND '92 the New York State legislature passed bills that would have provided real help to the mentally ill living in the community. The legislation mandated that money saved by reducing the state hospital population be used for community programs— like group homes and day treatment programs. For each hospital bed eliminated, about $100,000 would go to community programs. (One less hospital bed would mean four new group home beds or a dozen new apartment beds.)

Governor Mario Cuomo opposed these bills and they died with little notice. The governor said in tough budget times he could not afford to have his hands tied on how to spend such revenues.

The governor tried to kill similar legislation in 1993, but this time he was in for a surprise. This time there was an extraordinary outcry. It is hard to say precisely why the public reaction was so different in 1993. Maybe the economy was a little better. Maybe the country was a little more hopeful about tackling its domestic problems, as reflected by the election of Bill Clinton. Maybe New Yorkers were a year wearier of being badgered on the streets by crazy homeless people.

For whatever reason, when Governor Cuomo announced that once again he would veto the mental health community reinvestment bill, there was an uproar. The advocates and the mentally ill staged demonstrations statewide—and this time they were covered by the press. Even loyal Democrats, like Steven Sanders, chairman of the state assembly's mental health committee, took on Cuomo publicly. Newspaper editorial writers and columnists attacked the governor for making such eloquent speeches about helping the nation's poor but failing to take care of New York's poor.

I wrote a column for *The New York Times* voicing these criticisms, and the morning it appeared, Sunday, July 11, 1993, Governor Cuomo called me at home and spent a half hour defending himself.

The governor claimed the bill had too many flaws, but he had to be embarrassed. His son Andrew had just been named by the Clinton Administration as an assistant secretary of the U.S. Department of Housing and Urban Development, with responsibility for homelessness.

Backed into a corner, the governor responded honorably. He worked to make the legislation better and did. On December 30 at Fountain House, an excellent New York City day treatment and housing program for the mentally ill homeless, Mario Cuomo signed the 1993 Community Reinvestment Bill. For the first time, New York State set up a schedule to close public mental hospitals—five of them, by 1997. The $210 million saved would go to community care.

News accounts called it landmark legislation, and it was. Never again in New York will the nineteenth-century lunatic asylum dominate public mental health care.

ACKNOWLEDGMENTS

WHILE A NOVEL comes out of your head, a work of nonfiction comes out of everyone else's head and by the time it is done, an awful lot of people are owed a serious debt of gratitude.

Linda Slezak, director of Melillo's group home program, knew me solely from my newspaper columns, but when I broached the idea for *9 Highland* her immediate reaction was, "Sounds wonderful." It is a testament to how much she believes in what she does and the kind of human being she is. For two years I sat at her staff meetings, listening in on every imaginable crisis. Never was I asked to leave a meeting. Only once did she request that I not include an incident in the book. And then, right after she asked, she apologized and kept saying, "forget it." (The incident is included). At the start of the project, when I was struggling to build an intimacy with my subjects, Linda gave me guidance, pointing me to important, yet subtle dramas at 9 Highland that I was too new to see on my own. Then, once I'd burrowed in and found my characters, Linda left me alone. A journalist could ask no greater favor.

Linda's supervisor, Dr. Dan Vogrin, director of the Melillo clinic, was the same way, even when my reporting brought pressure on him from colleagues.

Maureen Coley, manager of 9 Highland, had to learn to function with a reporter in the house. Privacy issues could have created major problems for both of us, but Maureen has an abundant amount of good sense. I'd inquire whether I could go along when she visited Jasper on a locked ward. "We'll just call Jasper and ask," Maureen would say. She treats everyone with dignity, even reporters.

I owe more than the normal amount of thanks to my agent, Barney Karpfinger. Though I'd been writing on the subject for several years for the *Times*, it was Barney who first believed a group home could make an important book. (Barney is the kind of guy who takes election day off to drive elderly Democrats to the polls.) Dan Frank, my editor, was the second believer. In his editing he was gentle but vigilant, pointing me toward the necessary changes, then waiting patiently for me to conclude the same.

I'm appreciative to my editors at *The New York Times*, particularly Joe Lelyveld, for giving me a leave to report *9 Highland*, and then hiring me back parttime so I could feed my family while I finished the manuscript.

My good friend Barry Bearak, whose writing I admire enormously, read the early versions of the book and told me what worked—and more important, what did not. It is a rare friend who will tell you the truth. Another longtime friend, Eric Rieder, a lawyer, guided me past some worrisome legal spots.

I owe special thanks to Ed Brown, a fine social worker, who has influenced this book in more ways than I can say. And to Dr. John Rivard for helping me describe the miracles of modern medicine accurately.

This book was written while my wife Sandy Keenan, a sportswriter, and I tried to care for our three boys—all under the age of five at the time. It was Sandy who knew when it was time to stop taking notes and start writing.

My largest thank you is reserved for the residents of 9 Highland, who made me welcome. People ask what it was like hanging out at a group home so much. I had a wonderful time. I laughed a great deal and was quite often moved.